KINESIOLOGY

MOVEMENT IN THE
CONTEXT OF **ACTIVITY**

KINESIOLOGY

MOVEMENT IN THE CONTEXT OF **ACTIVITY**

DAVID PAUL GREENE, PhD, MS, OTR
Associate Professor,
Department of Occupational Therapy,
Colorado State University,
Fort Collins, Colorado

SUSAN L. ROBERTS, MDiv, OTR
Tucson Unified School District,
Tucson, Arizona

with 258 illustrations

illustrations by
David Paul Greene, PhD, MS, OTR,
and Avtar Dunaway, OTR

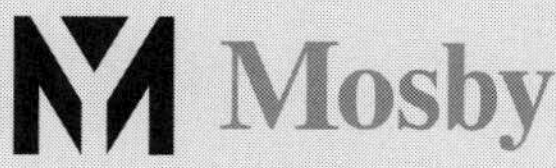

St. Louis Baltimore Boston Carlsbad Chicago Minneapolis New York Philadelphia Portland
London Milan Sydney Tokyo Toronto

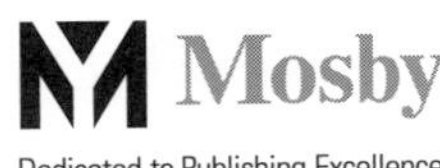

Dedicated to Publishing Excellence

Publisher: John Schrefer
Executive Editor: Martha Sasser
Senior Developmental Editor: Amy Christopher
Project Manager: Linda McKinley
Production Editor: Kristin Risley
Designer: Renée Duenow
Manufacturing Manager: Dave Graybill
Cover Photo © PhotoDisc, Inc.

Printed in the United States of America
Composition by Top Graphics
Printing/binding by Maple-Vail Book MFG Group

Mosby, Inc.
11830 Westline Industrial Drive
St. Louis, Missouri 63146

Library of Congress Cataloging in Publication Data

Greene, David Paul.
Kinesiology : movement in the context of activity / David Paul Greene, Susan L. Roberts ; with illustrations by David Paul Greene and Avtar Dunaway.
p. cm.
Includes index.
ISBN 1-55664-416-7
1. Kinesiology. 2. Human mechanics. 3. Occupational therapy.
I. Roberts, Susan L., 1951- . II. Title.
QP303.G74 1999
612.7'6—dc21 98-45273
CIP

99 00 01 02 03/9 8 7 6 5 4 3 2 1

To all those who in reading this book
will heighten their understanding of kinesiology
not at the expense of a larger world view.

DPG

To all the people whose lives have touched mine
and deepened my appreciation for infinite variety in the human spirit.
Some of their courage was passed on to the characters in this book.

SLR

Foreword

O ***ccupation is the foundation*** of the practice of occupational therapy. Work and productive activities, play and leisure, and activities of daily living are all occupational performance areas comprising occupation. Understanding the meaning of occupation greatly contributes to its use as a therapeutic mechanism for change. In occupational therapy, change is what the process is all about. Occupational therapy practitioners advocate change in others. We talk about change as transformation.

Kinesiology: Movement in the Context of Activity provides a wonderful resource for better understanding one component integral to occupation—human movement. What David Greene and Susan Roberts have achieved in their text is to provide the occupational therapy student and practitioner with an engaging approach to the understanding of human movement in a person-environment context. The authors have explored the kinesiology of the upper and lower extremities in this text and have included clear explanations of both normal kinesiologic function and pathokinesiology of the wrist and hand. Learning kinesiology and biomechanics is made more comprehensible through the incorporation of clinical problems throughout the text in the form of ongoing vignettes. The authors also have demystified and deemphasized algebra and trigonometry without compromising understanding—no easy feat!

I believe this textbook will be especially successful in facilitating the student's understanding of kinesiology and biomechanics. Each chapter includes a content outline, a list of key terms, and problem-solving exercises. "A Closer Look" boxes provide an in-depth look at more complicated and difficult-to-understand topics. In addition, the material in each chapter is brought to life through numerous illustrations.

The rigor required to become a competent, ethical, and skilled occupational therapy practitioner seems to increase daily as we face an ever-changing and complex health-care environment and evolving occupational therapy theories and models that support evidence-based outcomes. I applaud the authors for providing us with *Kinesiology: Movement in the Context of Activity*. This text is an important addition to the student's library and will support the practitioner's lifelong continuing competency.

Karen Jacobs, EdD, OTR/L, CPE, FAOTA
Clinical Associate Professor,
Department of Occupational Therapy,
Boston University,
Boston, Massachusetts

Preface

K*inesiology and biomechanics* are frames of reference that can be used to analyze human activity. They have always been foundations for occupational therapy practice. Oftentimes practitioners have attempted to use kinesiology and biomechanics as their sole frames of reference, much to the detriment of those they seek to help. In this book, we explore the intricacies of kinesiology as it relates to the practice of occupational therapy. Our intent in every lesson is to maintain a perspective in which the relative significance of the details are viewed in the context of the larger life experience. Clinical problems are presented throughout the book as problems encountered by *individuals.* Although the immediate focus may be on the biomechanical aspects of the problems, the individuals encountering the problems are presented in a more holistic light.

In Appendix H, these individuals' situations are summarized in brief, narrative form. The "characters" are fictional compilations of people we have known, and many appear more than once throughout the course of the book. They are listed in Appendix H in alphabetical order by first name, allowing quick reference to the "bigger picture" in each case. We have attempted to present some diversity of age, race, and ethnic background in this cast of characters.

The clients and practitioners presented in the book reflect a variety of OT settings. Occupational therapists alternate with assistants in the vignettes and portray realistic clinical roles. In most instances the roles are interchangeable, but evaluation activities usually feature therapists rather than assistants because evaluation is chiefly a therapist's role. Although we often refer to assistants as *OT assistants,* the term *OT practitioner* is used to refer to individuals, both therapists and assistants, who engage in OT practice.

Overview of Chapters

Section One of this book is composed of five chapters and provides background information from other fields pertaining to philosophical issues and contributions to the kinesiologic aspects of occupational therapy. Chapter 1 defines the role of kinesiology and biomechanics in current OT practice. Chapter 2 provides some basic vocabulary and concepts for discussion of the human musculoskeletal system and mechanical physics. Chapter 3 looks at how gravity affects movement, whereas Chapters 4 and 5 explore linear and rotary forces and movement.

The final four chapters of the book comprise Section Two, in which concepts presented in the first half of the book are applied to regions of the human musculoskeletal system. Chapter 6 explores the head and torso. Chapters 7 and 8 look at the upper extremity, both proximal and distal, and Chapter 9 introduces the reader to the lower extremity.

Each chapter begins with an outline and a list of key terms. Chapters contain "A Closer Look" boxes that expand on various topics presented in the book to aid the reader's comprehension. Each chapter also concludes with applications in the form of questions to be answered or problems to be solved. All answers and related discussions are included in Appendix C. Readers are encouraged to work through each application, solving the problems as best they can before consulting Appendix C for the answers.

There are 12 appendixes at the end of the book. In addition to the listing of characters (Appendix H) and answers to the chapter applications (Appendix C) already mentioned, these appendixes include a conversion table from English to metric equivalents, a diagram of body segment parameters, a brief review of mathematics, a table of trigonometric functions, a listing of commonly used formulas in biomechanics, a journal article, a brief illustrated review of muscle anatomy, instructions for the creation of finger and wrist models, learning objectives, and laboratory activities. A glossary also is provided to aid in the understanding of complex terminology.

How We Solve Problems Based on Kinesiology

The problems presented throughout the book encourage readers to apply specific kinesiologic and biomechanical principles to human activity. Each scenario follows a logical progression so that the reader learns information in much the same order that an OT practitioner would follow to solve a clinical problem. These problems usually require that the reader draw a diagram to organize the information and solve some basic mathematical equations. This is the point at which many readers, both OT students and practitioners, become intimidated.

Detailed and lengthy solutions are included in Appendix C for those interested in specific trigonometric solutions. OT practitioners can and do sometimes work with engineers, whose knowledge and understanding of mechanics permits use of the precise mathematics necessary in the designing of complex adaptive equipment, orthotics, and ergonomic industry tools. Understanding how mathematics works in biomechanics can help OT practitioners identify the relevant data needed to solve clinical problems, especially those that may require teamwork with bioengineers or orthotists.

We recognize, through years of experience teaching this subject, that the majority of students will not pursue the more complex mathematically based solutions. Instead, this stage of complexity is too often an invitation to disengagement, and many students retreat from common sense at the first sight of sines and cosines in algebraic formulas. The traditional approach to kinesiology emphasizes the use of trigonometry to solve problems. This has led to a general opinion among OT practitioners that what they learned in their kinesiology courses was good for school but is impractical for use in everyday practice.

In truth, every situation presented in this book and most biomechanical challenges in daily practice can be reasoned through with sound kinesiologic thinking *without ever* looking up a sine or cosine. We have tried to deemphasize algebra and trigonometry in an effort to encourage *all* readers to think completely through the problems as presented and not get sidetracked by less-familiar material. Pictorial (graphic) solutions have been used throughout this text, and only absolutely necessary mathematics have been included.

We have used kilograms instead of newtons as the unit of force in the presentation of applications. This is not by oversight or in error because we have explained the difference in these units in Chapter 3 and provided examples for their proper conversions. Our use of kilograms as units of force follows our intention to present information in terms common to the experience of the readers and the therapists and assistants they observe during fieldwork.

This nontraditional approach has been used to provide tools for clear thinking and to emphasize that these are concepts and thought processes important to our full understanding of real client situations on a daily basis in clinical practice. This is *not* something you do "only in school."

David Paul Greene
Susan L. Roberts

Acknowledgments

Many people were helpful to us while we wrote this book. Without their assistance and support, writing would have been much more difficult and far less enjoyable.

Our developmental editor, Amy Christopher, wisely suggested that biomechanics should be more interesting. This, added to our desire to expand readers' views beyond mere biomechanics, yielded the addition of fictional clients. These clients were fortunate enough to have a very real team of people who were not only interested in the client's progress but willing to accept phone calls at home, often late at night. All these people shaped the lives of the fictional clients and ensured that this book would look at more than just body parts and principles of physics.

Barbara E. Brown, OTR, offered a wealth of treatment suggestions for almost every character, especially those clients with spinal cord and hand injuries. Ellen Buenaventura, MD, considered how particular diagnoses and complications might affect various clients, especially children. Melissa Price, PhD, suggested that if one of our characters, Eduardo Ybarra, taught his son carpentry, this may help him recover from depression. Sharon Kutok, SLP, provided the essential information that allowed Bernice Richardson, another character, to resume her singing career. Mary Raye Hestand, MBA, provided detailed consulation on the character Xavier Morales and would have been happy to shoot a few baskets with him on the court if he had been a real person. Finally, Joel Cannon, PhD, served as our contact in the world of theoretical physics, ensuring the integrity of the information as we attempted to explain basic but complicated concepts in understandable terms.

Linda Larson, COTA, and Noelle Everhart, COTA, made it possible for Susan to spend time concentrating on the book without worrying that students were going without OT services. Ellen Buenaventura kept the house running and provided meals when writing consumed entire days.

Over the years, students in David's biomechanics classes unknowingly contributed to this text through their thoughtful questions. Donna Wills Greene served as the major sane influence for David, taking care of everything, *including* the "kitchen sink," while experiencing the adventures of temporarily raising two young boys alone.

David Paul Greene
Susan L. Roberts

Contents

KINESIOLOGY

MOVEMENT IN THE CONTEXT OF **ACTIVITY**

Multidisciplinary Basis for the Understanding of Human Movement

SECTION **OUTLINE**

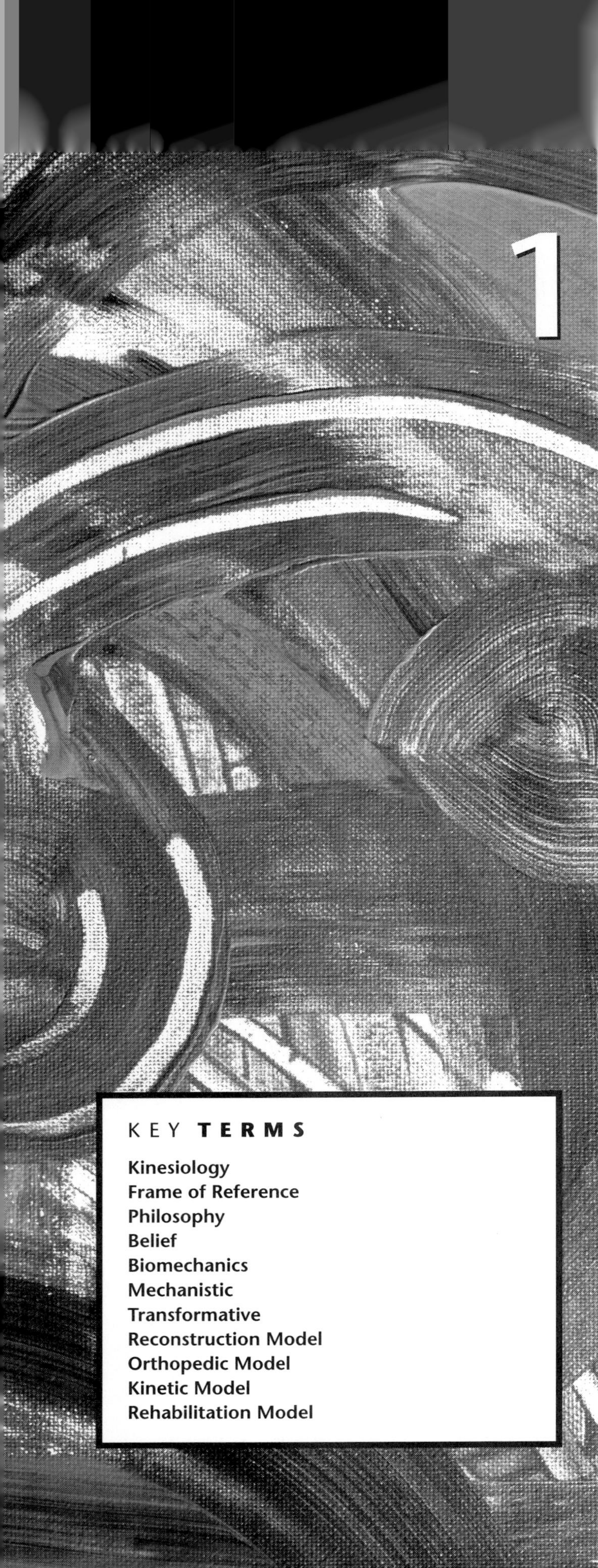

1

Biomechanics, Kinesiology, and Occupational Therapy

A Good Fit

KEY **TERMS**

Kinesiology
Frame of Reference
Philosophy
Belief
Biomechanics
Mechanistic
Transformative
Reconstruction Model
Orthopedic Model
Kinetic Model
Rehabilitation Model

CHAPTER **OUTLINE**

BELIEFS AND DEFINITIONS

MECHANISTIC AND TRANSFORMATIVE PHILOSOPHIES

A BIOMECHANICAL FRAME OF REFERENCE
Limitations of Biomechanical Approaches

INTEGRATION OF BIOMECHANICS WITH MODELS OF PRACTICE

SUMMARY

The 8-year-old** third grader with cerebral palsy struggles to raise his head when introduced to the occupational therapy (OT) assistant visiting his classroom to make equipment modifications. He presses his head against the back of his wheelchair and holds it there unsteadily while the teacher explains, "**Jason's biggest problem is that he won't pay attention and keeps ignoring us. He's always looking down at his lap tray. We've been giving him a sticker if he holds his head up and pays attention for 5 minutes. If he can get five stickers in one day, he can go on our weekly field trip, but he just won't try hard enough."*

Reminded of his failures, Jason begins to cry.

• • •

*"I don't care what you people in rehab say about **Mrs. Smith** being strong enough, it takes two of my aides to get her off the toilet!" complains the head nurse at the weekly review of residents in Maple Grove Skilled Care Facility.*

The OT practitioner remembers Mrs. Smith was fearful of falling and had difficulty leaning forward when standing for transfers from her wheelchair. It took a lot of coaxing and reassurance to get her up.

"Why don't we bring her into therapy for a few weeks and see if we can get her into our dance group, as well as work with your aides to show them some ways to get her to stand up more easily," the OT practitioner suggests.

• • •

OT practitioners use their understanding of movement to solve these and other clinical problems. They apply principles of biomechanics and kinesiology as part of their assessments and treatment plans. The school therapist will readjust Jason's wheelchair to enable him to hold his head up more easily. OT practitioners in the skilled nursing facility will begin engaging Mrs. Smith in activities that provide vestibular stimulation through movement to decrease her fear of falling, enabling her to lean forward and decrease her effort to stand.

Kinesiology provides the best means of solving these problems because of the unique blend of fields that converge in this area of study. Kinesiology is the study of movement from the perspective of three physical sciences: musculoskeletal anatomy, neuromuscular physiology, and biomechanics. The complexity of these three fields often makes their introduction into activity analysis an exercise in examining the trees that make up the forest (A Closer Look Box 1-1).

BOX 1-1

A **CLOSER** LOOK

Defining Kinesiology and Biomechanics

The terms kinesiology *and* biomechanics *often are confused. The* biomechanical frame of reference *commonly referred to in treatment settings involves aspects of kinesiology that include functional anatomy of the musculoskeletal system, neuromuscular physiology, and biomechanics. OT educational programs offer courses that typically blend content from these three areas into courses called* kinesiology, biomechanics, *and* human movement.

The following definitions from Stedman's Medical Dictionary[8] *are among the clearest. They may be helpful for understanding that the two sciences are inseparable:*

Kinesiology. The science of the study of movement and the active and passive structures involved

Biomechanics. The science of the action of forces, internal or external, on the living body

Kinesiology is the study of movement. Biomechanics forces us to look at how forces affect movement. Biomechanics is one perspective for the study of movement.

As OT practitioners, we must recognize that kinesiology is a fascinating topic but is never the whole story. Focus on a specific movement or adaptation must be done with recognition of the larger environment. An understanding of movement can only lead to successful adaptations when it is integrated into real-life activity and applied to individual environments.

An OT practitioner who saw Jason could write two very different evaluation notes. Focusing primarily on kinesiology, the OT practitioner may write the following:

> This is an 8-year-old boy with cerebral palsy. He has limited head and neck extension secondary to severe spasticity. Abnormal tone has resulted in flexion contractures of the elbows and wrists. Control of the head and neck and wrist extension are severely limited.

A change of focus, based on performance in the school environment, might lead to a very different evaluation:

> Jason is an active 8-year-old boy. He is a third grader in a regular classroom and is having difficulty in class because of poor head control secondary to cerebral palsy. His inability to lift his head from the lap tray interferes with his ability to

*The names presented in this text appear in bold italics on first mention in each chapter. See Appendix H for more information.

participate in class. He also experiences flexion contractures of the elbow and wrist secondary to severe flexor spasticity, making it difficult for him to use his upper extremities to reach and grasp as his classmates do.

Both evaluation notes contain the important details. The first demonstrates a keen sense of biomechanics and kinesiology, but the document shows little insight into the significance of these problems. The latter is more representative of the bigger picture. It presents a view that embraces the importance of meaningful activity that can lead to successful role function. An OT practitioner's point of view affects the way assessments are conducted and treatments performed. It is the practitioner's **frame of reference**. Many factors shape an OT practitioner's frame of reference, and understanding them is an essential part of professional development.

Beliefs and Definitions

Perspective shapes the way we define the limitations and possibilities of any problem. Our viewpoints are defined by our philosophies about life and the way we integrate these beliefs into OT models of practice. A **philosophy** affects an individual's perceptions of experience and is broad based. Related theories, models, and frames of reference may restrict our views, even though they are considered consistent with our overall philosophies.

OT practice is based on the **belief** that purposeful activity (occupation), including its interpersonal and environmental components, may be used to prevent and treat dysfunction to promote maximal functional adaptation.[13] Kinesiology, the study of movement influenced by active and passive structures, includes **biomechanics**, the study of internal and external forces. Together, they represent two restricted views of purposeful activity and adaptation, helping OT practitioners to understand movement in the context of the musculoskeletal system only.

Because kinesiology and biomechanics are restrictive frames of reference, OT practitioners must question how these approaches fit within the philosophy and definition of the profession. If it is based solely on scientific collections of techniques and protocols, intervention is therapeutic only in the narrowest sense. We must have a broader view of therapy than its effect on range of motion, strength, and endurance.

As OT practitioners, our focus goes far beyond movement for movement's sake (for example, flexing the arm to move through full range of motion). Our focus also goes beyond functional movement because even this may be little more than movement to fulfill the function of the particular joint. Our primary concern for movement involves movement within the context of activity.

Environmental supports and barriers, specific skills, and occupational demands representative of real-life environments have tremendous effects on individual performance. Kinesiology fits when its more restrictive viewpoint for intervention is anchored in the context of meaningful activity and the effect of activity on role function. Kinesiology is simply a valuable tool for assessment and treatment of an individual with movement-related difficulties.

Fundamental details of a situation are crucial, and we must thoroughly understand them to perform the unique service that is OT practice. We must know, for example, the specifics of splinting, including the necessity of a perpendicular force and the danger of forces applied at angles other than 90 degrees. The ultimate value of this intervention, even if the biomechanics are correct, is that it facilitates individual adaptation. Every detail must help the individual to perform the necessary and desirable role functions that are meaningful to that individual's life. Biomechanics is the means to the end.

To understand how we use kinesiology in OT practice, we need to define it and understand its place in our beliefs about human movement. Kinesiology, and even more so biomechanics, has its roots in a branch of physics based on the belief that individuals function like complex machines. This belief system, mechanistic philosophy, shaped the study of science and medicine for many centuries. In the twentieth century, a newer system, transformative philosophy, has gained precedence over mechanistic philosophy. Transformative philosophy made many new discoveries and theories possible. How do these philosophies continue to affect our understanding of functional activity?

Mechanistic and Transformative Philosophies

Aristotle and his contemporaries recorded an interest in the analysis of human motion in the fifth century, BC. They developed a view of the human musculoskeletal system as a mechanism involving levers, forces, and a center of gravity. In the early part of the sixteenth century, Galileo, considered the father of modern science, combined his observations of the world with mathematics. Descartes, his contemporary, outlined a mechanistic philosophy that separated mind from matter. Both men were considered radical thinkers. Galileo was threatened with torture unless he renounced his belief that the Earth revolved around the sun. He spent the last decade of his life under house arrest because his ideas were considered so dangerous. Descartes took heed and became more circumspect about publishing his work.

Nonetheless, the work of both Galileo and Descartes

influenced Sir Isaac Newton. In the latter half of the sixteenth century, he constructed a system of mechanics that became the foundation of classic physics. In 1703, he was knighted for his work. The science and technology that grew out of mechanistic philosophy spawned the Industrial Revolution of the nineteenth century.[3,6,14]

Mechanistic philosophy separates mind from body. Subscribers to this viewpoint see human beings as compositions of interrelated components. Time is linear and evolutionary. The past becomes a focus for management of future events. Relationships between people and objects are interfacing parts of a larger machine. When the machine is managed and maintained, it functions at peak efficiency. Conflict, trauma, and other difficulties are interpreted as breakdowns. People, communities, or objects at the center of these breakdowns become victims who may not be restored to working order. Those who choose to intervene with a mechanistic philosophy use a managerial style to coordinate the isolated parts.[1,2,9,10]

Newtonian physics was not seriously challenged until Einstein's work in the twentieth century. Einstein's theories and the advent of nuclear technology caused major upheavals in both science and philosophy. As a result, new sciences and philosophies developed.[6]

For example, scientists trying to understand the chaotic phenomena of both weather and cardiac rhythms developed a new field of mathematics. The mathematics of chaos provided a means for understanding events that previously had been unpredictable. They found that relatively insignificant changes at particular moments produced global changes later. It was as if a butterfly flapping its wings in China could produce rainstorms in Iowa.[7]

The mathematics of chaos reflected and influenced a new philosophy. **Transformative** philosophy was born of radical changes in the twentieth century. Individuals who subscribe to the transformative philosophy see others as integral members of a large and interdependent open system. Time is relative; new emerges from old, and both are changed. Human relationships make dynamic, infinitely unique patterns and harmonies. Conflict, trauma, and difficulty serve as catalysts for creative adaptation. Individuals and communities who adapt and change are like artists who find dynamic and harmonious places within their environment.[1,2,9,10]

A Biomechanical Frame of Reference

Although OT practice evolved in the mechanistic model of medical management, most contemporary OT practitioners define problems in terms of creative adaptations. OT models of practice based on biomechanics still have an important place in the history of the OT profession.

In 1918, psychologist Bird T. Baldwin organized an OT department at Walter Reed General Hospital in Washington, DC. He began routine measurements of joint motion and muscle strength to develop a method of evaluation and treatment. From these measurements, he developed a set of problem-solving steps known as the **reconstruction model.** Baldwin believed that voluntary activities, graded and adapted to specific muscles and joints, would result in a return of function. Whenever contemporary OT practitioners increase resistance or complexity in an activity, they build on the knowledge this model provides.

In the first half of the century, OT practitioner Marjorie Taylor used anatomy, physiology, pathology, and kinesiology to develop the **orthopedic model.** She believed that treatment activities should be specific to muscle and joint problems. OT practitioners use this model whenever they tailor an activity to strengthen a specific muscle group or increase the movement in specific joints.[12]

In 1950, physicians Sidney Licht and William R. Dunton, Jr. wrote an OT textbook outlining the **kinetic model.** Licht believed that OT practitioners needed to become more scientific. To this end, he developed many working definitions of OT practice that are still valuable. He promoted activity analysis and reported on many kinds of adaptive equipment.[12]

OT models based on biomechanics have provided practitioners a means to do the following:

1. Outline and define musculoskeletal problems
2. Develop exercises and activities that restore and maintain function
3. Design and fabricate adaptive equipment to meet functional activity goals
4. Measure functional musculoskeletal progress in treatment

Biomechanics can be used to research the effects of activity on the musculoskeletal system. It provides an approach that is most useful in hand clinics, centers for physical rehabilitation, work-hardening clinics, and ergonomics. Biomechanics, although often useful, reduces the focus of treatment by isolating parts.

LIMITATIONS OF BIOMECHANICAL APPROACHES

Biomechanics emphasizes the mechanics of the musculoskeletal system. It does not address the cognitive, emotional, and social aspects of human occupation. Kinesiology, although it encompasses the psychomotor aspects of movement, still falls short of balancing performance components of individual function with the environment in which a person operates. Kinesiology has not provided a comprehensive framework for OT practice. The confusion of OT with physical therapy has resulted from a single-minded focus on using activities, including exercise, to improve and maintain musculoskeletal function.

OT practitioners must use kinesiology to fuel their problem-solving engines and then move on to the next step. An individual's improved musculoskeletal function, made possible through biomechanical applications, should contribute to a functional occupational role. Improved musculoskeletal function isolated from the occupational contexts of self-care, work, and play* has no place in OT practice. Because our profession stresses a holistic approach, we must use biomechanics within other models of practice.

Integration of Biomechanics with Models of Practice

Kinesiology provides a structured way of evaluating movement in activity. Movement generally involves the musculoskeletal system, and it should be addressed as part of any OT evaluation. Biomechanics provides a lens through which the OT practitioner can examine movement in activities. Biomechanics guides the practitioner to provide interventions that emphasize remediation of specific body parts. Although this focus is far removed from occupational function of the individual, when blended and used within current models of practice, biomechanics is an essential part of contemporary OT practice.

OT theorists have developed many models of practice that are more closely related to transformative philosophy. Jean Ayres' theory of sensory integration postulates that small changes in the processing of sensory input produce global adaptive responses. Lorna Jean King elaborated on Ayres' work to develop a model of adaptive responses for the understanding of patterns of change and growth. Mary Reilly and Gary Kielhofner used open systems models to describe human activity. These models assume that growth and change are interdependent, not linear. Their belief in the uniqueness of individual experience results from a transformative rather than mechanistic philosophy. Even in these transformative models of practice, the understanding of movement depends on principles of biomechanics.

*Play encompasses a broader range of human occupation than recreation. "Under Reilly's leadership, the 'play lady'[5] was taken out of the closet, and a new generation of leaders and scholars in the profession were inspired to reclaim play as a fundamental concept in OT practice and to make it an object of research."[11]

The **rehabilitation model** highlights adaptations toward function in meaningful activity, not remediation of specific body parts. Anne Fisher's expansion of this model[4] identifies four domains of function: level of independence, level of effort, degree of efficiency, and degree of safety. This provides a broader range of information for the understanding of motor and processing skills. Mechanistic frames of reference, like biomechanics, can be guided under this model; therefore, specific thinking from a more restricted viewpoint occurs in the context of solving problems associated with meaningful activities.

Summary

Biomechanics provides a key to understanding levels of independence, effort, efficiency, and safety. As a part of kinesiology, an understanding of biomechanics better equips the OT practitioner to solve problems and offer suggestions leading to improved function in relevant contexts.

Kinesiology equips OT practitioners with tools to formulate a problem and arrive at a solution. That solution must be relevant to an individual's everyday life. For example, a device that improves proximal interphalangeal flexion may work brilliantly, but it cannot give an individual a functional grasp at work unless it is used. OT practitioners have responsibility for not just solving a problem but ensuring that the solution can be incorporated into daily life. The latter responsibility offers our profession its greatest challenges and rewards.

OT practitioners use kinesiology to design and modify adaptive equipment, evaluate the safety of home and work environments, and create therapeutic activities and exercise programs. Most OT practitioners try to determine how a piece of equipment, modified work station, or trip to the mall enables an individual to participate more fully in the community. Like the butterfly in China that sets off a weather pattern leading to rain in Iowa, OT practitioners expect their little bit to go a long way.

REFERENCES

1. Cannon K: *Black womanist ethics,* Atlanta, 1988, Scholars Press.
2. Cannon K: *Katie's cannon: womanism and the soul of the black community,* New York, 1995, Continuum.
3. *The concise Columbia encyclopedia,* New York, 1995, Columbia University Press.
4. Fisher A: *Assessment of motor and process skills,* ed 2, Fort Collins, Col, 1997, Three Star Press.
5. Florey LL: An approach to play and play development, *Am J Occup Ther* 25:275-280, 1971.
6. Fritjof C: *The Tao of Physics,* New York, 1984, Bantam.

7. Gleick J: Chaos: *Making a new science,* New York, 1987, Viking.
8. *Illustrated Stedman's medical dictionary,* ed 24, Baltimore, 1982, Williams & Wilkins.
9. Levine RL, Fitzgerald HE: *Analysis of dynamic psychological systems, vol 1: basic approaches to general systems, dynamic systems, and cybernetics,* New York, 1992, Plenum Press.
10. Mead GH: *Movements of thought in the nineteenth century,* Chicago, 1936, University of Chicago Press.
11. Parham LD, Fazio LS: *Play in occupational therapy with children,* St Louis, 1997, Mosby.
12. Reed K: *Models of practice in occupational therapy,* Baltimore, 1984, Williams & Wilkins.
13. American Occupational Therapy Association: *Reference manual of the official documents,* Bethesda, Md, 1996, The Association.
14. Trager J: *The people's chronology,* New York, 1995, Henry Holt.

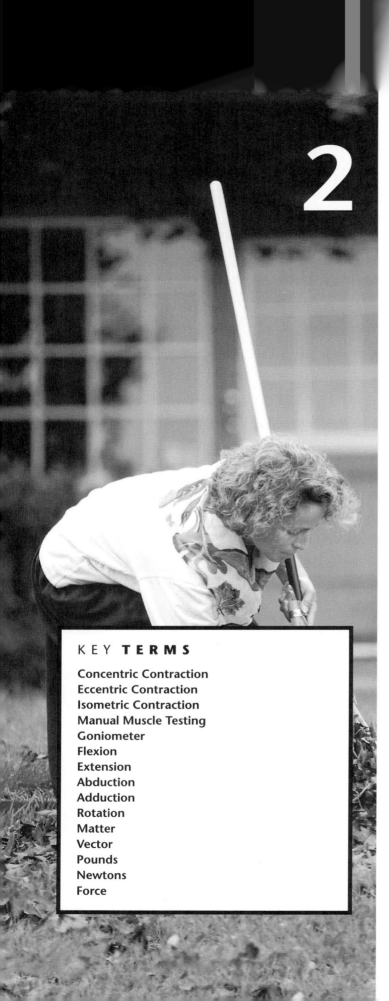

2 The Study of Human Movement

Concepts from Related Fields

KEY **TERMS**

Concentric Contraction
Eccentric Contraction
Isometric Contraction
Manual Muscle Testing
Goniometer
Flexion
Extension
Abduction
Adduction
Rotation
Matter
Vector
Pounds
Newtons
Force

CHAPTER **OUTLINE**

M*edicine and physics* converge in the study of biomechanics and kinesiology. Each discipline has its own perspective and language. Learning some vocabulary and concepts of each discipline is necessary for the OT practitioner to travel in both these worlds and apply knowledge from each discipline to functional activity.

The language of medicine is rich with words that describe unique physiologic conditions and minute areas of anatomical geography. These words are derived from Greek, Latin, and a variety of other languages.

Although medical terms often are confusing to the uninitiated, the ability to say in one word what otherwise would take several phrases is useful. This chapter explores terms commonly used to describe human movement and diagnoses that deal with abnormal biomechanics and kinesiology.

The terms rooted in physics are equally as valuable as those in medicine. Physics describes the world and its relationships with mathematics. These relationships help explain the past and predict the future. Biomechanics is based on the concepts of mechanical physics, which is the study of motion in gases, liquids, and solids.

Although you may know many of the terms relating to the musculoskeletal system, we may be applying them in new and unfamiliar ways. A review of gross anatomy, neuroanatomy, motor control, and muscle physiology may be necessary to solve the problems presented in this text. Further reading and study of physics is most useful to OT practitioners, who must apply mathematics to human motion regularly. We offer the brief summary of the following concepts as a guide. This list is not comprehensive.

Concepts from Medicine

In medicine, the ability to identify specific areas of the human body is essential. The body is most often envisioned in anatomical position, that is, upright with the face, feet, and palms facing forward. The head is superior to the shoulders because the head is above, or higher than, the shoulders. The shoulders are inferior to the head because they are below the head when the body is vertical. Those parts closer to the front of the body are anterior, and those near the back are posterior. Medial body parts lie near the middle of the body, and lateral parts lie near the right or left sides of the body. Arms and legs are extremities, and they connect to the trunk at their proximal ends. Fingers and toes are located at the distal ends of the extremities. Tissues close to the surface are superficial to underlying, or deep, tissues.

THE CENTRAL NERVOUS SYSTEM

The brain and spinal cord comprise the central nervous system (CNS), which controls all the body's activities. The brain is divided into three major anatomical parts: the cerebrum, cerebellum, and brain stem. The cerebrum receives sensory information and processes it to produce body responses, including movement. The cerebrum is divided into two hemispheres. Fibers that transmit impulses from each hemisphere cross from one side to the other in the corpus callosum and other smaller pathways, allowing one side of the brain to communicate with the other. Generally, each hemisphere receives sensory information from and controls movement of the opposite side of the body. The cortex is the superficial layer of the cerebrum and processes information for all tasks that require conscious thought. Two strips of cells run from ear to ear over the superior part of the cortex. Each strip contains a separate cell population—one for processing of sensory information and one for direction of motor performance.

The cerebrum contains other important centers for processing of sensory information and organization of subcortical motor responses, which do not require conscious thought. The cortex and corpus callosum surround the limbic lobe and basal ganglia. Cells that collect in the limbic lobe govern behavior and emotion. In the basal ganglia, cells pool to coordinate complex motor responses to environmental stimulation.

The brain stem connects the cerebrum to the spinal cord. It contains a number of differentiated cellular structures. The thalamus and hypothalamus regulate breathing, digestion, alertness, hormonal balance, and temperature control.

The cerebellum rises out of the brain stem to form a separate structure. The cerebellum chiefly regulates muscle tone and equilibrium, or balance, reactions. It also coordinates voluntary motor acts.

The spinal cord carries information to the brain from the body and to the body from the brain. Cells that carry specific kinds of information are grouped together to form pathways known as *tracts*. The spinal cord is the location of the reflex arc, through which motor responses to some external stimuli are carried out before sensory impulses reach the brain.

THE PERIPHERAL NERVOUS SYSTEM

The peripheral nervous system (PNS) is an extension of the CNS, and neither system can operate independently from the other. Individuals studying the body arbitrarily have differentiated these systems to understand how they work.

Information is carried to and from the CNS via nerve fibers that have cell bodies in the brain and spinal cord or in special structures called *ganglia.* Ganglia are collections of nerve-cell bodies that lie outside the CNS. Afferent nerve fibers carry impulses from the body tissues to the spinal cord and brain. Efferent fibers carry information from the brain to muscles and glands. Somatic nerves carry impulses to and from muscles. Visceral nerves transmit impulses to and from organs and glands.

Spinal nerves branch out from the spinal cord in an organized pattern. Their organization makes it possible to identify which segments of the spinal cord are responsible for specific areas of sensation and muscle movement. In several locations, spinal nerves are grouped into a network to form the plexus. A plexus is composed of motor and sensory fibers innervating various structures. The cervical plexus, located in the neck, innervates structures in the neck and shoulder. The brachial plexus, located under the shoulder in the axilla, supplies the upper extremities. Lumbar and sacral plexuses supply the lower extremities.

Cranial nerves are peripheral nerves that branch out directly from the brain and brain stem. There are 12 pairs of cranial nerves. All these nerves except the tenth cranial nerve innervate structures in the head and neck. The tenth, or vagus, nerve primarily innervates organs and other structures in the thorax and abdomen.

The CNS controls organs and glands through a system of visceral efferent fibers and ganglia known as the *autonomic nervous system (ANS).* Nerve fibers that carry messages from the body's organs are not considered part of the ANS. These visceral afferent fibers run alongside the nerves of the ANS and go directly to the CNS, not to ganglia. The CNS interprets the sensory information and directs the response. The ANS then carries these reaction messages back to the organs and glands.

The ANS is divided into two parts that balance control of bodily functions. The parasympathetic fibers originate in the brain and lower portion of the spinal cord (craniosacral) and connect with secondary fibers in ganglia located throughout the viscera. These fibers conserve and build up energy and calm the body, for example, slowing the heart rate and facilitating digestion. The sympathetic fibers and ganglia emerge from the middle (thoracolumbar) position of the spinal cord. They respond to environmental crises and produce an excitatory effect on the body known as the *fight-or-flight reaction.*

CONTROL OF MOVEMENT

The nervous system controls movement in the head, neck, trunk, and limbs through impulses generated in the brain's motor centers. These impulses are initiated either by a conscious intention to move or in response to incoming sensory impulses. Impulses reach the CNS from sensory receptors in the skin, muscles, and related tissues. Motor responses depend on the destination of the sensory fibers.

Skin contains an assortment of sensory end organs that produce withdrawal responses when stimulated. Skeletal muscles contain muscle spindles. These sensory organs are receptive to prolonged muscle stretch (tonic response) and rapid changes in length (phasic response). Stimulation of a muscle spindle most commonly results in contraction of the muscle. However, golgi tendon organs are tension-sensitive receptors that protect muscles from tearing. When stimulated, they inhibit muscle contraction.

Under certain conditions, motor responses to muscle spindle stimulation appear exaggerated. Too much muscular activity occurs, and skeletal muscles are unable to relax. An unyielding contraction of the muscle on one side of a joint limits desired movement in the opposite direction. This imbalance and movement disturbance generally is seen as an abnormality in muscle tone, a condition that requires intervention to help the individual regain normal motor control and movement.

Responses to sensory receptors also can occur without conscious thought. They follow reflexes, which are subcortical pathways. Pathways that make a complete sensory-to-motor connection in the spinal cord are spinal reflexes. Spinal reflexes provide protective responses to noxious stimuli or muscle spindle stretching. Pathways that make connections in the brain stem are brain stem reflexes. These reflexes regulate muscle responses to gravity acting on the body. Brain stem reflexes also regulate head movements that affect the entire body.

Righting reactions are complex interconnections that travel pathways to higher levels of the brainstem. These responses primarily involve positioning the head in relation to gravity. They respond to stimulation of the semicircular canals, or labyrinths, and the visual pathways. Equilibrium reactions require connections among the cortex, basal ganglia, and cerebellum. They involve adjustments of the entire body to changes in its center of gravity.

Bones

The skeletal system is composed of more than 200 bones. Although bones are rigid, bony tissue is dynamic and changes throughout life. The most obvious of these changes is the ossification of cartilage that occurs during a child's early years. An infant skeleton has a smaller percentage of bone than that of an adult because the entire skeleton has not changed from cartilage to bone. This change occurs over time. Centers of cartilaginous growth, or epiphyseal plates, allow bones to grow throughout childhood and into an individual's early 20s. Stress from carrying weight, movement, or trauma all stimulate bony tissue growth. Bone continually remodels itself throughout life because the skeleton provides not only structure but also storage for calcium. Bone is absorbed, and new bone is laid down when needed.

Joints

A joint is the articulation of two adjacent bones. Diarthrodial joints have a fluid-filled space between the two or more bones. Articulating surfaces are covered with smooth hyaline cartilage, and a strong ligamentous capsule surrounds the whole joint. Elbows, knees, hips, and shoulders are diarthrodial joints. Because they are so mobile, diarthrodial joints are referenced frequently in biomechanics and kinesiology.

Amphiarthrodial joints allow only slight movement and are composed of adjacent bones connected by cartilage. Symphysis joints located between vertebral bodies and the temporary joints between the epiphysis and the shaft of a long bone are examples of amphiarthrodial joints. Synarthrodial joints are immovable joints involving a fibrous interface between bones, for example, the suture joints of the skull.

Muscles

Muscle tissue is unique in its ability to contract. Three varieties exist: smooth, cardiac, and skeletal. Skeletal, or striated, muscle is of the most interest in biomechanics and kinesiology. Muscle fibers are the cellular units that make up muscles. Their measurements increase or decrease depending on the intracellular buildup or removal of contractile proteins (A Closer Look Box 2-1).

Skeletal muscle strength depends on the thickness of its cross section. Genetics determines the number of fibers contained in muscle. Larger, stronger muscles contain thicker fibers, not a larger number of fibers.

The length of the muscle fiber determines the distance a muscle can contract or expand. Shorter muscles (shorter fiber lengths) contract less distance (excursion) than longer muscles. Generally, muscle fibers can shorten to and can be stretched 50% longer than their resting lengths.

Skeletal muscles vary greatly in shape and fiber configuration. The attachment of muscles to bones via either broad, fleshy attachments or concentrated, tendinous insertions determines the gross shape of the muscle and its force for movement. The biceps brachii and the lumbricals in the hand are fusiform muscles. All the fibers in fusiform muscles run from the origin to the insertion.

BOX 2-1

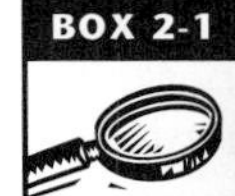

A **CLOSER** LOOK

Contractions Versus Contractures

Contractions *and* contractures *are two words with almost identical spellings, but they describe two very different concepts. A contraction occurs in a skeletal muscle. It is a process that depends on the expenditure of energy. In a concentric contraction the muscle fibers shorten, but in an eccentric contraction, they lengthen. A contracture describes a state of being, not a process. In a contracture, the resting length of the tissue has become physically shorter than at a previous time. Contractures occur in muscle and joint ligaments that are inadequately stretched over time or in skin that is scarred by second- and third-degree burns. A contraction is a normal muscle movement, but a contracture is a lack of movement caused by a pathological process.*

Pennate and bipennate muscles have fibers that attach to a central tendon, which bridges the gap between the fiber's other attachments and gives them the appearance of a feather. Pennate and bipennate muscles like the interossei and long flexors of the digits have short excursions because of their short lengths. However, their thick cross sections provide impressive strength.

Muscles may spread out in broad sheets like the pronator quadratus and trapezius or assume unique shapes like the deltoid and serratus anterior. Some muscles, like the latissimus dorsi and pectoralis major, twist between attachments, allowing separate muscle parts to act differently.

Muscles are connected intimately to the skeletal system through tissue called *fascia*. The fascial sheaths surrounding bundles of muscle fibers and entire muscles continue along the tendons that attach muscle to bone.

Muscle fibers are contracted through a chemical process involving oxygen and adenosine triphosphate (ATP). The primary source of oxygen in muscle tissue is myoglobin. Like hemoglobin in the blood, myoglobin contains oxygen bonded to iron, which produces the characteristic red color. Muscles with fibers that contain high concentrations of myoglobin are red muscles. They consist of slow-twitch fibers and rely on high concentrations of myoglobin and a rich blood supply. Postural muscles that must work for prolonged periods without becoming fatigued are typical red muscles. Muscles with low concentrations of myoglobin are white muscles. They are composed mostly of fast-twitch fibers and contract rapidly, like the flight muscles of birds. These fibers contract quickly but for limited amounts of time because of their lower concentrations of myoglobin.

Muscle activity

Several types of contractions are common to all skeletal muscles. When a muscle moves, one attachment usually remains stationary while the other attachment moves. ***Concentric*** contractions cause muscles to shorten (Figure 2-1). **Eccentric** contractions occur when muscles attempt to shorten but are stretched by an overpowering external effort (Figure 2-2). In **isometric** contractions the contractile mechanisms are activated, but no appreciable change in length of the fibers or movement of the attachment ends results. Isometric contractions occur when some force in the opposite direction equally balances the effort of the contraction.

The amount of force generated in different contraction types often is misunderstood. When we move weight we easily can control, the greatest force involves a concentric contraction, then an isometric contraction, and finally an eccentric contraction. This follows the reasoning that to lift (concentric), we must overcome; to hold (isometric), we must balance; and to lower with control (eccentric), we must let the weight overcome the muscle by pulling upward slightly less than the weight being lowered.

When the weight being manipulated is at the maximum limit of control, the ratio changes. Therefore the greatest force is associated with eccentric contractions and the least with concentric contractions; isometric contractions remain in the middle. We can lower more weight (eccentric) than we can hold (isometric) and hold more than we can lift (concentric).

Every action involves more muscles than those primarily responsible for a particular movement. Muscles that act to produce a specific movement are prime movers, or agonists. Opposing muscles are antagonists. Antagonists must relax to allow agonists to move. When agonists and antagonists contract simultaneously to stabilize a joint, it is a cocontraction. To protect joints, antagonists stop movement at the end of a range of motion. When gravity is the primary force initiating movement, antagonists control movement through eccentric contraction.

Muscles that act together to produce specific movements are working in synergy. If a muscle performs more than one action, another muscle must neutralize one of the actions via stabilization. The combination of wrist extension and finger flexion in grasp provides one example of this concept. If the wrist extensors did not stabilize the wrist in extension, the finger flexors would flex both the fingers and the wrist, diminishing the strength of the grip.

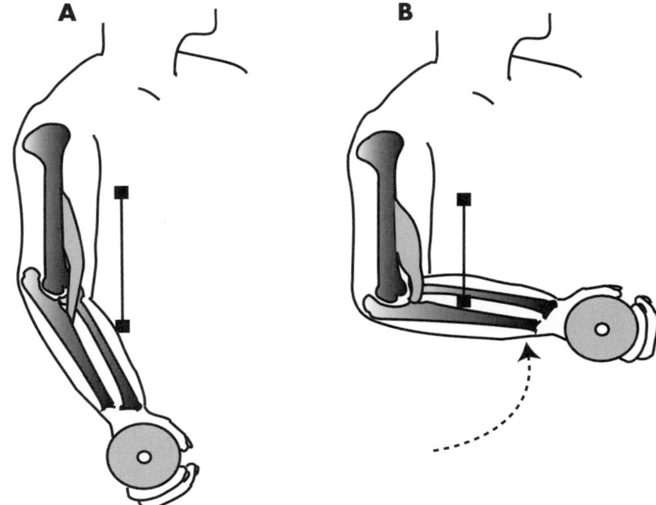

FIGURE **2-1**
Concentric contractions cause muscles to shorten. The muscle begins the contraction at a longer length **(A)** than the length at completion **(B)**. The distance traveled by the moving end of the muscle is called *muscle excursion.*

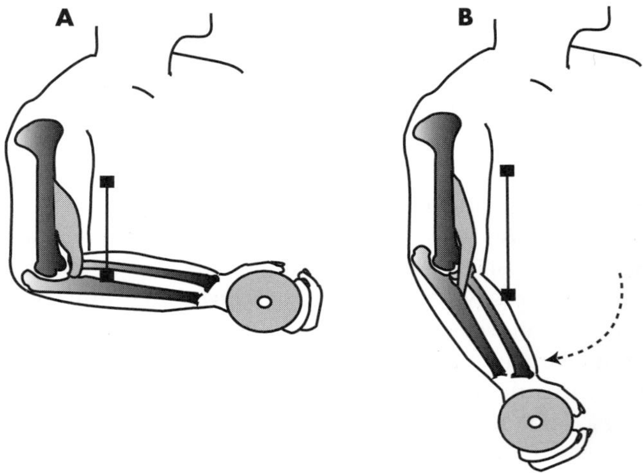

FIGURE **2-2**
In eccentric contractions, the muscle attempts to shorten against an overwhelming force in the opposite direction. The muscle begins in its shortened length **(A)** and, while attempting to shorten, is pulled longer **(B)**.

In this example, the finger flexors are agonists for grasp, the wrist extensors are synergists (stabilizers), and the finger extensors are antagonists to grasp. Some muscles also function as supporting muscles that hold the trunk and proximal parts of the limbs in advantageous positions. For example, the back extends, the shoulder adducts, and the elbow flexes when the hand grasps to unlock the door.

Slow, active movement involves continuous muscle tension throughout a range of motion. Ballistic movements are strong, rapid contractions completed primarily through momentum. These movements can be controlled through contraction of antagonistic muscles. When ballistic movements are not controlled, they are stopped passively by muscles, ligaments, and other joint tissues at the end of a range of motion. Ballistic movements that are passively controlled put joints at more risk for injury than ballistic movements that are actively controlled with antagonistic muscles.

Muscle strength

Muscle strength can be measured with force gauges (grip and pinch strength dynamometers) or by the application of graded resistance in **manual muscle testing (MMT).** MMT evaluates muscle groups responsible for pure motions. Single muscles are isolated when possible. An individual moves through a specified range of motion against the resistance of gravity, that is, the weight of the body part moved. Resistance may be added at the endpoint of the range. If full movement against gravity is not possible, the resistance of gravity is eliminated (minimized) through positioning, and the subject attempts to move again.

MMT is measured on a 6-point scale of 0 to 5, with 0 as no movement and 5 as normal strength. A measure of 1 is trace, or palpable contraction; 2 is poor, or insufficient strength to lift the weight of the body part through the entire active range of motion; 3 is fair, or the ability to lift the weight of the body part through its active range of motion; and 4 is good, or the ability to hold the weight against some but less than normal resistance.

Muscle strength grading in MMT is subjective. Practitioners have questioned the consistency of scoring. Some earlier studies indicated a high degree of reliability among experienced practitioners, but more recent work has demonstrated otherwise.*

Regardless, MMT remains a universally used technique in the assessment of muscle strength. Muscles can be measured individually or in functional groups. The relatively inexpensive techniques are simple to learn, and a variety of textbooks explain testing in great detail. (Guidelines for the examination of isolated muscle functions are provided in later chapters.)

Muscle tone

Observation and palpation (feeling the muscles) are used to assess muscle tone. Hypertonia, or increased muscle tone, makes muscles feel very firm and causes increased resistance to passive stretching. Spasticity is severe when resistance to quick stretching occurs in the first third of a range of motion. Resistance in the second third is moderate, and resistance in the last third is mild. Hypertonicity can be observed when responses to resistance involve muscles on the opposite side of the body and muscles located above or below those being tested on the same side. Rigidity is uncontrollable resistance throughout a range of motion.

Hypotonia, or low muscle tone, is a condition in which muscles feel soft and mushy and are unable to give or sustain resistance. Hypotonicity is most easily observed in the postural muscles. An individual with excessively poor sitting or standing posture may have hypotonicity. Such disturbances in muscle tone invalidate MMT grades.

MUSCULOSKELETAL MOVEMENT

Joint movement is measured with a **goniometer** (Figure 2-3). A goniometer is placed directly over the axis of motion in the joint and can measure a full 360 degrees of rotary motion. Most joints exhibit a range of motion within 180 degrees. Paired motions such as flexion and extension occur at each joint and are measured within a single plane or surface. Movement is universally viewed as occurring in three planes, or along three surfaces, to ensure accurate and valid measurement and clear communication.

The movement in each plane occurs around a central axis that is always oriented perpendicular to the plane, as if the axis were sticking out of the plane like a flagpole sticking out of the ground. Each pure motion is measured in only one plane, although functional motion can occur in a number of planes.

Figure 2-4 shows an individual divided into parts by each of the three planes. The sagittal plane divides the body into right and left halves. Rotary movement in this plane (**flexion** and **extension**) is centered on an axis oriented left to right. Vertebral flexion and extension occur within this plane. Flexion and extension of joints such as the shoulder, elbow, and wrist occur in planes of the same orientation drawn parallel to the sagittal plane.

Abduction and **adduction** are movements that occur in the frontal plane. This plane divides the body into front and back halves, and movement is around an axis running front to back, or anterior to posterior.

Rotation occurs in the transverse, or horizontal, plane, which divides the body into upper and lower halves. The axis for movement in this plane always is oriented in an up-to-down position. As in flexion and extension, movements in the frontal and transverse planes occur in either one of the planes shown in Figure 2-4 or parallel planes of the same orientation.

*Lawson and Calderon[2] found consistency among practitioners in two of four muscles tested. Freese and others[1] conducted a larger study that demonstrated low consistency in all four muscles tested, even when adhering to a strict testing protocol.

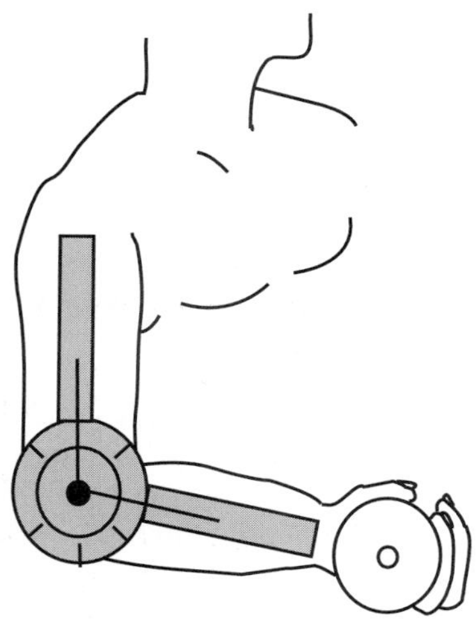

FIGURE **2-3**
Goniometers measure joint position and range of motion.

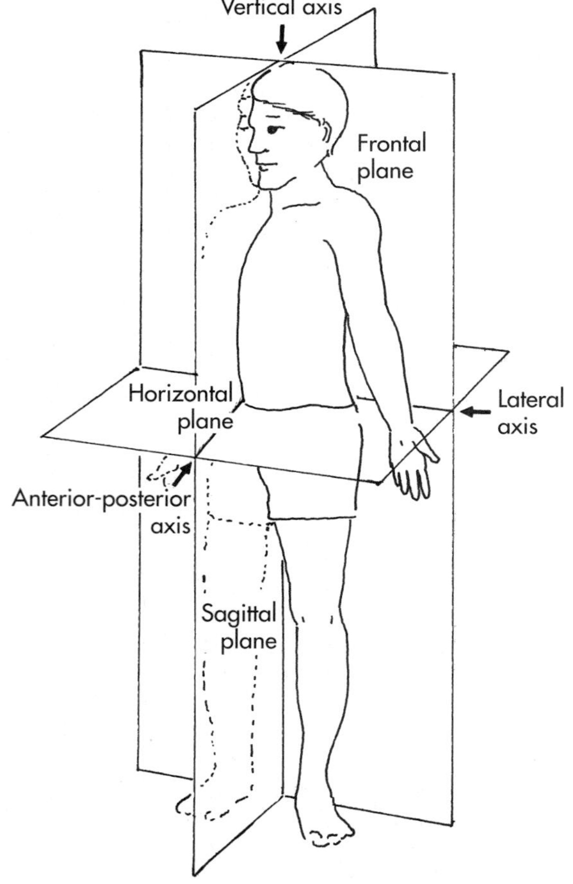

FIGURE **2-4**
The human body is divided into three anatomical planes, each of which has an axis around which movement takes place.

Goniometry may be used to measure the extent of active and passive joint motions within these planes. Active motion occurs when an individual voluntarily moves a body part. Passive motion occurs when someone or something moves the body part.

MEDICAL DIAGNOSES AFFECTING MOVEMENT

Any pathological condition that affects the nervous system or the musculoskeletal system has some effect on movement. How movement changes varies according to the condition and the individual involved. A brief look at some conditions that can affect movement follows.

Many different pathological processes, from traumatic injuries to illnesses, can affect the CNS. When the head receives severe blows or rocks forward and backward violently, damage to the cerebrum results.* Damage that occurs after intracerebral bleeding or clotting is called a *cerebral vascular accident* (*CVA*) or *stroke.* A variety of illnesses, such as multiple sclerosis, which affects the myelin sheath covering nerves, can cause damage to CNS tissues.

In all cases, damage to the cerebrum affects voluntary and involuntary movements. Generally, when either the left or the right hemisphere is affected, movement on the opposite side of the body is restricted. Damage to cerebellar structures affects muscle tone and coordination. Spinal cord damage affects muscle use and sensation below the level of the lesion. Damage can be mapped according to the affected ranges of sensory and motor loss.

Damage to peripheral nerves affects individual muscles and areas of sensation. Peripheral nerves can be cut, crushed, or attacked by viruses, bacteria, and the body's immune system response. Peripheral nerve fibers have the ability to regenerate, unlike CNS structures. If the nerve cell body is intact after injury, recovery of muscle use and sensation sometimes is possible.

Metabolic problems, trauma, and disease all can result in skeletal disorders, which affect movement. Some conditions such as scoliosis occur because of abnormally formed but healthy bone tissue. In scoliosis the vertebral bodies form a wedge shape, causing abnormal spinal curvatures. Muscle imbalance, severe weakness, and lack of adequate trunk support also can cause scoliosis. In addition, scoliosis may have an idiopathic cause (no known reason).

Scoliosis can become so severe that it compromises the heart, lungs, and other organs. Although surgery may provide the only permanent solution, careful posi-

*Infants in particular are susceptible to this form of trauma. Their neck muscles are insufficient to stabilize the head, and even brief shaking can cause brain damage.

tioning that provides lateral support to the trunk may slow the progression of the curvatures.

Other diseases may alter bone development and thus movement. Osteogenesis imperfecta is an example of a disease that affects the metabolic formation of bone tissue and makes the bone more susceptible to fracture. Fractures or other trauma to the epiphyseal plates in growing children may disrupt or halt bone growth. Damage to a bone's blood supply can lead to avascular necrosis and progressive bone deterioration.

BOX 2-2

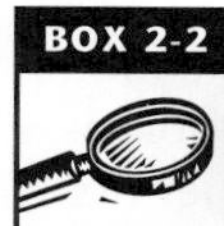

A **CLOSER** LOOK

Range of Motion Precautions After Hip Surgery

Hip-replacement surgery, or total hip arthroplasty, repairs the hip joint but leaves it vulnerable. If an individual moves the wrong way, the surgery can be undone in a moment. Hip precautions differ slightly depending on the surgical approach used, but the following are usually recommended after total hip arthroplasty:

- *No hip flexion beyond 90 degrees*
- *No hip internal rotation past the neutral position*
- *No hip adduction past the neutral position*

Osteoporosis affects bone through a gradual decrease in calcium content. The bone becomes weaker until it is so weak that it fractures during normal shifts in body weight and muscle contractions. Weakened bones place older adults with age-related osteoporosis at greater risk of fractures from falls.

Both biomechanics and kinesiology play parts in the treatment of fractures. Normal muscle forces can contribute to the misalignment of fractured fragments and must be considered in splinting or range-of-motion restrictions. Such restrictions are critical after hip fractures, especially when fractures are treated by surgical replacement of the hip joint components, or total hip arthroplasty (A Closer Look Box 2-2).

Damage to joints also may restrict movement. Fractures that cross the joint line, that is, extend to the joint surface, may result in limited joint motion after the fracture has healed completely. Ligaments severely damaged through dislocation may produce chronic joint instability or predispose the joint to stiffening and decreased range of motion from osteoarthritis.

Rheumatoid arthritis, in contrast, causes joints to become loose and unstable. The joints may undergo subluxation under normal use and muscle pull, causing misalignments such as ulnar drift (Figure 2-5, *A*). Boutonniere misalignment consists of hyperflexion in the proximal interphalangeal joint (Figure 2-5, *B*). Swan neck is hyperextension of the proximal interphalangeal joint, which may occur with volar subluxation (Figure 2-5, *C*). Each condition commonly leads to secondary joint contractures involving the distal interphalangeal

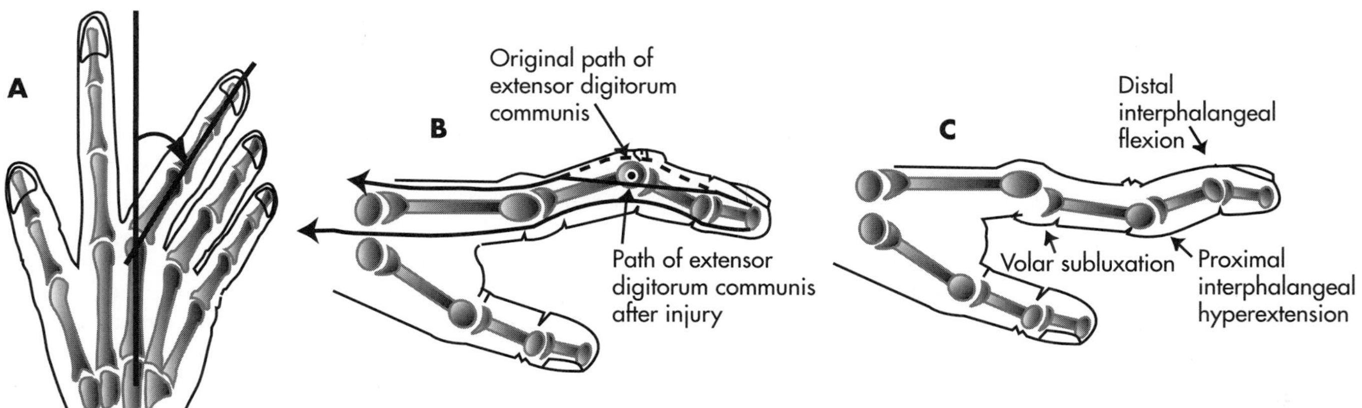

FIGURE **2-5**
A, Ulnar drift occurs after displacement of the extensor digitorum tendon in the ulnar direction. The index finger is normally aligned, whereas digits 3 through 5 exhibit 45 degrees of ulnar deviation at the metacarpophalangeal joints. **B,** Boutonniere involves a buttonhole tear in the extensor aponeurosis and inability to actively extend the proximal interphalangeal joint. **C,** Swan neck exhibits hyperextension of the proximal interphalangeal joint and may occur with volar subluxation of the metacarpophalangeal joint.

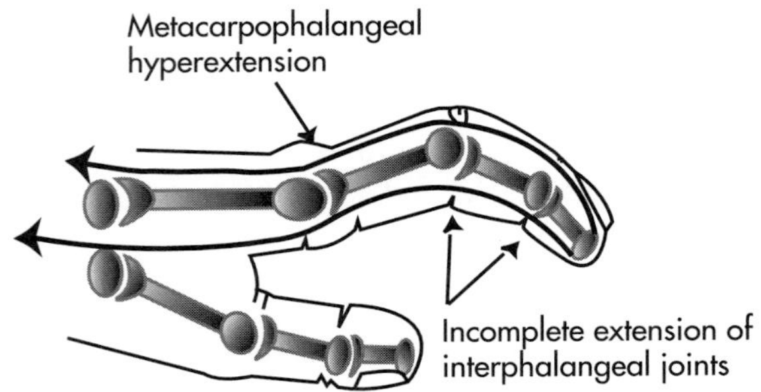

FIGURE **2-6**
The hallmark of intrinsic minus hand ("claw") is metacarpophalangeal hyperextension with incomplete interphalangeal extension.

joints. (These four conditions are more fully explored in later chapters.)

A pathological condition of the joint also can occur after a CVA when the weight of the affected arm stretches the joint capsule and separates the head of the humerus from the glenoid fossa. Joints usually are assessed using goniometers to measure range of motion, but medical practitioners may describe shoulder subluxation in terms of the distance developed between joint surfaces.

Tendons and muscles also are subject to movement-related pathological conditions. Boutonniere consists of a buttonhole tear in the elaborate extensor tendon of the extensor digitorum communis muscle. The proximal interphalangeal joint protrudes through the hole when the finger is flexed. As the tendon falls from the posterior to the anterior side of the joint axis of motion, the individual is unable to straighten the finger, even though the extensor muscle is contracting (see Figure 2-5, *B*).

Imbalances in muscle function can make specific movements difficult or impossible. For example, if the intrinsic muscles of the hand are weak or no longer functioning, the extensor digitorum communis muscle is unable to extend the finger completely. When the extensor contracts, the interphalangeal joints extend, but the metacarpophalangeal joint hyperextends. Over time, metacarpophalangeal hyperextension increases and interphalangeal extension becomes less complete; the result is a condition called *intrinsic minus* (Figure 2-6).

Repeated use of the tendon causes tendinitis, or inflammation of the tendon. The resulting swelling is usually painful and sometimes results in severe crowding of tissues and reduced blood flow. When this happens, nearby nerves may be damaged. For example, frequent and forceful flexion of the fingers and wrist can lead to tendonitis. This in turn can cause nerve compression in the wrist, or carpal tunnel syndrome.

Concepts from Physics and Engineering

When physicists talk about a body, they are referring to a collection of matter. A body may be incredibly small like the protons and electrons that make up an atom or very large like the sun. The human body is a collection of matter. Because *body* is a generic term, in physics it must have specific modifiers to prevent confusion.

Space, time, and mass are all quantified to describe their relationships with one another. Different systems of measurement develop in different cultures. Most Americans use the English system, but the scientific community worldwide uses the metric system. This book uses the metric system for all measurements. (Appendix A contains a complete conversion table for English and metric systems.)

SCALAR QUANTITIES

A scalar quantity is one that can be measured by an instrument or a scale. Scalar quantities are static. These quantities tend to stay in one place, which makes them easy to measure.

Measures of space

Length, area, and volume are spatial measurements. In the metric system, space is measured in millimeters, centimeters, and meters. The English system measures space in inches, feet, and yards. Length is a linear, one-dimensional measure of distance (centimeters, meters, inches, and miles). Area is a planar, or two-dimensional, measure of a flat surface (square centimeters or square feet). Volume is a cubic measure of three dimensions (cubic centimeters, liters, cubic inches, quarts, and gallons).

Measures of time

Time presents a fourth dimension. The basic unit of measurement for both the metric and the English systems is the second.

Measures of mass

Matter is composed of molecules made up of atoms, which consist of neutrons, protons, and electrons. The chemical composition of a substance and the closeness of its molecules determine the quantity of mass. For example, a hydrogen atom has only 1 proton and electron pair, whereas larger atoms like carbon, nitrogen, and oxygen have 6, 7, and 8 proton-electron pairs. Potassium, calcium, and iron have 19, 20, and 26, respectively. As OT practitioners, we rarely consult a periodic table to discover the number of proton-electron pairs in a particular element, but we do encounter matter daily and should be familiar with this concept.

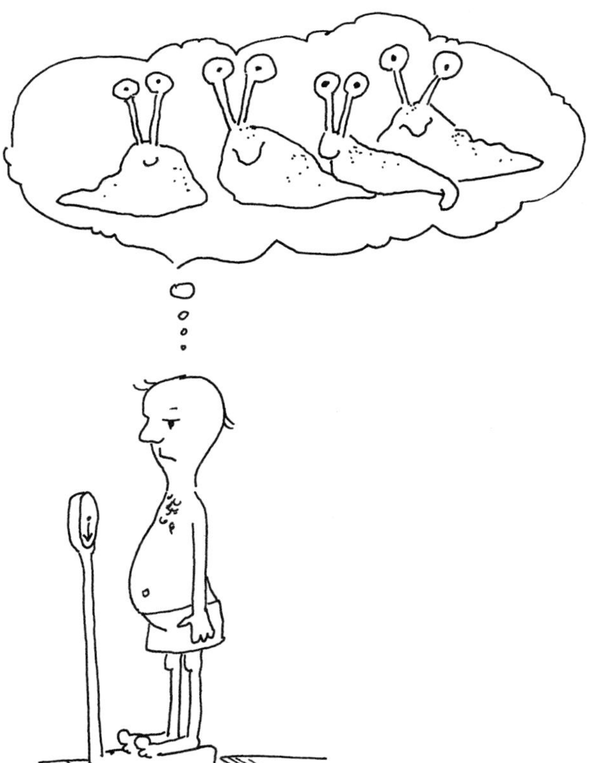

FIGURE **2-7**
One possible reason the British measurement system did not flourish.

The arrangements of these elements within solids, liquids, and gases affect the mass of the different substances. Molecules in solids are closely packed. In liquids they move freely around each other, and in gases they bounce around and keep their distance from everything else. Water is in a class by itself. Body substances are composed mostly of hydrogen, carbon, and oxygen compounds, but their slightly different chemical compositions determine their mass. Fat, for example, is less dense than bone and muscle, both of which have more calcium and iron in their compositions.

In the metric system, mass is measured in grams. In the English system, it is measured in slugs (Figure 2-7). For example, 1 slug equals 32 pounds.

VECTOR QUANTITIES

A **vector** indicates movement. It can be measured only at a specific moment in time because it constantly changes. Arrows that indicate a starting point (point of application), magnitude, and direction represent vectors. A simple arrowhead drawn on the end of a line converts a haphazard mark into a story indicating a specific force, specific point at which it was applied, and specific direction in which it is moving. Without the arrowhead, it is a mere line.

Measures of physical movement

Movement involves a starting point, motion in a specific direction, and distance traveled. Taken together, this is displacement, which is a vector quantity. Velocity is the rate at which displacement occurs. When we divide displacement *(s)* by time *(t)*, we can express velocity *(v)* as an equation:

$$v = \frac{s}{t}$$

When velocity increases, the change occurs over time, and the amount of that change is acceleration. Acceleration *(a)* can be calculated by subtracting an initial velocity *(u)*, from a final velocity *(v)*, and dividing the result by time *(t)*.

$$a = \frac{v-u}{t}$$

Measures of weight

Weight reflects both mass and the pull of gravity on that mass; therefore weight is a force. Gravity always pulls toward the center of the Earth. For example, individuals stand on the Earth's surface with their feet toward the Earth's center and experience gravity as a downward pull, a vector quantity. Gravity is a constant factor; therefore as mass increases, weight increases. In the English system, weight (a force) is measured in **pounds.** In the metric system, force and weight are measured in **newtons,** named after Sir Isaac Newton. He first realized that gravity gives mass its direction when an apple landed on his head (Figure 2-8).

Measures of force

In physics a **force** is defined as something that causes an object to be deformed or moved. Forces are measured in metric newtons or English pounds. The force muscles produce is the most common force encountered in this text.

Drawing muscles as vectors is somewhat different than drawing muscles in an anatomical drawing. The length of a vector is determined by the specific amount that a muscle pulls. Vectors drawn to represent muscles indicate a pull from the attachment where the force has its effect (that is, insertion) toward the other attachment (that is, origin), which implies a tendency toward movement in that direction. Because these arrows indicate the amount of force, they may be either longer or shorter than the muscle itself. Vectors can be drawn from the origin or the insertion of the muscle depending on which

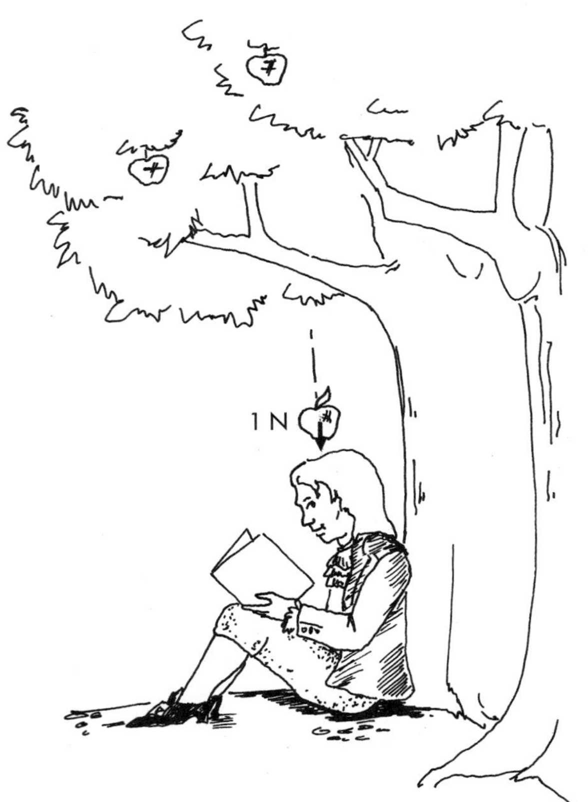

FIGURE **2-8**
As Sir Isaac Newton discovered, gravity produces movement at a constant rate of acceleration.

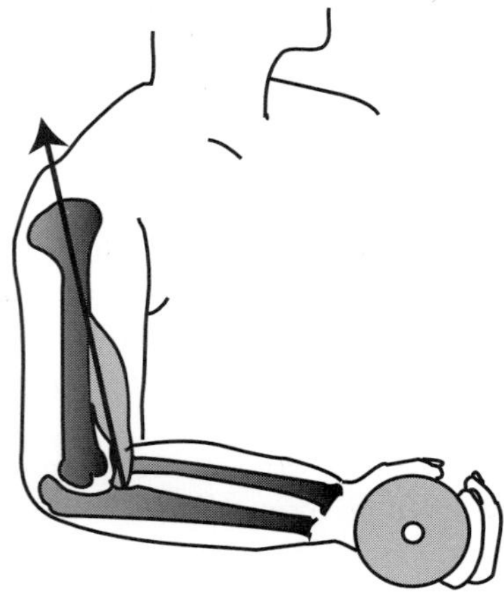

FIGURE **2-9**
A vector drawn to represent the pull (force) of a muscle must be drawn from the moving attachment, through the muscle fibers, and toward the stationary attachment.

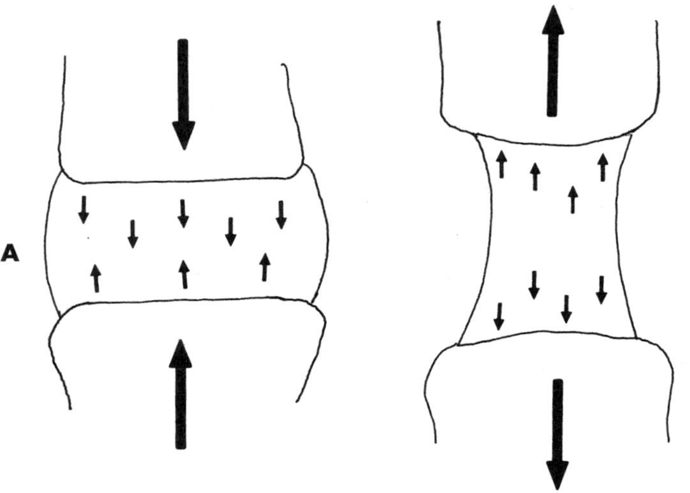

FIGURE **2-10**
Normal forces are perpendicular to surfaces pushing together as compressive forces **(A)** or pulling apart as tensile forces **(B)**. Stress occurs in the materials on which forces act.

direction the force is moving, but the arrow always follows the direction of muscle fibers (Figure 2-9).

Normal forces are forces directed perpendicularly toward or away from a surface area. Normal forces that push two surfaces together are compressive forces (Figure 2-10, *A*). Normal forces that pull two surfaces apart are tensile forces (Figure 2-10, *B*). Forces that act parallel to the surfaces are shear, or tangential, forces (Figure 2-11).

Gravity is a normal force. Reaction forces, another type of normal force, produce an equal and opposite response to gravity or other forces. Muscle forces act in a variety of ways with reaction forces.

Measures of stress

Stress is different from force. Stress is found in the material on which forces act. Tensile forces on the knee produce tensile stress in the tissues of the knee joint. The amount of stress is determined by the division of the amount of force by the specific quantity of tissue. Stress is measured in units of Pascals (Pa), or newtons per meter squared (N/m^2).

Measures of friction

Friction is similar to stress. To determine friction (F), multiply a normal force (N) times a coefficient (μ) that is unique to the material in question:

$$F = \mu N$$

For instance, the coefficient of cartilage in a synovial joint is essentially 0, whereas the coefficient of a crutch tip on rough wood is about 0.70 to 0.75 (Figure 2-12). The closer

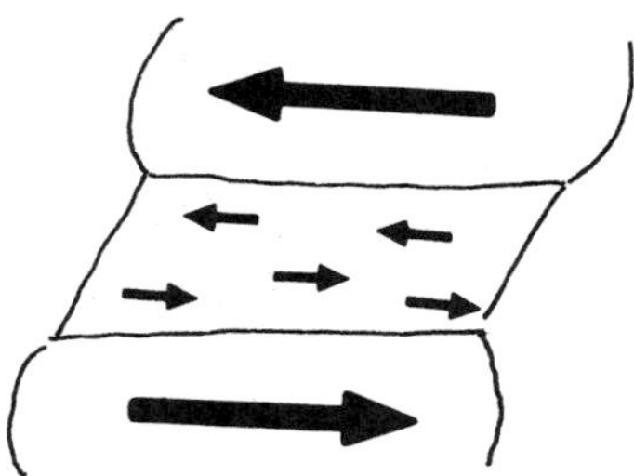

FIGURE **2-11**
Shear forces are parallel to the surfaces they affect.

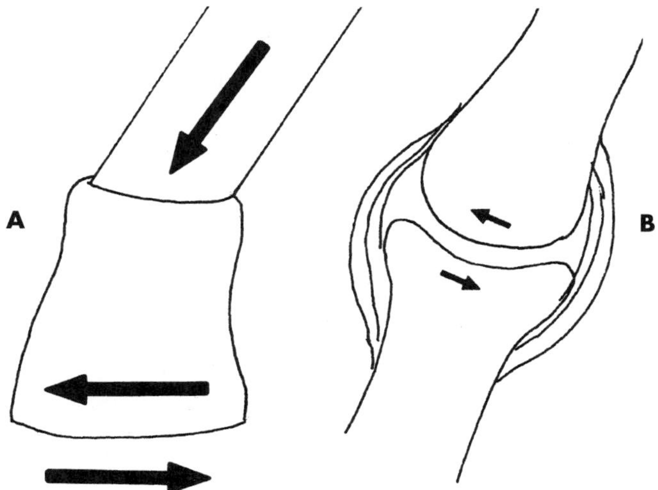

FIGURE **2-12**
Friction is determined by the nature of the surface material. The friction between rubber and wood **(A)** is much greater than that between two cartilaginous surfaces coated with synovial fluid **(B)**.

the coefficient gets to 1.0, the more force is needed to move the material across a specific surface.

Measures of work

Work is calculated by the multiplication of weight by distance by the number of repetitions. For example, to measure the amount of lifting work needed to do a job, use the following formula:

$$L = mg \times h \times r$$

Here, L represents lifting work, mg represents mass times gravity (weight), h represents the height of objects lifted, and r represents the number of repetitions. To find the amount of hauling work done on a job, use the following formula:

$$H = mg \times d \times r$$

H represents hauling work, d is the distance traveled, and r is the number of repetitions.

Summary

OT practitioners must be familiar with medicine and physics to understand and apply principles of biomechanics and kinesiology to functional activity. The vocabulary and concepts outlined in this chapter are part of every problem presented in the chapters that follow. Most OT students are comfortable with medicine, but for many, physics is strange territory. However, physics should become more familiar as its concepts are applied to human activity.

Applications

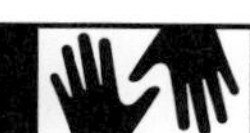

APPLICATION **2-1**

Appreciating Mass and Gravity

Thinking about mass and gravity separately is difficult. Although our body mass changes throughout life, the Earth's gravity does not. Our only indication of changing mass is gravity's effect on it—this is our weight. To appreciate mass, we must remove the effect of gravity:

1. Obtain samples of two vastly different elements: lead (a fishing weight) and aluminum (foil).
2. Crumple a piece of aluminum foil to equal roughly the size of the fishing weight.
3. Compare the two weights by feel.

Which is heavier? Because gravity affects both equally, what accounts for the difference in weight?

APPLICATION **2-2**

Identifying the Active Muscle

Understanding which muscles are active in different movements and contraction types first requires that we believe what medical books tell us is happening really is happening. We are oriented to basic function in gross anatomy. Without realizing it, most of us develop a bias that flexors flex and extensors extend. Therefore we believe that when we observe elbow flexion as a movement, the elbow flexors are the active group. This is far from the truth.

In some cases, activity in the wrong group may be disastrous. For example, if you slowly lower a bowling ball from above your head to the top of your head, the elbow moves from extension into flexion. You conclude that if you see elbow flexion, the elbow flexors must be active. *Don't* activate the elbow flexors. The ball will accelerate and hit your head.

To better appreciate which muscles are active, try this activity. Hold a heavy book above your head with your elbow fully extended. Lower it slowly about half the distance to the top of your head. At this point the elbow has flexed through about 45 degrees of motion. Hold it there and think about the active group:

1. Palpate the belly of the triceps and compare this feeling to that of the biceps. Which muscle is active? As you hold it, which muscle gets sore?
2. Now raise the book two times and palpate the two muscles one at a time each time you raise the book. Which muscle is active?
3. Now lower it slowly two times and again determine the active group.
4. Repeat these steps with the opposite hand and measure the origin-to-insertion distance for the long head of the triceps (infraglenoid tubercle to the olecranon). Now move into flexion, stopping at 45 degrees. Again measure origin to insertion. What happened to the distance as you slowly flexed the elbow? Which muscle was active? What kind of contraction was this?
5. As you hold the book steady with a partially flexed elbow, what happens to the origin-to-insertion distance for the triceps long head? Which muscle is active? What kind of contraction occurs?
6. As you raise the book back into full elbow extension, what happens to the triceps long head origin-to-insertion distance? Which muscle is active? What kind of contraction is implied?

See Appendix C for solutions to Applications.

REFERENCES

1. Freese F and others: Clinical reliability of manual muscle testing middle trapezius and gluteus medius muscles, *Phys Ther* 67(7):1072-1076, 1987.
2. Lawson A, Calderon L: Interexaminer agreement for applied kinesiology manual muscle testing, *Percept Mot Skills* 84(2):539-546, 1997.

RELATED READINGS

Behrman RE and others: *Textbook of pediatrics,* Philadelphia, 1996, WB Saunders.

Fiorentino M: *Reflex testing methods for evaluating CNS development,* Springfield, Ill, 1973, Charles C Thomas.

Fritjof C: *The Tao of physics,* New York, 1984, Bantam.

Gowitzke BA, Milner M: *Scientific bases of human movement,* ed 3, Baltimore, 1988, Williams & Wilkins.

Leveau BF: *Biomechanics of human motion,* ed 3, Philadelphia, 1992, WB Saunders.

Norkin CC, Levangie PK: *Joint structure and function: a comprehensive analysis,* ed 2, Philadelphia, 1992, FA Davis.

Rasch PJ: *Kinesiology and applied anatomy,* ed 7, Philadelphia, 1989, Lea & Febiger.

Williams PL, Bannister LH: *Gray's anatomy: the anatomical basis of medicine and surgery,* ed 38, New York, 1995, Churchill Livingstone.

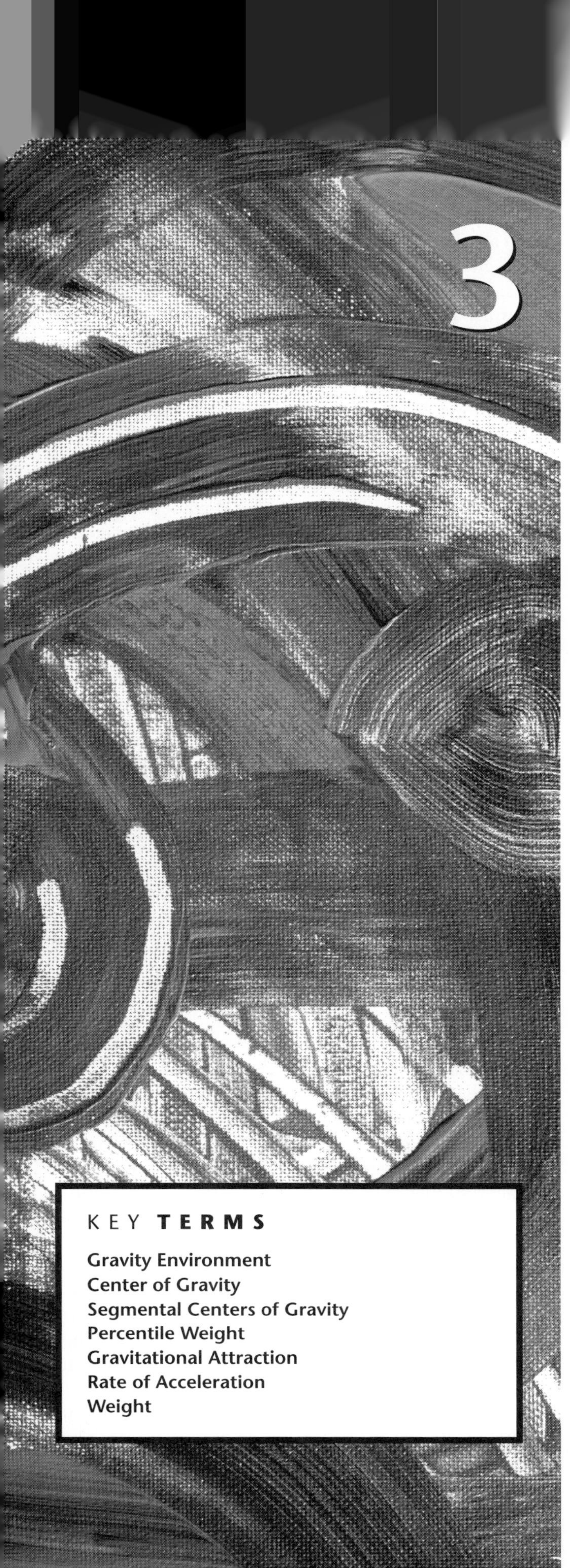

Gravity

A Constant Force

CHAPTER **OUTLINE**

KEY **TERMS**

Gravity Environment
Center of Gravity
Segmental Centers of Gravity
Percentile Weight
Gravitational Attraction
Rate of Acceleration
Weight

G***ravity is the most basic of forces.*** We feel its constant tug on our bodies even before birth. From infancy we struggle to stand upright and break free of its pull. We drop toys off our high chair trays in one of our earliest experiments with gravity. Gravity is so much a part of our daily experiences that we seem to intuitively know how it works.

We know that skiers and parachutists move in the same direction—down. If we throw a bowling ball and a baseball out the window at the same time, we expect them to land on the ground at the same time. We know that rockets break free of the Earth's pull of gravity because they have tremendous power. The space shuttle orbits our planet because it is held there by gravity, just as the moon orbits the Earth, and the Earth orbits the sun. We take these facts for granted.

If we had stated these beliefs 500 years ago, we could have been persecuted or put to death.* Even 400 years ago, students and professors argued ideas about gravity that seem like common sense to us today.

In the late sixteenth century, Galileo explored movement with a series of experiments in which he rolled objects down ramps. From these experiments, he developed laws of uniform acceleration, which state that objects of differing sizes and weights travel at equal speeds. In 1592, his ideas were so radical that he was forced to leave his teaching position at the University of Pisa.

Because Galileo was a mathematician, his laws of uniform acceleration were written as mathematics equations. Some 20 years after Galileo's death, Isaac Newton used Galileo's formulas to develop the law of universal gravitation. His genius was not just to explain why objects always fall to the ground but to extrapolate that gravity is an underlying force affecting all movement, celestial and earthbound. Newton's laws of motion help us understand forces and their interactions. These laws have become part of our general experience with gravity. We readily accept that gravity produces a constant force on matter (A Closer Look Box 3-1).

Gravity and the Development of Movement

Gravity affects all movement. Gravity exerts physical effects on bodies to the extent that all movement on Earth in some way or another is affected by the **gravity environment.** Voluntary movements are neuromuscular responses to external stimuli, including gravity's downward pull. Movement in the gravity-free environment of space versus the gravity-diminished environment of the moon is radically different.

In early life, gravity is both a stimulus and a barrier to movement. Infants must overcome its effects to raise their heads, reach out, crawl, and stand. Gravity also stimulates mechanisms (reflexes) within the body that result in movement. It is the primary stimulus to muscle stretch receptors (muscle spindles) that results in muscle contractions, yielding trunk and limb movements. Gravity makes an infant's environment rich with experience in movement.

When a baby lies in the prone position with the head unsupported, gravity pulls on the head and produces head and neck flexion that stretches the neck extensors. Gravity stimulates and resists contractions in the extensor muscles. A baby lying in a supine position with the head unsupported experiences gravity pulling the head into extension. Neck flexors are stretched, stimulated, and resisted. For a baby in the same position with the back of the head supported, gravity forces rotation of the baby's head to the left or right, stretching, stimulating, and resisting the flexor and extensor muscles involved. Over time the infant gains the strength and experience to control head movement voluntarily.

Development proceeds in response to the environment. Movement caused by gravity in one direction typically leads to movement by muscle contraction in the opposite direction. When the infant begins to prop on the elbows in the prone position, gravity pulls down on the upper trunk, stretching the shoulder girdle muscles (scapular protractors) and upper back and neck extensors. This stimulus results in responsive contractions, and the baby develops an ability to suspend the upper trunk away from the floor or mat.

As the child matures and can sit and stand upright, gravity affects the trunk and lower-extremity muscles. When the child leans forward, gravity pulls the trunk into more flexion, stretching and stimulating the trunk and hip extensors.

These examples highlight the importance of gravity on stretch reflexes, but gravity has more subtle effects. The delicate vestibular mechanism of the inner ear (labyrinth) is sensitive to gravity's downward pull on small crystals of calcium carbonate (otoliths) located there. Movements of the head stimulate hair cells in gelatinous material surrounding the otoliths and in the fluid of the semicircular canals. The hair cells transmit messages to the brain, which becomes aware of the head movement. They also produce a variety of eye, trunk, and limb movements known as *labyrinthine reflexes*.[2,3]

In all these examples, gravity's effect on body segments is concentrated around the center of gravity, a central

*In 1600, Giordano Bruno, an Italian priest and scholar, was burned at the stake for speculating that the stars were like the sun. He believed planets might circle the stars and be held together by the same forces that cause the Earth to revolve around the sun.

BOX 3-1

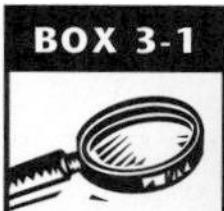

A **CLOSER** LOOK

Galileo and Newton

Galileo and Newton explained their ideas with mathematics. Galileo found that whenever he rolled a ball down a ramp, it traveled faster as it reached the bottom of the ramp. He could measure the rate of acceleration (a) *by subtracting the initial velocity* (u, *the distance traveled divided by time, as in miles per hour) from the final velocity* (v) *and dividing that by time* (t). *He found that objects always accelerate at the same rate:*

$$a = \frac{(v - u)}{t}$$

If objects are dropped from a tall building, they all experience the same rate of acceleration, 9.8 m/sec^2.

Newton took Galileo's ideas a step further. He said that all bodies of matter are attracted to each other and that the force of gravity (F_g) *can be measured in the multiplication of a constant* (G) *by the masses of the two objects* (m_1m_2) *divided by the square of the distance between them* (r^2):

$$F_g = \frac{G\,(m_1m_2)}{r^2}$$

Because the Earth is so large, its pull is much stronger than any other mass in our environment. This pull is a gravitational constant. On Earth that constant is 9.8 m/sec^2. The force of gravity always is measured as mass times acceleration. The consideration of mass and the acceleration of gravity together is weight, a force produced by gravity on our mass:

$$F = ma$$

We can determine how gravity affects us when we measure the mass of any object and multiply that by the average rate of acceleration of all objects on Earth, 9.8 m/sec^2, which is often rounded to 10 m/sec^2 for convenience.

If we went to the moon, the average rate of acceleration would be different and we would multiply mass by a different rate of acceleration. In video clips of moon walks from the days of the Apollo explorations, the rate of acceleration due to gravity on the moon is clearly less than that on Earth. Objects descend to the moon's surface more slowly. The slow-motion appearance of human movement on the moon is due to this lesser effect of gravity in that environment.

We appreciate gravity's effect on us daily when we stand on a scale and read our weight. In this case the multiplication of mass by the constant for the acceleration of gravity has been done in the calibration of the scale. The number value we read in pounds reflects the multiplication of slugs (mass) by the constant, 32 ft/sec^2 (9.8 m/sec^2).

point. OT practitioners use this point in diagrams to represent the effect of gravity.

Gravity and the Human Body

Gravity's force acts on a body's **center of gravity** by pulling it down toward the center of the Earth. In uniform bodies like balls and cubes the center of gravity is easy to find because it is located in the exact center of the object. Bodies have three dimensions; therefore the center of gravity is in the exact center of the three planes, each of which divide the object into equal halves.

Figure 3-1 shows an orange cut three ways to demonstrate these planes. It is cut first from top to bottom into front and back pieces and again into left and right pieces. The third cut is from side to side, dividing the fruit into top and bottom sections. Each cut represents the surface of a plane. The two top-to-bottom planes intersect to

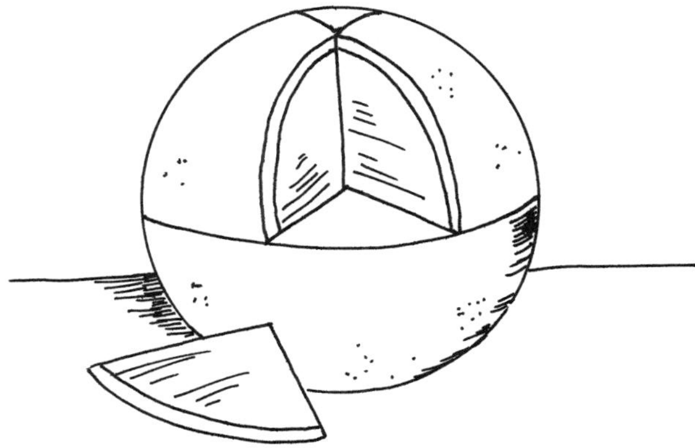

FIGURE **3-1**
An object's center of gravity is the point at which the vertical and horizontal planes meet.

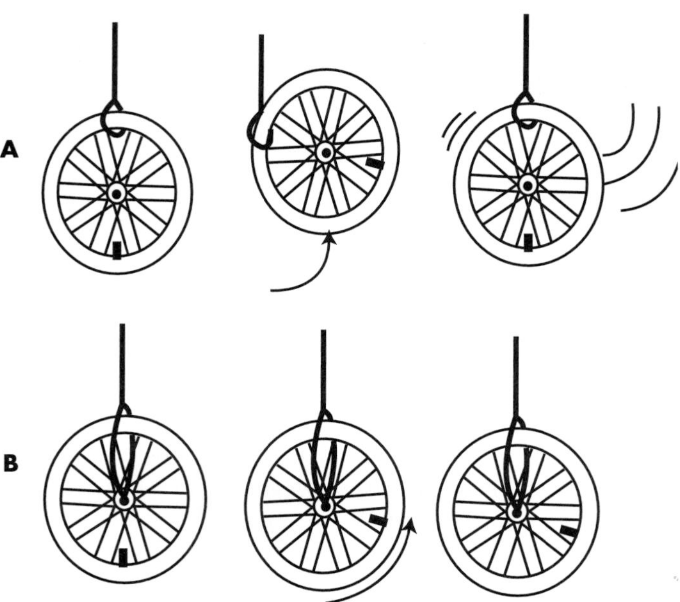

FIGURE **3-2**
A, A bicycle wheel suspended from a point other than its center of gravity falls to its most stable position. **B,** When the rim is suspended from the center of gravity, the wheel stays in any position into which it is rotated.

BOX 3-2

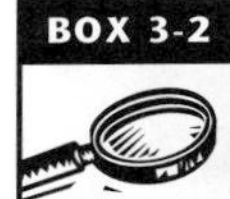

A **CLOSER** LOOK

Vectors Representing the Pull of Gravity

Gravity is a force and must be drawn as a vector. Use these general guidelines to indicate vectors representing gravity when you diagram an activity:

1. *Use a small circle to indicate the center of gravity.*
2. *Draw a line from the circle to indicate the direction of gravity's pull. The line is always perpendicular (90 degrees) to the ground.*
3. *Draw an arrowhead on the end of the line to indicate the direction in which gravity pulls. The arrow is always on the end of the line closest to the Earth and points toward the center of the Earth.*
4. *Make the length of the line proportional to the body's weight. It helps to write down the scale so that you don't forget it. For instance, 1 cm = 10 N. The scale converts distance (1 cm) to a measure of weight/force (10 N).*

form a central line, and the third plane intersects this line at its center. This is the center of gravity.

The human body is not uniform, but its center of gravity is found in much the same way. The body's sagittal plane divides it into left and right halves, its frontal plane separates front from back, and its horizontal plane forms top and bottom sections. Like the orange, a person's center of gravity is the point at which the three planes meet.

A body's center of gravity is known also as its *balance point.* Mobiles suspend objects from strings connected to each object's balance point. As the mobile moves, the objects may shift position but remain balanced. The subtle changes in movement make the mobile appear to float. Objects suspended from points other than their centers of gravity remain stationary.

For example, in Figure 3-2, *A,* a bicycle wheel hangs by a cord tied around its rim. The part of the rim attached to the cord is always the highest point. We can elevate another part of the rim, but once we release it, the wheel falls back into its original position.

However, if the string is attached to the wheel's axle (the center of gravity) as in Figure 3-2, *B,* it does not matter how we move the wheel. Wherever we release the wheel is where it remains. The wheel is balanced and thus at rest.

Any analysis of activity must account for the force of gravity acting on the person and tools or other objects involved. The force of gravity always has its effect at the body's center of gravity and should be drawn from that point and directed straight down (A Closer Look Box 3-2).

CENTERS OF GRAVITY

Our center of gravity changes when we move. The human body almost constantly is moving, and its center of gravity constantly is changing. When we stand upright, our center of gravity lies in the abdominal cavity, about 6 inches above the pubic symphysis. As the arms and legs move, this center of gravity shifts, and in some instances, it may be located outside the physical body (Figure 3-3).

To determine the center of gravity for the entire body, we must locate each body segment's center of gravity. Then we tabulate the cumulative effect of these **segmental centers of gravity** to locate a new center of gravity.

OT practitioners also use segmental centers of gravity when analyzing the forces that operate on a specific body part, for instance, when they design orthotic or adaptive equipment. When human body segments are diagrammed this way, they are free body diagrams. Vectors can be drawn to indicate individual muscles, other forces, and the force of gravity acting on a specific segment at its center of gravity.

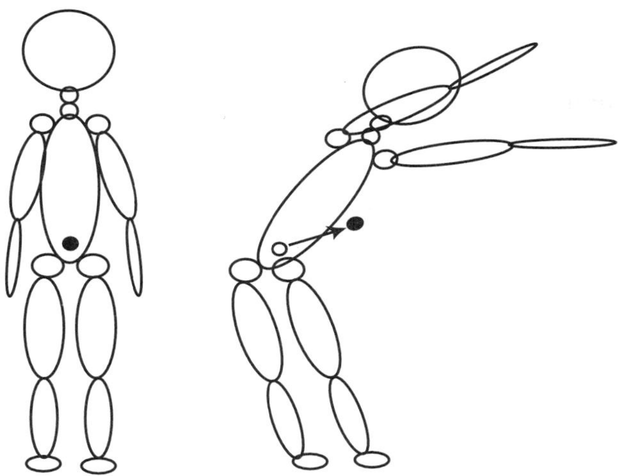

FIGURE 3-3
The center of gravity of the entire body is influenced by body position. With the arms raised and the trunk arched to the left side, the center of gravity moves upward and leftward.

TABLE 3-1
Proportional Percentages of Body Segments to Total Body Weight*

BODY SEGMENT	% OF TOTAL BODY WEIGHT
Head and neck	7.9
Trunk with head and neck	56.5
Upper arm	2.7
Forearm	1.5
Hand	0.6
Thigh	9.7
Lower leg	4.5
Foot	1.4

*Modified from Dempster WT: *Space requirements of the seated operator,* WADC technical report 55-159, Fairborn, Ohio, 1955, Wright-Patterson Air Force Base.

The center of gravity in a nonuniform object is closer to the end with the greatest mass. For example, the forearm is more bulky proximally; therefore we would expect the center of gravity to be more proximal than distal.

However, we can be more specific than this. The percentage of total body mass for each body segment already has been determined through research.[1] (Table 3-1 gives each body segment's **percentile weight,** and Figure B-1 in Appendix B shows the center of gravity in terms of a percentage of distance from either end of a line running proximal to distal.) OT practitioners use this information to draw the center of gravity for each body segment on a drawing or an actual person.

As an example, an OT practitioner works with an individual learning to eat independently. As this individual prepares to scoop food from a bowl, the forearm is flexed to about 90 degrees. To determine the center of gravity of the forearm, first measure the distance from the olecranon process to the styloid process of the ulna (25 cm in this individual). Then multiply that distance by the percentage value from Appendix B, Figure B-1 (43% from the olecranon process or 57% from the styloid process). The product of 25 cm and 0.43 is 10.8 cm. Start at the olecranon and measure 10.8 cm down the forearm. Place a dot on the forearm to represent its center of gravity (Figure 3-4). A vector representing the pull of gravity on the forearm would begin at this point.

The segmental method of determining center of gravity can be applied to the entire person in a specific position. One method is to take a photograph and superimpose it onto a graph. Another method is to make a scale drawing on a grid. (Figure 3-5, *A* shows a scale drawing of a 60-kg individual standing on one leg to reach into an overhead cabinet).

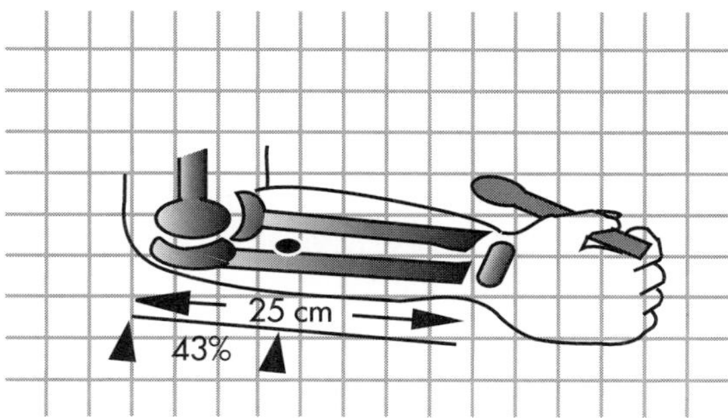

FIGURE 3-4
Multiply the length of the forearm by the percentage from Figure B-1 to determine the forearm's center of gravity.

To determine the center of gravity for this entire body, measure the length of each segment. Next multiply the percentage amount from Appendix B as before to determine where along each segment the center of gravity falls. Mark these centers of gravity with small circles that correspond to x and y coordinates on the grid (Figure 3-5, *B*). Then mark and plot each bony segment.

The body's center of gravity is a combination of the centers of gravity of all its parts. Because the x and y coordinates tell us the specific segmental positions in relation to the center of gravity of the entire body, we use these coordinates to adjust the body's center of gravity. We multiply the proportion of weight for each segment (see Table 3-1) by the x and y coordinates to obtain that segment's center of gravity. Each segment moves the center of gravity up or down and left or right in proportion

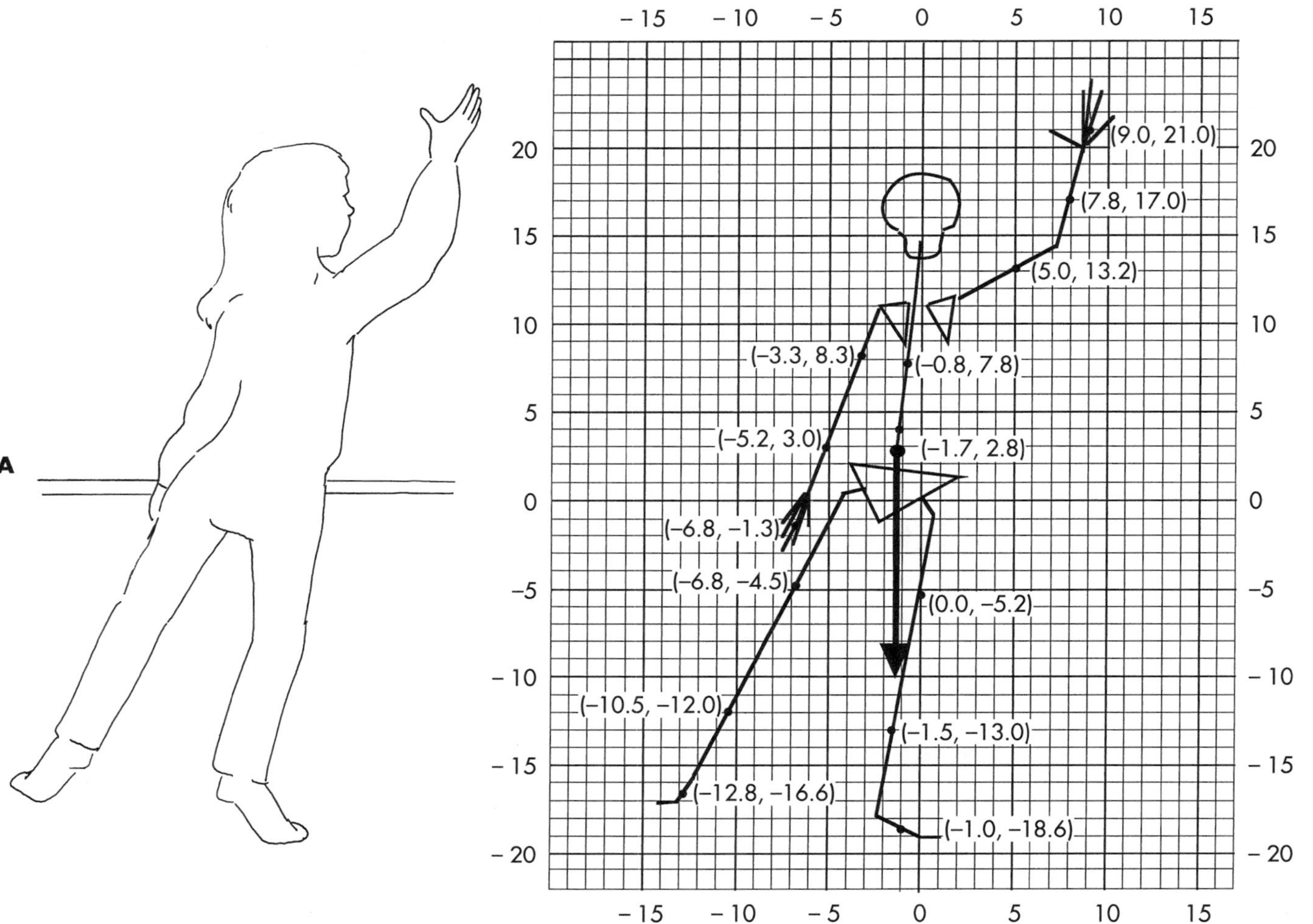

FIGURE **3-5**
A, An individual weighing 60 kg stands on the right leg to reach an overhead cabinet. **B,** This motion changes the body's center of gravity in response to the proportion of body weight and its distance from the body's midline. In this case the center of gravity shifts upward. If this person were leaning far enough forward, the center of gravity would fall outside the body.

to that segment's weight and position. (Table 3-2 shows the calculations involved in determining the center of gravity for the body shown in Figure 3-5, *B*). This process involves combination of individual segmental effects to determine the center of gravity for the entire body. In Table 3-2 the location of the center of gravity of the entire body corresponds to x coordinate −1.74 and y coordinate 2.88. The largest dot in Figure 3-5, *B* marks this individual's center of gravity. A vector represents the force of gravity acting on total body mass. (Remember, the combination of mass and gravity's effect equals weight.)

An individual's center of gravity sometimes is altered by the adaptive equipment and tools the individual uses. This becomes clear when we analyze wheelchair design for an individual who has had both lower extremities amputated. The lower extremities, when present, shift the center of gravity in the anterior direction for an individual in a wheelchair (Figure 3-6). A lack of lower extremities shifts an individual's center of gravity posteriorly. If the wheelchair's design does not accommodate the posterior shift, the chair may tip over. (We will explore this scenario when we discuss stability.)

Mass, Weight, and Acceleration

We have considered gravity and its effect on objects. We now turn to gravity's daily effect on us as we move our bodies and use tools.

Newton said all objects are attracted to each other and the strength of that attraction is in proportion to the object's mass. Because the mass of the Earth is so large, it

TABLE 3-2
The Center of Gravity

BODY SEGMENT	% BODY WEIGHT (EXPRESSED AS DECIMAL)	X COORDINATE	PRODUCT (% BODY WEIGHT × X COORDINATE)	Y COORDINATE	PRODUCT (% BODY WEIGHT × Y COORDINATE)
Head and trunk	0.565	−0.8	−0.45	7.8	4.41
Right upper arm	0.027	5.0	0.14	13.2	0.36
Right forearm	0.015	7.8	0.12	17.0	0.26
Right hand	0.006	9.0	0.05	21.0	0.13
Left upper arm	0.027	−3.3	−0.09	8.3	0.22
Left forearm	0.015	−5.2	−0.08	3.0	0.05
Left hand	0.006	−6.8	−0.04	−1.3	−0.01
Right thigh	0.097	0.0	0.00	−5.2	−0.50
Right lower leg	0.045	−1.5	−0.07	−13.0	−0.59
Right foot	0.014	−1.0	−0.01	−18.6	−0.26
Left thigh	0.097	−6.8	−0.66	−4.5	−0.44
Left lower leg	0.045	−10.5	−0.47	−12.0	−0.54
Left foot	0.014	−12.8	−0.18	−16.6	−0.23
Product total*	N/A	N/A	−1.74	N/A	2.86

N/A, not applicable.
*The two product totals serve as the x and y coordinates of the body's center of gravity. x coordinate, −1.74; y coordinate, 2.86.

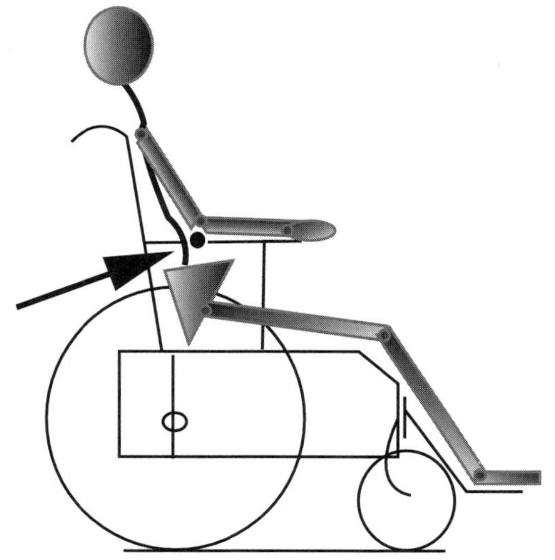

FIGURE **3-6**
The center of gravity for a person seated in a wheelchair is more forward and slightly higher than that of a person standing due to the forward and upward placement of the lower extremities.

overwhelms the smaller attractions that occur between objects on Earth. The pull toward the Earth that we feel when we jump is the pull of **gravitational attraction.** The Earth is so massive that all objects on it move toward its center. This pulling force of attraction changes in proportion to an object's mass, but its **rate of acceleration** remains constant.

Figure 3-7 shows a tall building in which each floor is spaced 4.9 m apart. If a bowling ball and a billiard ball are dropped off various floors, the following phenomena can be observed. When the balls fall from the first floor, they hit the ground in 1 second. When they fall from the fourth floor, they hit the ground in 2 seconds. When they fall from the ninth floor, they hit the ground in 3 seconds. They take 4 seconds to reach the ground from the sixteenth floor.

Note that the balls always land simultaneously and that the rate of acceleration follows a pattern. The rate of acceleration is proportional to the square root of the distance traveled. The average rate of acceleration caused by the Earth's gravitational field is 9.8 m/sec^2. This is rounded off to 10 m/sec^2, a constant, which is multiplied by the mass of an object to understand the force of gravity's attraction on that object. The force of gravity's attraction is the **weight** of an object. In the metric system this force is measured in newtons. One newton equals 9.8 kg-m/sec^2. The units demonstrate how to move from kilograms to newtons, multiplying the mass times the acceleration constant for gravity on Earth.

Weight often confuses us as OT practitioners. At home we read the number that appears on the bathroom scale. The units are pounds, and we understand this as a unit of weight. In the clinic we read the numbers written on wrist cuffs and engraved on free weights. These values are typically in units of kilograms. We also interpret these units as units of weight because they are labels on weights. The number of kilograms on weights in the clinic indicates a scalar measurement of the weight that is its mass.

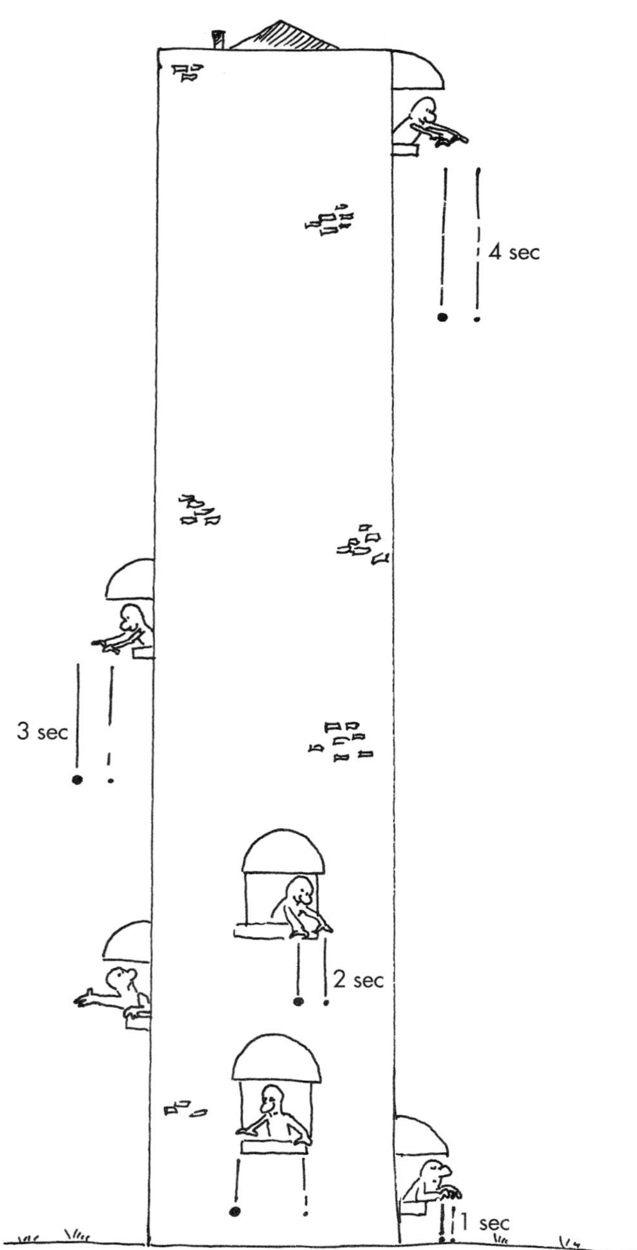

FIGURE 3-7
Gravity causes objects to travel toward the Earth at a constant rate of acceleration, 10 m/sec^2.

The actual weight is the effect of gravity on this mass and is considered a vector measurement because gravity pulls the mass downward. To convert the weight of an object labeled in kilograms to newtons, multiply mass (kilograms) by the constant for acceleration by gravity (10 m/sec^2).

BOX 3-3

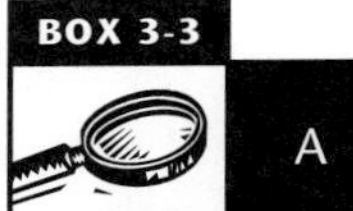

A CLOSER LOOK

Daily Encounters with Weight and Mass

In a clinical setting an OT practitioner responds to the question, "How much weight is George lifting?" by reading the number of kilograms marked on the weight. Few OT practitioners carry out the multiplication.

To understand and communicate the forces George uses to lift the weight, we must convert weight to the same measurement we use to describe muscle force. Muscle power is a force, and therefore kilogram amounts (mass) must be converted into measurements of force. To do this, multiply the kilogram amount (mass) by 10 m/sec^2. Keep in mind that if the weight is labeled in pounds, no multiplication is necessary.

The pound is the unit most often used in the United States to measure weight. In the British system of measurement, pound is used interchangeably to refer to both mass and force, even though slug is more correct for mass. Kilogram, the metric measure of mass, often is used interchangeably to represent both mass and weight, even though newton is the correct measurement unit for weight, a force[1] (A Closer Look Box 3-3).

Summary

Newton envisioned gravitational attraction like the attraction of magnets. Einstein envisioned space as a fabric in which large objects such as planets, stars, and black holes create deep pockets to draw smaller objects such as light rays inward on a curved trajectory. The conceptual models these mathematicians developed have kept physicists employed for centuries.

For our purposes the specific details of the conceptual models are less relevant. Objects are pulled downward to the Earth in direct proportion to their mass. Although the force of that attraction depends on mass, the acceleration of all objects is constant, which means a larger, heavier object falls to the ground just as fast as a smaller, lighter one. However, the heavier object requires more force to push it over the edge than the lighter one. We use these important concepts to visualize gravity's effect on movement by drawing objects with vectors that demonstrate gravity's ever-present influence.

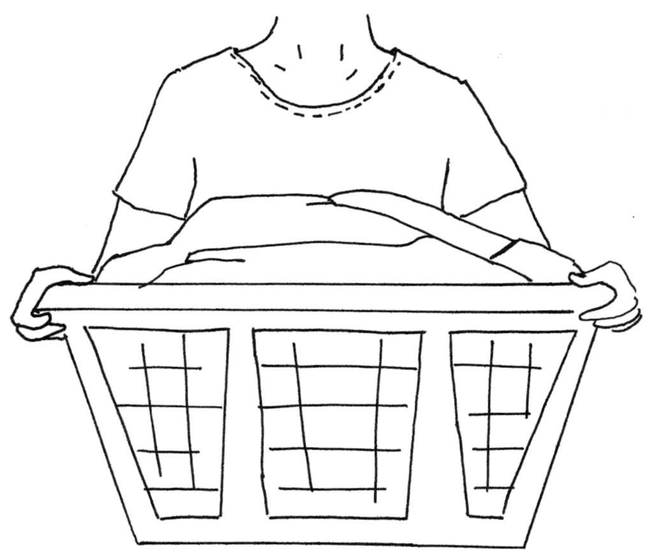

FIGURE **3-8**
This laundry basket weighs 10 kg. Converting kilograms to newtons, draw the vector representing its weight.

Applications

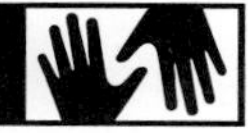

APPLICATION **3-1**

Creation of a Mobile

Make a mobile from three to five objects in the room. Hang the objects from a clothes hanger. Can you find each object's center of gravity? How do you know when each object is balanced? Which are easiest to suspend?

APPLICATION **3-2**

Scale Drawing of Your Lab Partner

On a scale drawing of your lab partner, find each body segment's center of gravity and mark it with a dot.

APPLICATION **3-3**

Vector Indicating Gravity's Effect on a Laundry Basket

Figure 3-8 shows a laundry basket weighing 10 kg. Converting kilograms to newtons, show the effect of gravity on the full basket. Also using newtons, show the effect of gravity on a basket that is half full, or 5 kg.

APPLICATION **3-4**

Force of Gravity Acting on a Spoon

The spoon in Figure 3-9 weighs 0.04 kg and is shown in three different positions. Converting kilograms to newtons, how is the force of gravity acting on the spoon drawn in each position? Does the center of gravity or its action on the spoon change as the position changes?

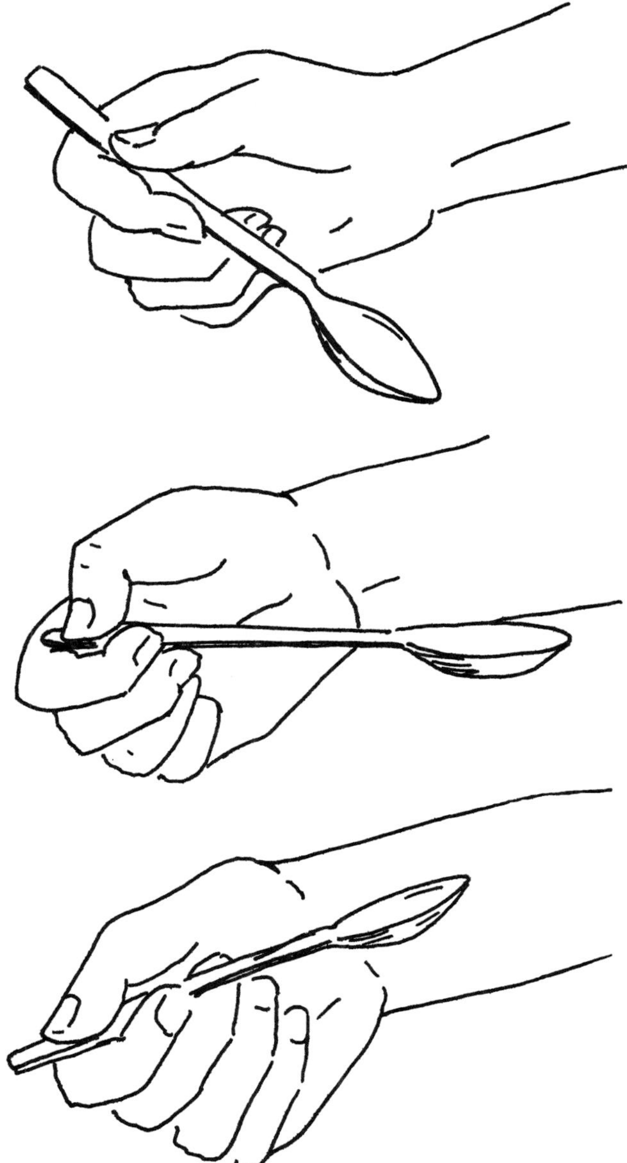

FIGURE **3-9**
This spoon weighs 0.04 kg. Converting kilograms to newtons, draw a vector representing the force of gravity in each position shown.

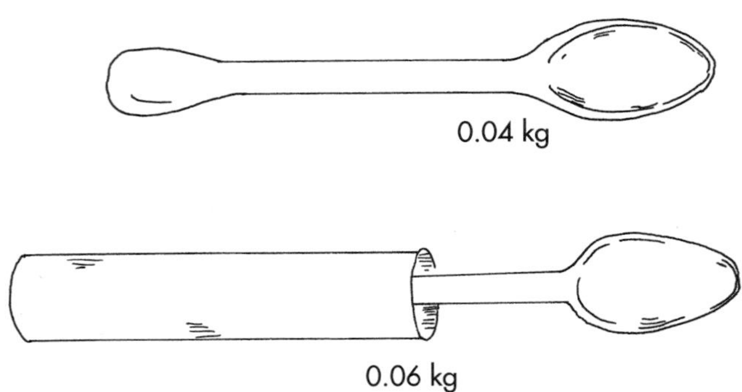

FIGURE **3-10**
The spoon without the adapted handle weighs 0.04 kg, and the spoon with the built-up handle weighs 0.06 kg. Converting kilograms to newtons, draw a vector representing the force of gravity in each spoon.

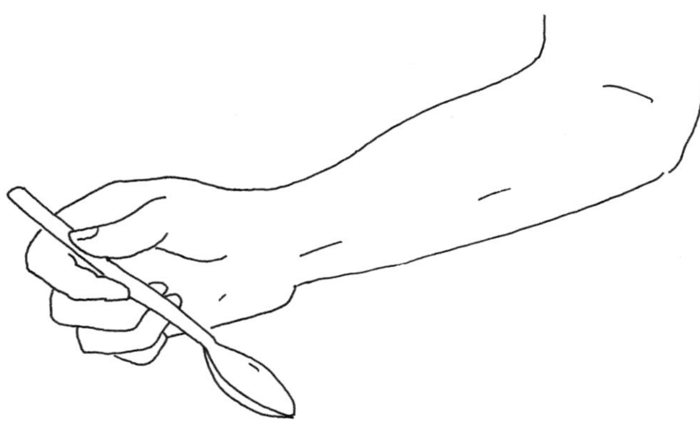

FIGURE **3-11**
A drawing of a forearm with a spoon. On your own drawing, use separate vectors to indicate the weight of the spoon and the forearm.

APPLICATION **3-5**

Force of Gravity Acting on Spoons of Different Weights

In Figure 3-10 a spoon with a built-up handle weighs 0.06 kg, and a regular spoon weighs 0.04 kg. Converting kilograms to newtons, how is the force of gravity acting on each spoon indicated in the diagram? Does weight affect each spoon's center of gravity?

APPLICATION **3-6**

Gravity Operating on the Forearm

Using the data from Application 3-5 and your own arm, draw a forearm with a spoon (Figure 3-11). Which has a greater gravitational force, the forearm or the spoon? How heavy would a spoon need to be to affect function of the forearm?

See Appendix C for solutions to Applications.

REFERENCES

1. Leveau BF: *Williams and Lissner's biomechanics of human motion,* ed 3, Philadelphia, 1992, WB Saunders.
2. McCance KL, Huether SE: *Pathophysiology: the biologic basis for disease in adults and children,* ed 2, St Louis, 1994, Mosby.
3. Williams PL, Bannister LH: *Gray's anatomy: the anatomical basis of medicine and surgery,* ed 38, New York, 1995, Churchill Livingstone.

RELATED READINGS

Fritjof C: *The Tao of physics,* New York, 1994, Bantam.

Krauss LM: *Fear of physics: a guide for the perplexed,* New York, 1993, Basic Books.

Luttgens K, Wells K: *Kinesiology: scientific basis of human motion,* ed 9, Madison, Wis, 1997, Brown & Benchmark.

Nordin M, Frankel VH: *Basic biomechanics of the musculoskeletal system,* Philadelphia, 1989, Lea & Febiger.

Norkin CC, Levangie PK: *Joint structure and function: a comprehensive analysis,* ed 2, Philadelphia, 1992, FA Davis.

Wiktorin CH, Nordin M: *Introduction to problem solving in biomechanics,* Philadelphia, 1986, Lea & Febiger.

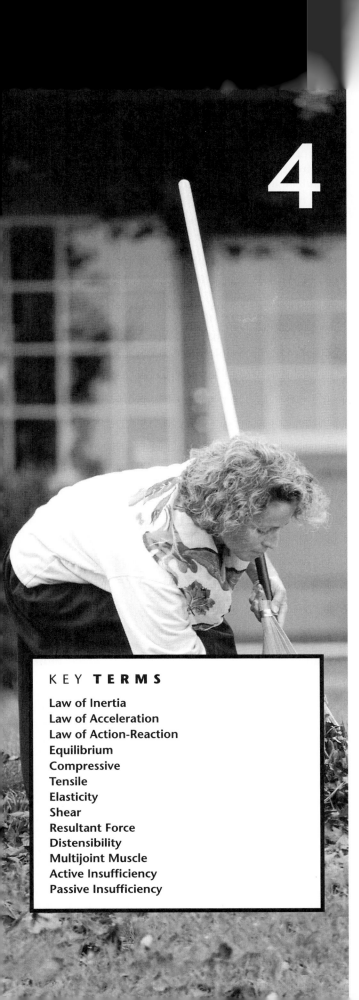

4 Linear Force and Motion

KEY **TERMS**

Law of Inertia
Law of Acceleration
Law of Action-Reaction
Equilibrium
Compressive
Tensile
Elasticity
Shear
Resultant Force
Distensibility
Multijoint Muscle
Active Insufficiency
Passive Insufficiency

CHAPTER **OUTLINE**

Forces are all around us. Though we cannot see them, we are as aware of their effects as we are of our own breathing. An apple falling from a tree to the ground and the collision of two automobile bumpers are examples of linear forces. They are considered external forces. Similar patterns of force, internal forces, exist within our bodies. The spindles that pull chromosomes to their respective poles in cell division and the substantial excursion of the sartorius muscle that results in forceful and rapid knee flexion are linear forces. This chapter explores the laws that govern motion caused by linear forces and details the effects of linear forces within the musculoskeletal system.

External Forces

External forces are forces that affect the body from the outside. Isaac Newton explained the effects of forces on objects in his three laws of motion. As OT practitioners, we observe Newton's laws at work every day. We relate what we see to the underlying principles involved to understand the observations more completely.

LAW OF INERTIA

Bernice Richards has quadriplegia and minimal control of the muscles balancing her trunk. She directs her electric wheelchair through the main thoroughfare of a shopping mall, and a child darts in front of her. As she stops the chair, she demonstrates Newton's first law, the **law of inertia.** As the chair quickly decelerates, Bernice continues moving forward, stopped only by her chest and pelvic seat belts.

This isolated event demonstrates a valuable lesson. Bernice, like other individuals with weak trunk muscles, needs seat belts to provide trunk support. Analyzing this event from a physics perspective increases our ability to generalize principles from previous chapters.

All matter has inertia, and a body in motion or at rest remains so unless acted on by an outside force (Newton's first law). We can appreciate the concept of momentum, but our experiences teach us that nothing lasts forever, including motion. We are accustomed to cars, bikes, and carts that are set in motion with a push and then stop. Therefore we think an object's natural tendency is to stop.

In truth, objects do not stop because of a natural tendency. Some outside force stops them, a force we cannot see. In many cases the force is friction, for example, the drag of the turned-off motor of the wheelchair and the resistance of the rubber tires on the floor. In other cases the object responsible is more obvious, as in the case of the seat belts. In Bernice's situation, when she stopped quickly, she and the wheelchair traveled together. An outside force, friction, slowed the chair, but Bernice's body continued moving forward. The force of friction on the chair did not affect Bernice's body. A separate, outside force, provided by the seat belts, stopped her body from continuing forward.

Understanding the event according to Newton's law allows us to extrapolate our understanding to different, perhaps less obvious situations and predict their outcomes.

What if Bernice didn't want a chest strap but needed some way to prevent herself from falling forward? If we understand the underlying principle, inertia, we can devise an alternative solution for Bernice. One possible solution is to focus on the force of gravity. We can tilt her seat and the back of her chair ("tilt-in-space"). When we tilt the chair backward, we increase the effect of gravity on Bernice's trunk. (We will examine this more closely in a later chapter.) For now, we must realize a variety of solutions exist to solve the same problem. We can recognize these solutions only when we look past the event and understand the nature of the problem.

LAW OF ACCELERATION

Newton's second law is the **law of acceleration.** When an instructor tells us that we must learn to apply the law of acceleration, we immediately imagine we must derive and solve algebraic formulas and lengthy word problems and draw complicated diagrams. The truth is most students and all OT practitioners apply Newton's second law every day.

Although this law often is stated in its algebraic form (force equaling mass times acceleration, or $F = ma$), the following example may make it easier to understand. It takes less effort to push a broken-down Volkswagen than a Cadillac. A Volkswagen, which has less mass than a Cadillac, requires less force to move (accelerate). Therefore the amount of force needed to move the Cadillac moves the Volkswagen farther faster.

Many applications of this law deal with the three variables—mass, force, and acceleration—by emphasizing mass. Objects that have more mass require more force to move (accelerate). If two objects, each with a different mass, are under the influence of one force, the object with the least mass moves first. This also applies to various regions of the body.

Eduardo Ybarra severed his radial nerve with a power saw while making his son a rocking horse for Christmas. An OT practitioner uses a splint to extend his wrist by pushing the fingers into extension. To the practitioner's surprise, his fingers overextend because they are lighter (have less mass) than the hand.

The same rule applies to ***Tony Adams,*** whose scapular stabilizers were paralyzed by a gunshot wound. When

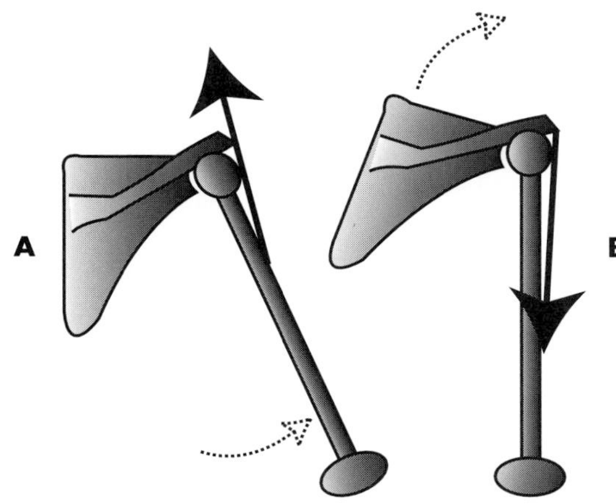

FIGURE **4-1**
A, The deltoid muscle moves its insertion and abducts the humerus when the scapula is stabilized. **B,** The deltoid muscle acts on its origin, the scapula, when the scapula is unstabilized.

his deltoid muscle contracts to abduct the arm at the shoulder, the result is an undesired downward movement of the scapula. Like any muscle, when the deltoid shortens, it can move either of its attachments. If the scapular stabilizers are paralyzed, attempts to abduct the arm result in scapular movement because the scapula is lighter (has less mass) than the entire upper extremity (Figure 4-1).

LAW OF ACTION-REACTION

Newton's third law is commonly referred to as **action-reaction.** Whenever a force acts on an object and that object remains stationary, an equal force acts on the object in the opposite direction. We often are unaware of these opposing forces in stationary objects until one force fails.

Imagine an individual sitting in a chair, listening to a speaker. Suddenly, this attentive listener appears to be thrown to the ground as the chair collapses with a loud bang. What happened? The listener's action (force of body weight downward) and the chair's reaction (force provided by the legs of the chair upward) are no longer equal because the structure of the chair has failed.

The listener's original force, body weight, takes over. This downward force was present the entire time but held in balance by the equal and opposite upward force of the chair's legs. It appears as if no actions are at work until the collapse. In truth, all is in equilibrium but not at rest. Newton's third law describes this condition of **equilibrium.**

OT practitioners use clinical applications of this law to make lateral trunk supports for Bernice's wheelchair. These supports counteract the effect of gravity on her otherwise unsupported trunk. Gravity's downward pull on Bernice's upright vertebral column results in lateral shifts that produce an S curve. If her spine is not supported, the curve can develop into scoliosis.

Lateral supports on Bernice's wheelchair help prevent formation of the S curve. Pads attached to the back of the chair's seat direct a medial force (reaction), which counterbalances the lateral movement of the vertebrae (action). If trunk movement is too strong, the support pad gives way. If the support pad pushes medially with too much force, the trunk is overcorrected and a lateral curve develops in the opposite direction. Unbalanced forces upset equilibrium.

Force equilibrium

The carefully placed supports that hold Bernice's trunk erect provide an example of a way to obtain equilibrium. The law of inertia applies: Her body remains at rest. The absence of lateral supports or poorly adjusted supports on Bernice's chair may lead to formation of an S curve, the result of unbalanced forces and a body in motion. Newton's second law (the law of acceleration) helps us understand situations in which equilibrium is upset. Is the force supplied by the lateral support pad sufficient to balance the mass of the vertebral column? Is the force of the pad too great and does it cause the vertebral segments to accelerate in the opposite direction?

Donna Nelson, a food server in a small Italian restaurant, encounters force equilibrium every day. Management wants its food servers to carry dinner orders out to the tables using large trays. Donna knows that to work at this restaurant, she must be able to hold the tray up no matter how heavy it is. Donna may not remember Newton's third law of motion, but her tips depend on her body's ability to respond to the law of action-reaction.

Donna encounters linear force equilibrium daily. Every time she carries her tray, her upper extremities provide a combined upward force that is equal in magnitude and opposite in direction to the downward-directed weight of the tray. If the tray's weight is the action, the upward force of her muscle contractions is the reaction (Figure 4-2).

When Donna carries the tray at shoulder height, she exhibits an isometric contraction. This contraction brings about equilibrium. Gravity or another force pulls a segment one way while the contraction in the opposing muscle balances the effect of that external force.

Donna uses a concentric contraction to overcome the external force of the tray's weight when she lifts it over her head to negotiate her way around another server, moving the tray out of equilibrium. She yields slightly to this external force when she lowers it back to shoulder height. The muscle force she uses to lower the tray is an eccentric contraction, which changes the system's equilibrium in the direction of the external force. (In the

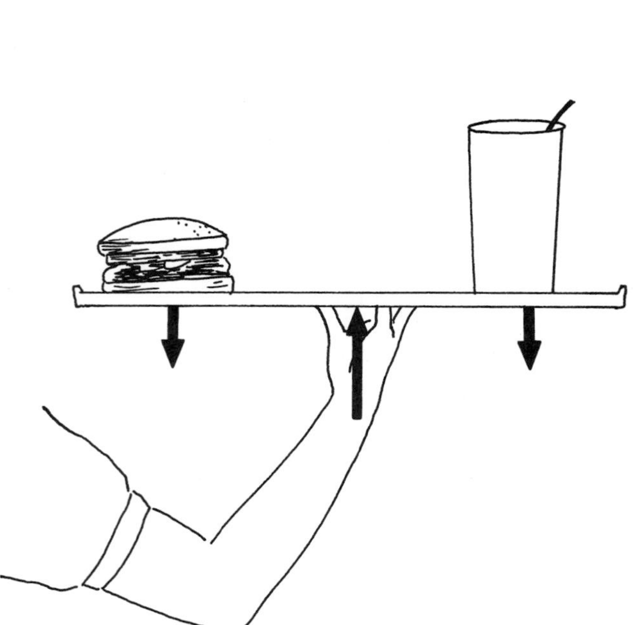

FIGURE **4-2**
Vertical forces upward and downward must be equal for the tray and its contents to remain stable (in equilibrium).

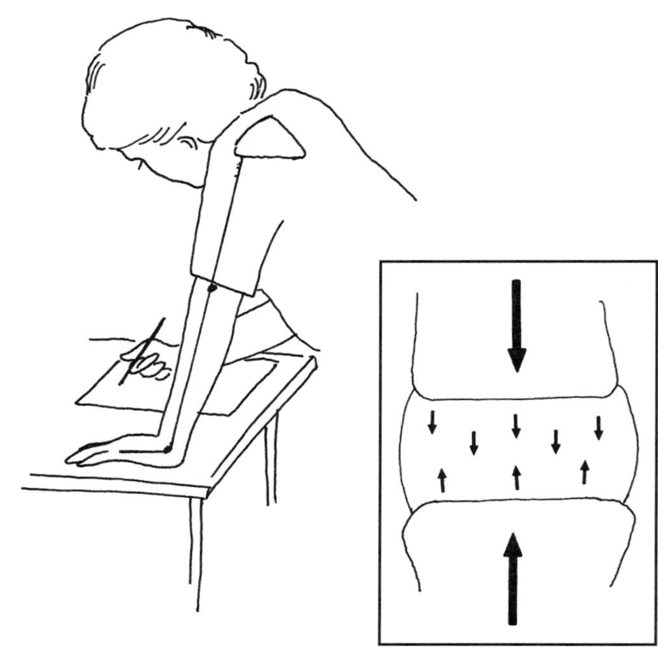

FIGURE **4-3**
An individual leaning on a table causes compressive forces to operate at the elbow and shoulder with corresponding compressive stress in joint tissues.

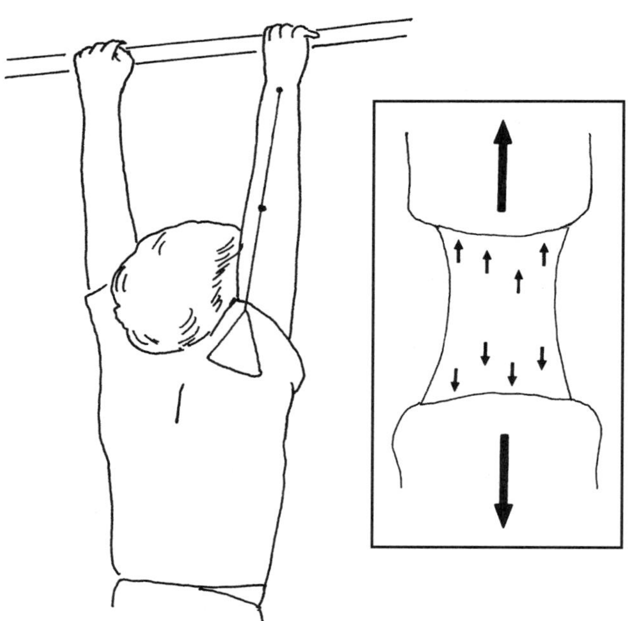

FIGURE **4-4**
An individual hanging on a bar causes tensile forces to operate at the elbow and shoulder with corresponding tensile stress in joint tissues.

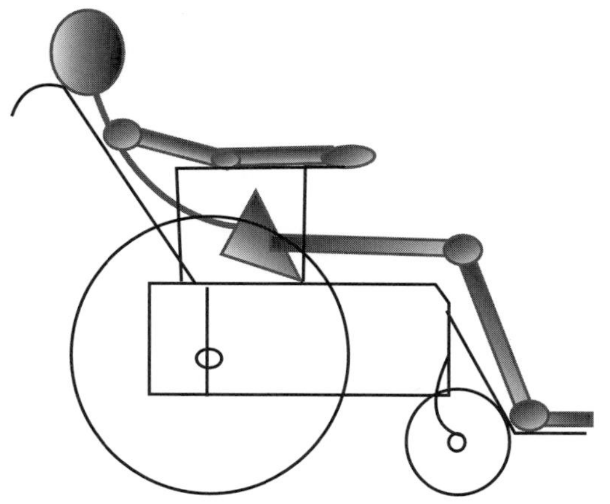

FIGURE **4-5**
Bernice's reclined position, combined with inadequate support, is dangerous. She may slide, and shear force may develop.

next chapter, we will see how Donna balances large orders and, more importantly, how she removes items without upsetting this balance.)

Normal forces

Normal forces are external forces that push joint surfaces together or pull them apart. In Figure 4-3 an individual leaning on a table pushes the surfaces of the glenohumeral joint together. In Figure 4-4 an individual hanging motionless from an overhead bar pulls these same joint surfaces apart. In each case the force is directed perpendicular to the surface on which it acts.

Anatomical structures alter their shapes in response to these forces. **Compressive** forces push tissues together, causing anatomical structures to become shorter and wider. **Tensile** forces pull tissues apart, causing anatomical structures to become longer and narrower. Anatomical structures usually return to their original shapes once the forces acting on them stop. The ability to return to its original shape is a structure's **elasticity.** When elasticity is exceeded, tissues can be injured.

Shear forces

External forces also can operate parallel to a surface. When the arm is raised above the head, the weight of the humerus produces a **shear** force on the glenoid fossa. Because of their orientation, shear forces also are called *tangential* forces. Shear and normal forces of the same magnitude have drastically different effects; shear forces can cause more damage to tissues. For example, Figure 4-5 represents Bernice in a recliner wheelchair. The reclined position, together with inadequate support, results in a dangerous shear force acting on the skin of her buttocks. In this position, Bernice may develop pressure sores, or decubiti.

Stress

When external force is applied to a material substance, like a joint capsule, it causes stress inside that material. Stress is a measure of force per unit area and is stated in metric pascals (Pa) or newtons/meter^2 (N/m^2). When stress inside human tissue exceeds the tissue's elasticity, tissue breaks down, causing injury.

Internal Forces

Internal forces are forces generated by tissue within the body. Our dealings with internal forces mainly involve those of muscle contractions. Muscle contractions generate linear forces, and we must understand the characteristics of these forces before we consider the anatomical movements they cause. (In Chapter 5, we will learn that the connection of these straight-line forces to articulated skeletal segments results in circular, or rotary, motion).

FORCE MAGNITUDE AND ORIENTATION

The forces of muscle contractions are represented as vectors (A Closer Look Box 4-1). Proper orientation and direction are crucial to an understanding of the function of these forces. A muscle force acts along the length of the muscle. Its orientation is parallel to the direction of the muscle fibers.

The number of active muscle fibers determines a muscle force's magnitude. The specific length of the vector, according to a chosen scale, represents magnitude. Graphic units of length equal specific units of force. A force drawn 3 cm long represents 30 N if the scale is 1 cm = 10 N.

In Figure 4-6 the brachialis muscle is shown at the elbow. The vector indicates a 450-N force. The force is in line with the fibers, which are nearly parallel to the humerus from origin to insertion.

In many muscles a tendon transmits force to the skeletal segment. The tendon may travel around various bony protuberances, completely reorienting the direction of the force by the time this force reaches the bony segment serving as its insertion. The force of the flexor hallucis longus (the long flexor of the great toe) is parallel to the tibia in the leg but parallel to the foot (90 degrees to the leg) at the point of the muscle's insertion (Figure 4-7). The tendon travels around and turns behind the medial malleolus, creating a pulley effect to flex the great toe. (See Chapters 7 and 8 for a discussion of how forces commonly can be redirected around pulleys that are within the hand.)

Some muscles have fibers oriented in different directions. The forces created by these fibers combine to form a **resultant force** that can be determined through care-

BOX 4-1

A CLOSER LOOK

Using Line Drawings to Organize Problems in Biomechanics

Line drawings accurately represent biomechanics in functional activity and do not require artistic skill. They can communicate information to bioengineers, physicians, orthotists, clients, and others involved in the treatment process. Biomechanics provides a framework in which OT practitioners can understand movement and the forces responsible for it. To organize information into a line drawing, follow these steps:

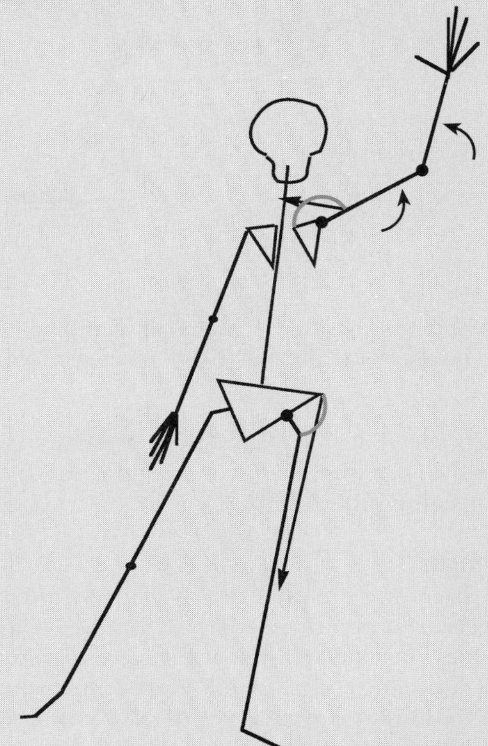

1. *Look at the body parts used in an activity. Observe the activity as a whole to determine where movement takes place. Note all important movements.*
2. *Identify which specific joints and active muscle groups play major roles in the activity. Some muscles and joints are less important than others. Joints and muscles that play major roles may change as the movements change.*
3. *Determine which plane or planes of motion provide the most information about the activity. The individual who makes the drawing determines the plane of view. A drawing of motion in the sagittal plane requires a view of the client from the side. Frontal-plane movement should be shown in a drawing that depicts the client from the front. Identify the plane of motion (the surface on which it occurs) and draw the segments with that plane on the plane of the paper. Different phases of an activity may require different views.*
4. *The line drawing should include the following relevant information:*
   a. *Movement of skeletal segments—Use curved arrows drawn from the point at which the segment begins to its location in the drawing to indicate moving segments.*
   b. *Joints—Use dots to indicate the axis of motion taking place. Each axis for the plane of movement drawn is oriented 90 degrees to the plane, sticking out of the paper like a pin; it appears as a dot on the paper.*
   c. *Muscles—Use light lines from the muscle's point of origin to its point of insertion, making sure to draw around any point about which the muscle is known to travel. For example, the middle deltoid is drawn around the tip of the shoulder [acromion], not through it, on the way from the insertion on the humerus to the origin on the acromion.*
   d. *Objects or tools—Use circles, squares, or other simple geometric shapes that approximate the object's size.*
5. *Determine where and how gravity acts on the human body and tools or other objects. Determine the segmental centers of gravity where needed and the center of gravity of the entire body using the methods described in Chapter 3.*
6. *Determine the forces that help move specific body parts, objects, or tools. Draw these forces as vectors scaled for magnitude, with an arrowhead pointing in the direction of force. Remember, the vector should be oriented parallel to the muscle fibers in the center of the muscle and should be drawn straight, even if the fibers curve around some anatomical pulley.*

Colored pens or pencils can help differentiate muscles, bones, and forces in a schematic drawing. Use a goniometer to measure joint angles.

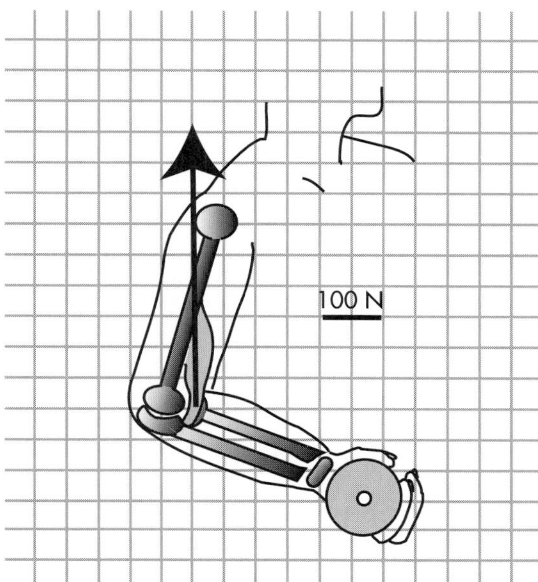

FIGURE **4-6**
A force of 450 N is generated by the brachialis muscle and indicated by the vector drawn to scale (100 N = 2 boxes).

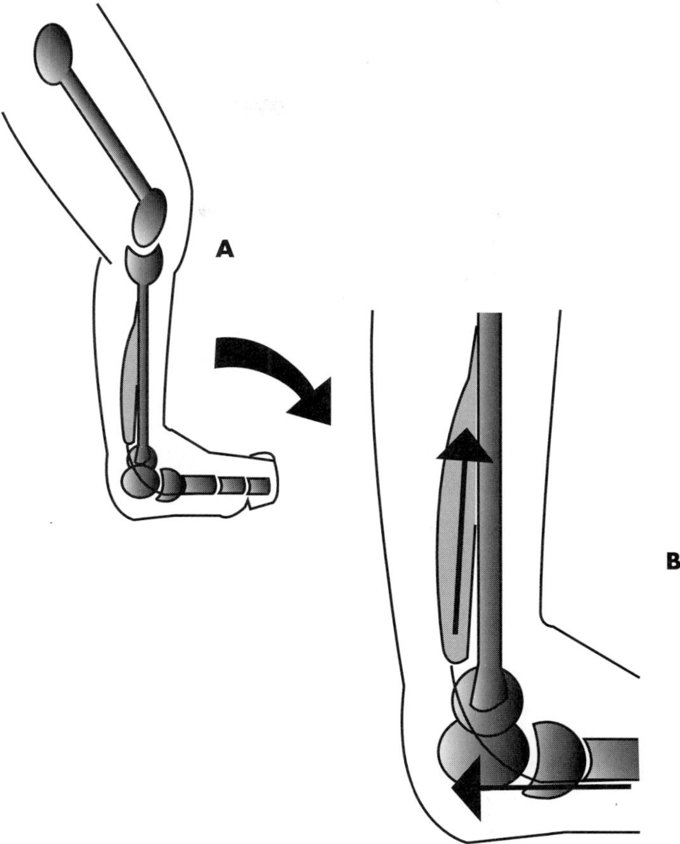

FIGURE **4-7**
A, The lower extremity. **B,** Close-up of the lower leg. The direction of the force as indicated by the placement of the arrowhead changes as the direction of the muscle fibers and tendon change around bony protuberances.

ful drawing. For example, the pectoralis major muscle has a fan shape. The active muscle fibers operating in it are all in the same plane but directed differently. To determine the resultant force and direction of contraction for all fibers of the pectoralis major, use the parallelogram method of graphic representation.

In this method, construct a parallelogram using two representative forces of this muscle as sides. (Figure 4-8 shows the two most contrasting forces in the muscle [the clavicular and inferior sternal fibers] represented as sides of a parallelogram.) A diagonal line down the center of the parallelogram represents the resultant force. This intersects the middle-lying fibers and gives us a general idea of the overall effect caused by simultaneous contraction of all fibers, or maximal effort.

FORCE DIRECTION

We also are concerned with the direction of forces. An arrow drawn from a muscle's insertion toward its origin implies the muscle moves the more distal part of the extremity. This happens only if the origin is stabilized. In Figure 4-6 the brachialis pulls a hand-held weight toward the shoulder, which is stabilized by scapular muscles. The force of flexion generated by the brachialis and other elbow flexors is oriented almost parallel to the humerus and directed proximally, pulling the distal insertion toward the origin.

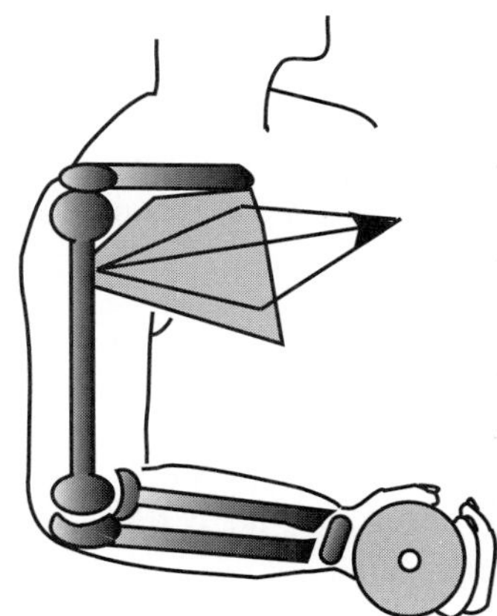

FIGURE **4-8**
The parallelogram method is used to determine the combined effect of muscle fibers of the pectoralis major. The resultant force is greater and travels in a different direction from the two component forces that represent divergent fibers of the same muscle.

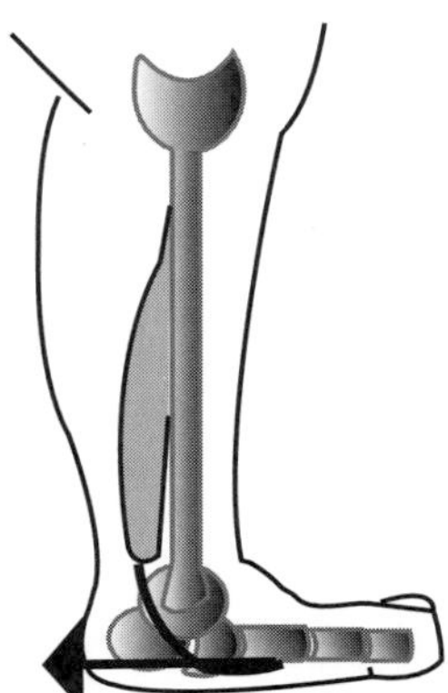

FIGURE **4-9**
The force vector continues in a straight path, although the muscle fibers curve around the ankle.

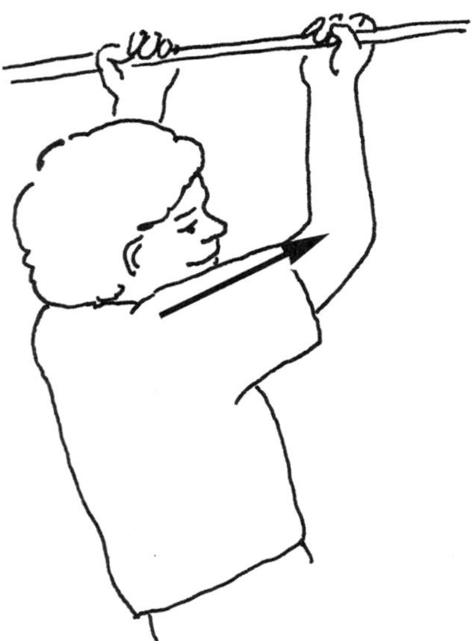

FIGURE **4-10**
When this individual pulls up on the bar, the wrist and hand are stabilized, causing the elbow flexors to bring the body closer to the forearm.

To represent the effect of force vectors in a drawing, draw a straight arrow from the moving part along the muscle fiber or tendon. Draw the arrow long enough to represent the magnitude (strength) of the force according to the chosen scale. If the muscle or tendon curves in its path, never follow the turn with the arrow; keep the arrow straight (Figure 4-9).

How we represent the direction of muscle contraction depends on which part—the origin or insertion—moves in the contraction. Human gross anatomy instructors generally teach students to think that when muscles contract, insertions always move toward origins. Figure 4-10 demonstrates how the elbow flexors pull the body toward a bar held in the hands. In this case the hand's grip on the bar stabilizes the insertion, which allows the origin to move. The direction of the force is proximal to distal, pulling the origin toward the insertion. The same is true in a push-up when the elbow extends to move the body away from the hand, which is stabilized by the floor, instead of the hand moving away from the body.

Tony, whose gunshot wound paralyzed some of his upward scapular rotators, provides an example of an individual with a muscle that moves its origin instead of its insertion. The bullet that barely missed his spinal cord damaged the ventral rami of cervical roots 3, 4, and 5, which supply a variety of nerves to scapular muscles. When his deltoid muscle contracts, it moves the unstabilized scapula instead of the upper extremity (via the humerus) in a contraction directed proximal to distal.

Muscle contraction types

When muscles contract, we know that the contraction works to approximate the two ends of the muscle. Stabilization provided by other muscle contractions or segments of attachment with larger mass than others determines which end moves. The force of the contraction is represented with an arrow drawn along the lines of the muscle fibers. The arrow points in the direction of the contraction and indicates which point—the origin or insertion—moves.

With a concentric contraction, one attachment moves closer to the other. Remember that whether the muscle shortens (concentric), stays the same (isometric), or lengthens (eccentric), it always attempts to shorten. The force is drawn the same way regardless of the type of contraction. We need to determine only which attachment moves, or in the case of isometric contractions, which attachment would move if equilibrium were disrupted.

Muscle force

Absolute strength, the maximum amount of force a muscle can exert, depends on the bulk or girth of the muscle's cross section (A Closer Look Box 4-2). Muscle girth depends on the amount of contractile protein packed into the muscle. A muscle's length at the time of contraction also affects force capability. The amount of force created depends on the state of overlap of the contractile proteins actin and myosin; overlap is determined by the length of the muscle at the time of contraction.[2] Therefore the amount of force a muscle with a specific cross section can generate when it contracts with maximal effort varies according to its length at the beginning of the contraction.

The resting length of the muscle fibers also determines a muscle's ability to shorten, or excursion (A Closer Look Box 4-3). Generally, a muscle can contract to half its length, but some muscles do vary. Consider muscle fiber length, not overall muscle length, to determine muscle excursion. Fusiform muscles like the

BOX 4-2

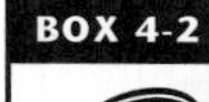

A CLOSER LOOK

Determining the Maximum Strength Capability of a Muscle

Common sense tells us that a larger muscle is a stronger muscle. If larger means more bulk and more bulk means a larger cross section, we can express strength more clearly. Measurements of bulk determine muscle strength.

*Researchers measure the strength of a muscle with special laboratory equipment, dividing the amount of strength by the cross section of the muscle to determine how much force can be produced per amount of bulk. Although 10 different muscles of different sizes would produce 10 different force values, dividing each force value by the cross section of the muscle always produces approximately the same answer, a constant. The constant commonly used for vertebrate skeletal muscle is approximately 100 N/cm², or 10 kg/cm².**

We use this constant to estimate the maximum force a muscle generates at the beginning of the contraction from its ideal resting length. Use this formula:

$$S = k \times cs$$

S is muscle strength, k is the constant (100 N/cm²), and cs is the muscle's cross section measured at a place in the belly of the muscle where a cut intersects all the fibers at 90 degrees to the length of the fiber. For example, if a pronator teres has a cross section of 3 cm², its force capability at optimum length would be 3 cm² × 100 N/cm² = 300 N. In comparison, a brachialis with a cross section of 6 cm² could produce 600 N of force.

*Different authors have reported the strength capability per cross section for human skeletal muscle.[1,3,4] The range of reported results is from 3.6 to 10 kg/cm².

BOX 4-3

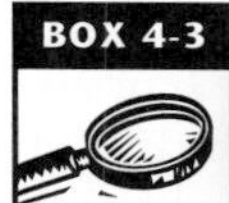

A CLOSER LOOK

Determining Muscle Excursion

As OT practitioners, we rarely need to determine active excursion, the distance through which a muscle contracts. However, when we measure active and passive range of motion, we indirectly measure active and passive excursion. Joints move because the agonist has sufficient active excursion to pull the joint through its motion. The antagonist must simultaneously have adequate passive excursion ***(distensibility)*** *to allow the joint motion.*

Approximate values for muscle excursion give us a deeper understanding of common range-of-motion measurements. Although experimental findings vary, average excursion is 50% of a muscle's longest length.[5] The longest length is the length of a muscle when the joints it crosses are moved fully in the antagonistic position. For the flexor digitorum profundus, longest length is a position of full wrist and finger extension.

We could calculate excursion from resting length if knowing the resting length of a muscle based on joint position were not so difficult. Positioning the muscle at its longest length and attempting an approximate measure of this length based on knowledge of the muscle's attachments provides a more reliable calculation. When Eduardo holds his upper extremity in full shoulder and elbow flexion, the long head of his triceps from the infraglenoid tubercle to the olecranon measures 35 cm. Based on the 50% estimate, we know that the maximum excursion would be approximately 17.5 cm.

biceps have fibers running the length of the muscle. If an individual's biceps muscle measures 15 cm from origin to insertion, this is the approximate length of the fibers. Pennate muscles like the long flexor of the thumb may measure 20 cm; however, actual fiber length may be only 4 cm because the tendon runs almost the full length of the muscle, and the fibers bridge from the bone to the tendon (Figure 4-11).

Excursion

Some muscle fiber shortening is required for each joint movement we observe. The more a joint moves, the greater the amount of shortening, or excursion, required. A **multijoint muscle** produces movement at more than one joint. It moves one or two joints at a time through full range of motion. It cannot move all its joints simultaneously because the amount this muscle must shorten (excursion requirement) is too great. If none of the joints are stabilized, the muscle shortens through all its excursion; however, the range of motion of the various joints remains incomplete. **Active insufficiency** describes a situation in which excursion of the muscle is too short and therefore cannot move all its joints.

Eduardo cannot grasp easily because of active insufficiency. When he tries to flex his fingers and close his hand around the handle of his hammer, his fingers cannot form a grasp forceful enough to pick it up. The flexor digitorum profundus contracts, but Eduardo no longer has active wrist extensors to prevent the wrist from flexing. As a result, the flexor digitorum profundus cannot flex the metacarpophalangeal and interphalangeal joints through full range. When a splint stabilizes Eduardo's wrist, the wrist no longer flexes and sufficient excursion remains to bring the metacarpophalangeal and interphalangeal joints through full range to grip the handle. Because of the injury to his radial nerve, Eduardo's flexor digitorum profundus is in active insufficiency when he attempts to grasp his hammer and lacks the shortening ability to move all its joints simultaneously.*

Insufficiency in the antagonist muscle also can cause incomplete movement or render the muscle unable to move at all. Antagonist muscles must allow every movement caused by an agonist muscle. For example, while the long finger flexor contracts, the long finger extensor stretches passively in the distal direction across the flexing joints. The extensor must be long enough to allow full flexion.

Directly after his injury, Eduardo's left forearm was placed in a cast that held his fingers in slight flexion, his wrist in about 15 degrees of extension, and his elbow in about 90 degrees of flexion. Eduardo's surgeon wanted to ensure that his radial nerve had sufficient time to heal. During that 5-week period, Eduardo used his hand very little. The combination of restricted use and inability of the wrist to flex and stretch the wrist and finger extensors led to shortening of the extensor digitorum tendons.

When Eduardo's cast was removed, his radial nerve had healed but radial nerve function had not returned. His grasp efforts continued to produce unwanted wrist flexion with the desired finger flexion. With shortened finger extensors, finger flexion for grasp was limited even sooner than before in the flexion range because of pas-

*When you try to push the clutch pedal fully down in a car in which the seat slips backward because the latch is broken, the resulting situation is similar to active insufficiency. The seat moves back before the clutch goes all the way to the floor. Knee and hip extension, or excursion, is adequate to push the clutch fully down only if the seat stays in position. The lock on the seat is like the muscles stabilizing the wrist in extension.

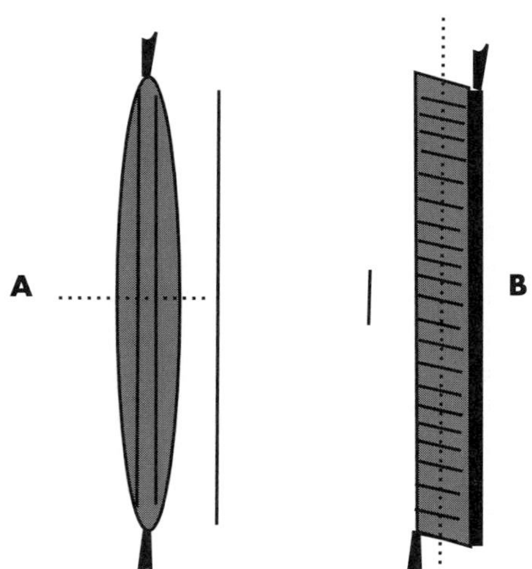

FIGURE **4-11**
Comparison of fusiform **(A)** and pennate **(B)** fiber length. The multiple solid lines within each muscle indicate actual fiber lengths. The two lengths are represented by the solid line to the right of **A** and to the left of **B.** These two muscles have generally the same gross length measured between tendon ends. Dotted lines indicate the different orientations necessary to measure a cross section, or where to cut each muscle to intersect all the fibers.

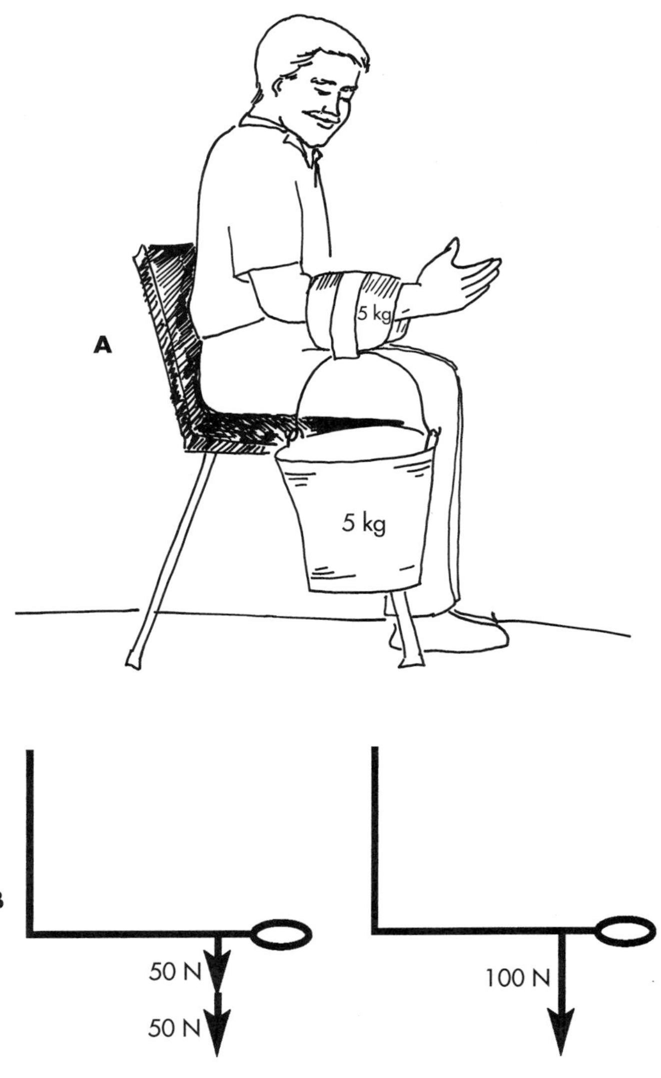

FIGURE **4-12**
A, A 5-kg bucket of sand is added to a 5-kg wrist weight to increase the amount of weight Spiros lifts. **B,** Converting kilograms to newtons, the 50-N force of the bucket added to the 50-N force of the wrist weight increases the force with which Spiros lifts to 100 N.

sive insufficiency of the long finger extensor. This passive insufficiency of the extensor digitorum muscle contributed to his inability to grasp the hammer.

Passive insufficiency restricts motion in the opposite direction because the muscle is too short to permit full movement. Active insufficiency involves insufficient shortening ability (active excursion), and passive insufficiency involves insufficient passive stretch (passive excursion). Both result in incomplete movement of some or all of the joints crossed by the muscles involved.*

MULTIPLE FORCES

We have explored external and internal forces separately. In contrast, suppose two or more forces act on a body simultaneously. For example, when we considered the various fibers of the pectoralis major, we saw that the forces they produce must be combined to determine how they act together. This combination of forces is a resultant force. The directions and amounts of the various forces involved determine the magnitude of a resultant force.

Forces along the same line

Forces acting along the same line of application always originate from a single point. They may act at some distance from that point, but the point always lies in a straight line with the force represented by the vector.

Force combination

When forces have the same point of origin and the same direction, we can add them. Many clinical applications of this combination can be made in work-oriented treatment programs. In Figure 4-12, ***Spiros Prasso*** exercises the elbow flexors as part of his regular strength-building circuit. He uses a 5-kg wrist weight. If a bucket of sand weighing 5 kg is attached to the wrist weight, the resultant force is the sum of both forces. If the vectors were drawn to scale (for example, 10 N = 0.5 cm) the resultant force would measure 5 cm:

$$50\text{ N} + 50\text{ N} = 100\text{ N}$$

When forces have the same point of application but opposite directions, we can subtract them.

In Figure 4-13, ***Henry Isaacs*** plays a board game requiring elbow and shoulder flexion to reach and position markers. An overhead pulley system provides the assistance Henry needs to lift a cast weighing 6 kg. The 5-kg weight on the pulley helps elevate the upper extremity. To determine the amount of assistance, convert kilograms to newtons and subtract the 50-N upward force from the 60-N downward force of the cast:

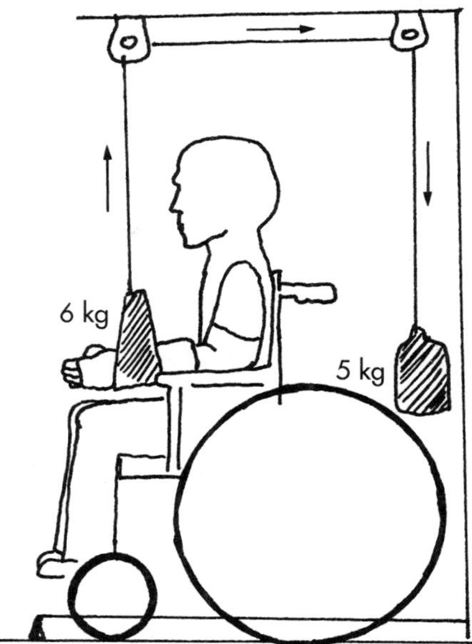

FIGURE **4-13**
The weight of a 6-kg cast on Henry's forearm is offset by the 5-kg weight applied through an overhead pulley.

$$60\text{ N} - 50\text{ N} = 10\text{ N}$$

The balance of 10 N lies in the downward direction; therefore Henry lifts with only 10 N of force instead of 60 N to move a game marker. The overhead pulley helps maximize Henry's available muscle strength.

Multiple force combination

We can combine more than two forces with the same lines of application by adding all the forces with the same direction and subtracting all the forces with the opposite direction. In Figure 4-14, each of five children tugging on a rope has different pulling power. On the right side, ***Zachary*** pulls with a force of 400 N, ***Yasmeen*** with 300 N, and ***Crystal*** with 100 N. On the left side, Tony pulls with 200 N and ***Karen*** with 500 N. Which side will win the tug of war?

To analyze this, set up the forces to act along the same line of application but in different directions; assign one direction positive values and the other, negative values. Orientation is based on the directions of x and y values on a graph. Vectors directed downward or to the left have negative values and those upward or to the right have positive values.

Following this system, assign those children pulling on the right side of the rope positive values and those on the left negative values to determine which side gen-

*Tight jeans or too many layers of clothing can restrict movement in the same way a shortened muscle can cause passive insufficiency. As muscles try to move the joints, the movement meets the resistance of cloth that cannot stretch any more, which restricts full movement. Movement beyond this point can cause cloth to tear.

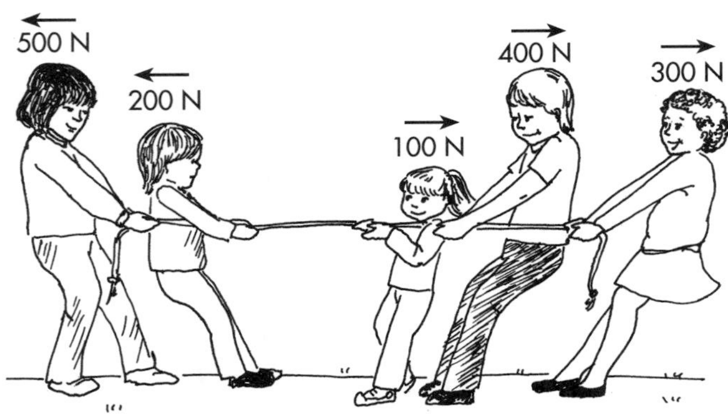

FIGURE **4-14**
Five children play tug of war. Which side will win?

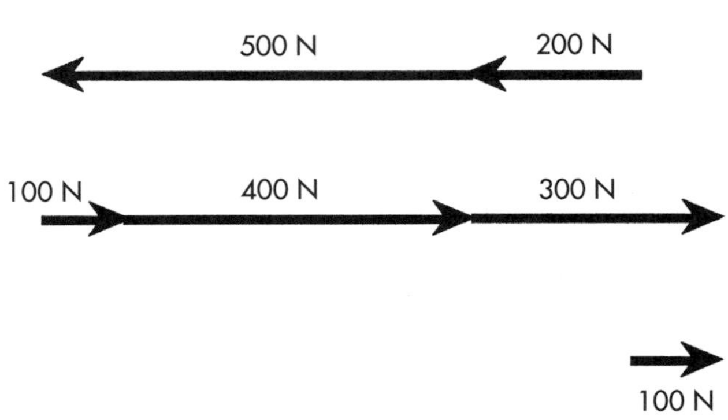

FIGURE **4-15**
The children on the right have a combined force of 100 N more than the combined force of the children on the left.

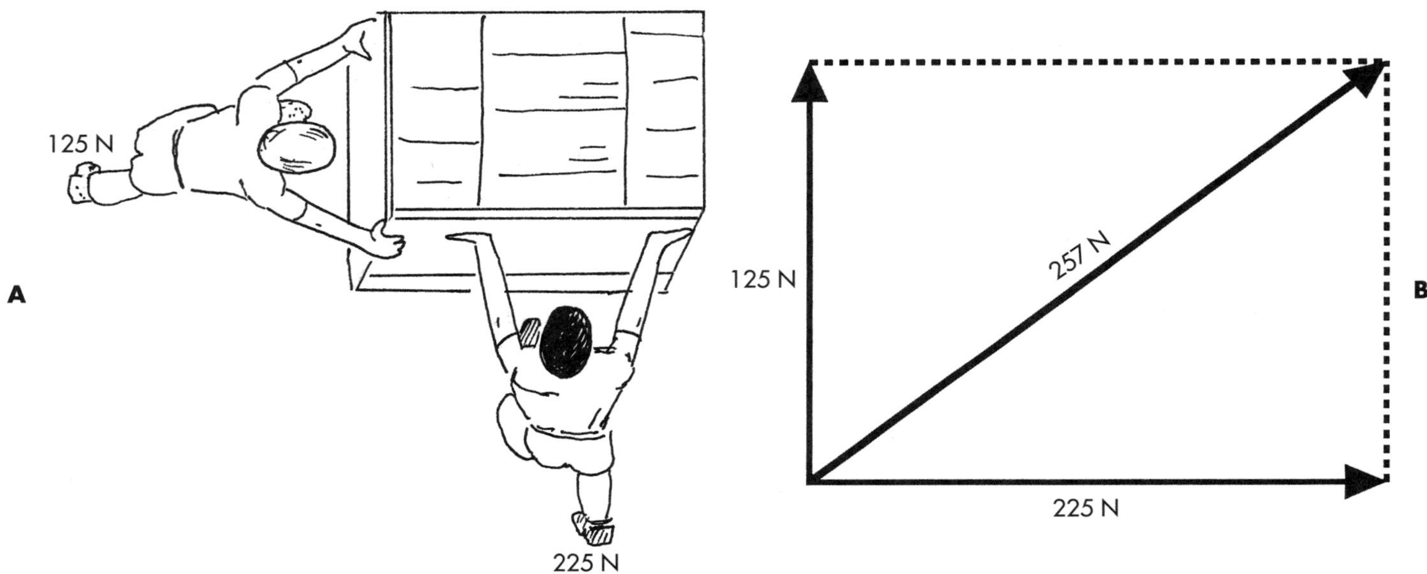

FIGURE **4-16**
A, Raul and George push a cart using 125 N and 225 N of force. **B,** The force diagram indicates that one person pushing the same cart must use 257 N of force.

erates the greater resultant force (Figure 4-15). If vectors were drawn to scale (for example, 100 N = 0.5 cm) and lined up next to each other, the vector to the right would be 0.5 cm longer than the combined vector to the left. Simple arithmetic provides the solution:

$$100\text{ N} + 400\text{ N} + 300\text{ N} + (-500\text{ N}) + (-200\text{ N}) = 100\text{ N}$$

We interpret the positive result as a net force of 100 N to the right. Zachary, Yasmeen, and Crystal won.

Forces acting on the same point but coming from different directions are concurrent forces. Two methods are used to find the resultant force of concurrent forces—the parallelogram and the polygon methods. We used the parallelogram method earlier to determine the resultant force of different forces active within the belly of the pectoralis major muscle. This method also is useful when we must determine the answers to questions of worker safety.

In Figure 4-16, ***George O'Hara*** and ***Raul Estrada*** must move a 1 m × 1 m × 1.5 m cart filled with metal parts. Raul pushes with a force of 125 N and George with a force of 225 N. The parallelogram method shows us how much force is needed to move the cart and how safe this task is when only one worker must move it.

The vector representing Raul's effort is 125 N upward. George's vector is 225 N to the right. Draw these vectors accurately and to scale; then draw two more sides of the same length parallel to each of the first two to form a parallelogram. Draw a diagonal line, which represents the direction in which the box will move and the magnitude of force necessary to move it. Measure the length of the diagonal vector to find the resultant force magnitude. The conversion of centimeters to newtons estimates the amount of force required for one worker to push the cart.

Although the measurement of the vector and conversion from meters to newtons provide a numerical answer, errors are involved in both drawing the vector and measuring its length. A more accurate value is necessary to answer the question of safety. Because these vectors intersect at 90 degrees, the Pythagorean theorem† can be used to determine an absolute value:

$$a^2 + b^2 = c^2$$
$$125^2 + 225^2 = c^2$$
$$15{,}625 + 50{,}625 = 66{,}250$$
$$c^2 = 66{,}250$$
$$c = 257 \text{ N}$$

When more than two forces are applied to an object, the polygon method is the method used to determine the combined effect. Arrows representing the forces are drawn sequentially, with the base of one to the tip of the preceding one. The arrow lengths are scaled in proportion to the force magnitudes. The orientations of the arrows correspond to the original directions of the forces.

In Figure 4-17, five individuals push a large ball. Raul pushes east with 300 N of force, George 45 degrees northeast with 150 N, Spiros north with 450 N, Eduardo 45 degrees northwest with 225 N, and Fred west with 75 N. In which direction will the ball roll? With how much force will the ball roll?

To determine the ball's final direction, draw the vectors accurately and to scale (for example, 1 cm = 50 N) and place the vectors end to end (Figure 4-18). The resultant force connects the last vector with the first vector. According to the scale, the resultant force should measure 14.5 cm, or 725 N. The vector representing this force points about 75 degrees northeast.

Use this same process to determine the effect of multiple forces on a digit in a splint. For example, ***Fred Jackson*** underwent surgery to replace a deteriorated metacarpophalangeal joint. As part of his postsurgical therapy program, he must wear a splint that provides rubber-band traction to the metacarpophalangeal joint in the direction of extension and radial deviation. The resultant force is the combination of two separately directed forces. In Fred's case the polygon method applies (Figure 4-19).

†The Pythagorean theorem states that in a right triangle (a triangle with one angle equal to 90 degrees) the square of the hypotenuse is equal to the sum of the squares of the two sides. If we know the length of the two sides, we can use algebra to determine the exact length of the triangle's hypotenuse.

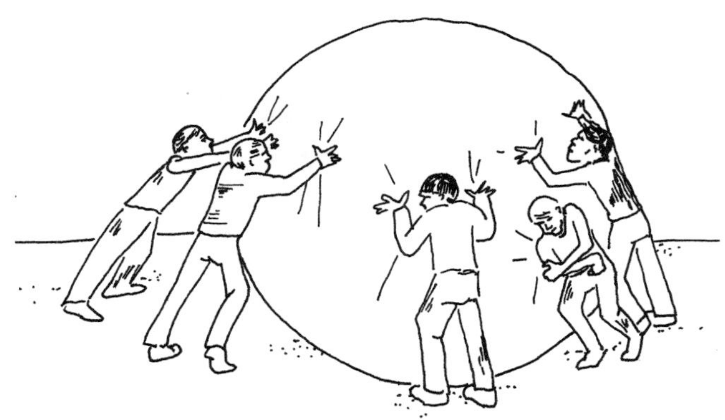

FIGURE **4-17**
Five individuals push a large ball with different amounts of force.

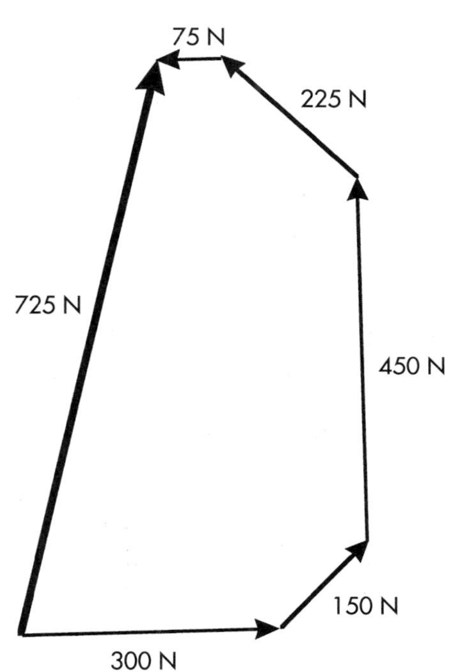

FIGURE **4-18**
The combined effect of the efforts moves the ball northeast with a force of 725 N.

Diagramming the separate forces makes it easier to understand what this splint does. The forces produced by the two rubber bands occur simultaneously; therefore the proximal phalanx is pulled on a diagonal resultant force that moves radially as it extends. Recognizing the resultant force as a combination of two separate, simultaneous forces allows us to make corrections in the final position. If one of the two forces is too great, for example, the proximal phalanx moves in a slightly different path. Correction involves only one force. Being able to

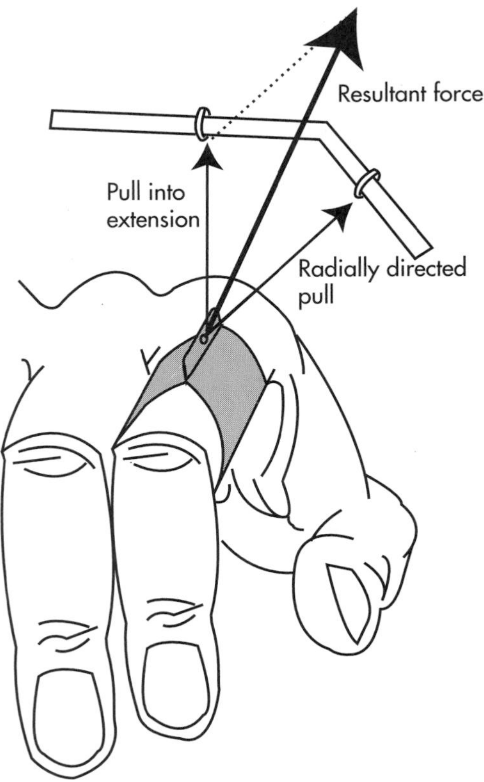

FIGURE **4-19**
In this splint the forces from the two rubber bands are combined to determine the resultant force. The force of each rubber band is represented by an arrow directed from the finger cuff toward the point of attachment of the rubber band.

break the resultant force down into components helps us visualize which force is too great. We then correct only that force. The OT practitioner who does not understand this process may know that the finger is moving in an undesirable way but attempt to correct the force through trial and error, a time-consuming and often frustrating endeavor.

Summary

The topics in this chapter all point to the need for us, as OT practitioners, to understand observations of functional activity. When we fail to understand what we see, we turn to other sources for ideas to solve our problems. We match our observation to a problem on a list and use the solution suggested by that particular protocol. This "cookbook" approach limits therapy to (1) finding a problem on a list, (2) using others' solutions, or (3) settling for a solution that does not exactly match the unique aspects of an individual's life.

Each observation represents a separate situation, and a few fundamental laws can explain many different problems. As we develop a greater sense of how these laws interconnect, our understanding of what we observe deepens and our solutions become more effective.

Applications

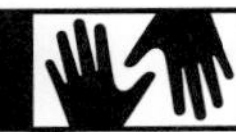

APPLICATION **4-1**
Adding Forces and Establishing Equilibrium

Donna carries a tray weighing 0.35 kg. It contains a soft drink weighing 0.5 kg and a sandwich weighing 0.3 kg. Converting kilograms to newtons, how much downward force must Donna match to hold the tray at shoulder height? Draw a graphic representation of this force, indicating the direction and magnitude of the force. Include arrows representing the force of gravity acting on the tray, soft drink, and sandwich.

APPLICATION **4-2**
Adding Forces

Spiros, advancing in his work treatment program, wears a 6-kg wrist weight and picks up a 7-kg bucket of sand. Converting kilograms to newtons, what is the downward force Spiros is required to overcome to lift both the wrist weight and the bucket of sand?

APPLICATION **4-3**
Finding the Resultant Force

Henry plays checkers using the overhead pulley. He wears the 6-kg cast, but the weight on the end of the pulley is 4 kg. Converting kilograms to newtons, how much downward force must Henry overcome to lift his arm?

APPLICATION **4-4**
Analyzing Forces by Direction and Amount

The children in Figure 4-14 have decided to play tug of war, boys against girls. On the right side, Zachary pulls with a force of 400 N and Tony with 200 N. On the left side, Yasmeen pulls with 300 N, Crystal with 100 N, and Karen with 500 N. Which side will win? Do you think this game will last longer than the last one? Why?

APPLICATION **4-5**
Combining Forces

George and Raul must move another 1 m × 1 m × 1.5 m cart filled with metal parts. It takes 350 N of force to move the cart this time. George can push only with a force of 225 N. How much harder must Raul push to make the cart move?

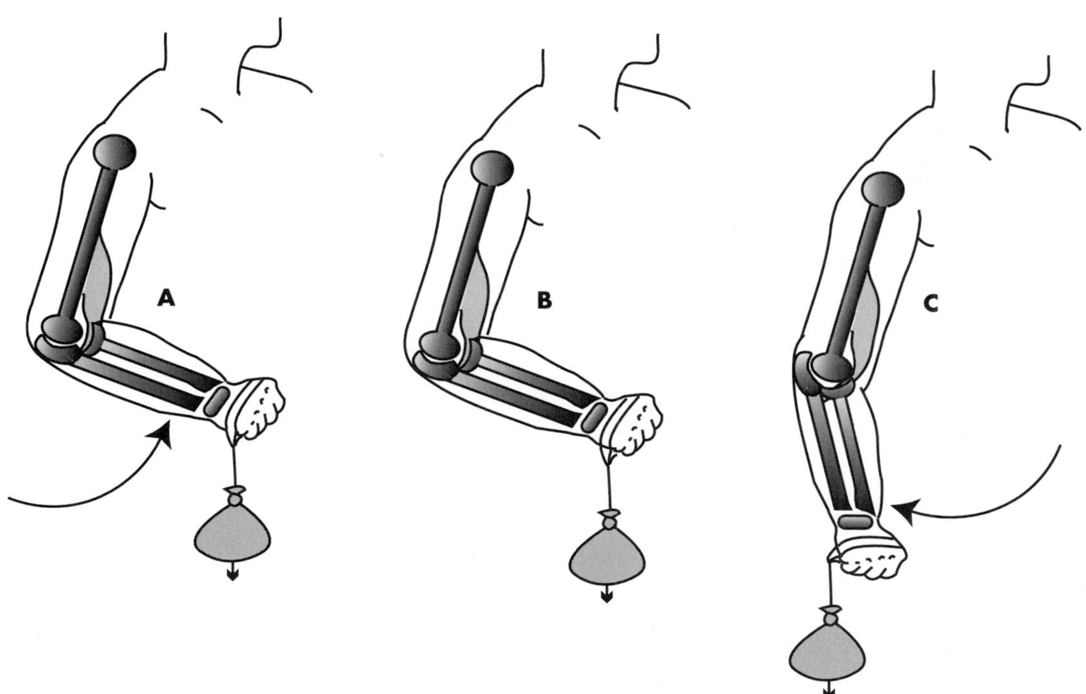

FIGURE **4-20**
Three contraction types: concentric **(A)**, isometric **(B)**, and eccentric **(C)**.

APPLICATION **4-6**

Combining Force Vectors to Determine the Resultant Force

The five individuals from Figure 4-17 push the ball again. Raul pushes 45 degrees northeast with 300 N of force, George north with 150 N, Spiros pushes east with 450 N, Eduardo 45 degrees southwest with 225 N, and Fred decides to sit out. In which direction will the ball roll and with how much force?

APPLICATION **4-7**

Determining Force Capability

Measure the girth of your lab partner's biceps and estimate the amount of force this muscle can generate.

APPLICATION **4-8**

Determining Excursion

Measure the long head of your partner's triceps at its longest length and estimate its maximum excursion.

APPLICATION **4-9**

Drawing Vectors Indicating Contractions

Look at the three drawings in Figure 4-20 and draw the vector for a contraction of the brachialis in each condition.

See Appendix C for solutions to Applications.

REFERENCES

1. Fick R: *Anatomie und Mechanik der Gelenke: Teil III spezielle Gelenk und Muskelmechanik,* Jena, 1911, Fisher.
2. Gordon AM and others: Variation in isometric tension with sarcomere length in vertebrate muscle fibers, *J Physiol* 184:170-192, 1966.
3. Haxton HA: Absolute muscle force in the ankle flexors of man, *J Physiol* 103:267-273, 1944.
4. Von Recklinghausen N: *Gliedermechanik und Lahmungsprothesen,* Berlin, 1920, J Springer.
5. Weber EF: *Ueber die Langeverhaltnisse der Muskeln im allgemeinen,* Leipzig, Germany, 1851, Verh Kgl Sach Ges d Wiss.

RELATED READINGS

Luttgens K, Hamilton N: *Kinesiology: scientific basis of human motion,* ed 9, Madison, Wis, 1997, Brown & Benchmark.

Nordin M, Frankel VH: *Basic biomechanics of the musculoskeletal system,* ed 2, Philadelphia, 1989, Lea & Febiger.

Wiktorin CH, Nordin M: *Introduction to problem solving in biomechanics,* Philadelphia, 1986, Lea & Febiger.

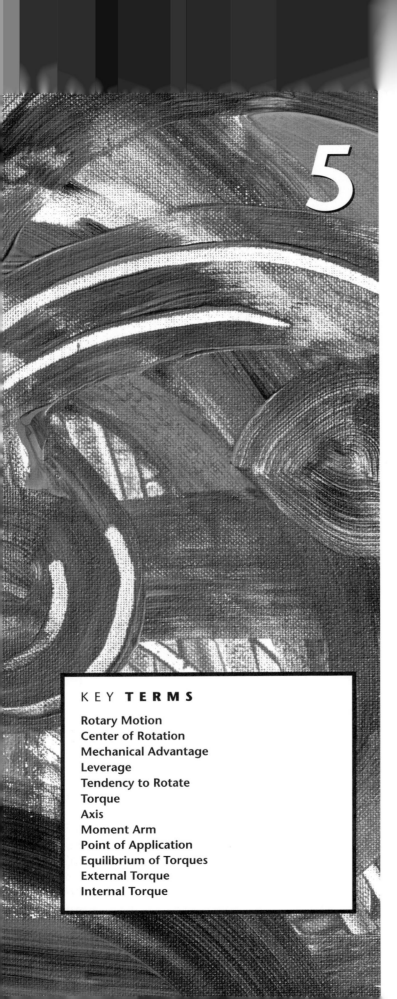

5 Rotary Force, Torque, and Motion

KEY TERMS

Rotary Motion
Center of Rotation
Mechanical Advantage
Leverage
Tendency to Rotate
Torque
Axis
Moment Arm
Point of Application
Equilibrium of Torques
External Torque
Internal Torque

CHAPTER OUTLINE

Like linear forces, we experience **rotary motion** every day without ever having to think about how it affects us. Examples of rotary motion are everywhere. They include swinging doors, turning doorknobs, and rolling wheelchair wheels. All these objects demonstrate motion around a central point. Once we understand what to look for, we realize that most skeletal movements are rotary as well.

For example, the brachialis is attached proximally to the humerus and distally to the ulna. When the humerus is stabilized and the brachialis contracts concentrically, the ulna moves the only way it will move—around an arc centered in the side-to-side axis of the elbow joint. The brachialis exhibits shortening (excursion) proportional to the amount the insertion moves in its arc. This movement, flexion, occurs because the brachialis is anterior to the flexion/extension axis; we say it has an anterior relationship (Figure 5-1). Elbow flexion is the rotary motion resulting from the linear force created by contraction of the brachialis.

In Chapter 4 we established the idea that the greater the force, the greater the effect on the movement of an object (Newton's second law). In this chapter, we see that the amount of force is only part of rotary motion. Only if another condition exists does a greater force produce a greater tendency toward rotation. That condition, distance of the force from the center of rotation, and the combined effect of the force and the distance are our major objectives.

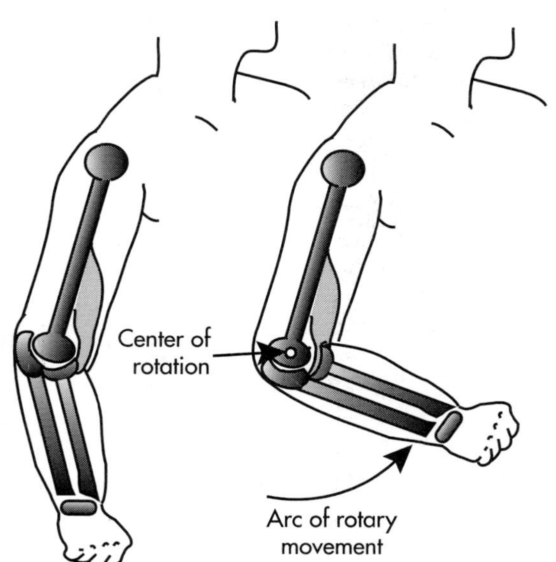

FIGURE **5-1**
The brachialis flexes the forearm at the elbow. The center of rotation is the side-to-side axis of the elbow. The forearm bones comprise the rotationally moving segment.

Rotary Motion

Rotary motion is fundamentally different from linear motion because it occurs in a circular pattern. Rotary motion of a skeletal segment occurs when the force of a muscle contraction is applied to a segment attached to another segment at a joint.

We are familiar with using linear movement to go somewhere. If all our movements were rotary, we would never go anywhere. Musculoskeletal segments move in circular paths, but the combinations of rotary movements at different joints take us from place to place in linear paths.

The rotary movements of the hands of a clock bring those hands to the same places again and again. Although they never go anywhere in terms of distance, they measure the passage of time, a linear concept. The clock demonstrates the fundamental characteristics of rotary motion (Figure 5-2). The clock's hands move in a circle around a central point. They change orientation, pointing up, right, down, then left. If we were to track different points on the second hand, we would notice these points appear to move at different speeds. In a drawing, the circumference of the circle traced by a point close to the center is less than that of a point on the end of the second hand. Because both points complete one revolution in 1 minute and the end point travels a greater distance in that time, the end point travels faster than the point closer to the center.

As we observe the movement of the second hand, three clear differences between rotary and linear motion emerge (Figure 5-3):

1. Rotary motion occurs in a circular path around a central point, the **center of rotation.** Linear motion occurs along a linear path, starting in one place and ending in a different place.
2. Objects that rotate change orientation during movement. Objects in linear motion remain in their original orientation throughout.
3. Two points in a segment moving in a circle move at different speeds, the point farther from the center of rotation moving faster than the other. Two points in a segment moving in a line from one place to another move at the same speed. Otherwise, the segment would rotate or break apart.

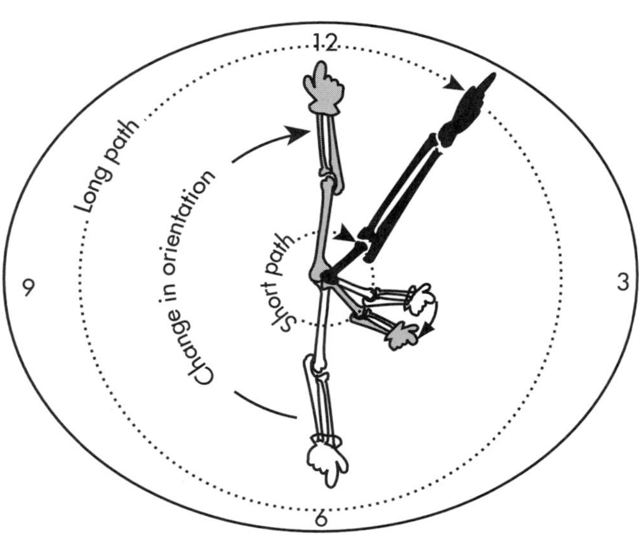

FIGURE **5-2**
The hands of this clock demonstrate the fundamental characteristics of rotary motion. They move in a circular path around a central point and change orientation as they move. The elbow point on the second hand moves at a slower speed than the wrist, which is farther from the center and moves through a greater circumference in the same time as the elbow point.

Tendency to Rotate

In rotary motion, both the force and the point of action of the force on the moving object are important. Opening and closing a door requires a certain amount of force. However, we may not always realize that where the force is applied also is important. For example, 4-year-old ***Crystal Turner*** tries to open a heavy glass door for the OT practitioner. Because she cannot reach the handle, Crystal pushes the glass toward the center of the door's width. When the door does not give way, she automatically moves her hands toward the door's swinging edge. Using the same force, Crystal succeeds.

We experience a similar event when we try to open a door on which the lock releases with a bar handle spanning the width of the door. (These are common in public places.) As we try to open the door, we find it easier to place our hand on the far end of the bar, away from the hinge. Attempts to open the door when we push closer to the hinge edge usually fail.

The tendency of a force to cause rotation is related to the spot at which the force is applied. Crystal and her brother experience this fundamental truth of mechanical physics on a playground seesaw. Because her brother is older and heavier than Crystal, he sits at the bottom

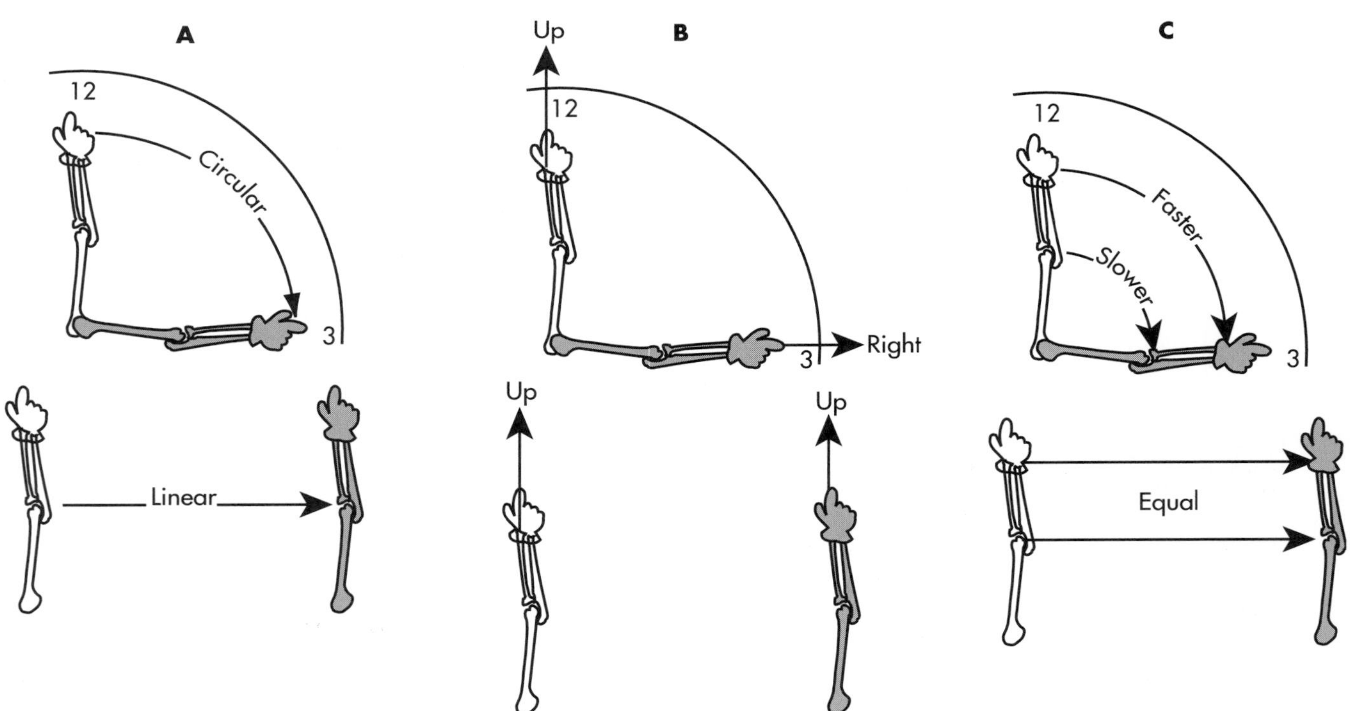

FIGURE **5-3**
Rotary motion has three unique characteristics. Movement is in a circular path **(A),** orientation changes **(B),** and movement occurs at different speeds depending on distance from the center of rotation **(C).**

and she sits at the top. The seesaw remains stationary until her brother moves along it closer to the pivot point.

A mechanical engineer may say that the brother's weight (center of gravity) must pull down closer to the pivot and Crystal's weight needs the **mechanical advantage** of pulling down farther from the pivot. This mechanical advantage is **leverage.** We gain leverage by moving the weight farther away from the pivot. Thus a lighter weight can be just as effective as a heavier weight. The lighter weight creates a **tendency to rotate** when it moves away from the pivot. Rotation depends as much on where a weight is applied—its distance from the pivot—as it does on the amount of force exerted.

The effectiveness of a force in causing rotation is the **torque** created by the force. Torque is the same as tendency to rotate. We know that the tendency of a force to cause rotation depends on the amount of force applied and the distance between the force and the pivot, or **axis,** the center of rotation. The formula to determine how much tendency toward rotation exists (value of torque) is torque (T) equals force (F) times **moment arm** (MA), the distance from the force to the axis (Figure 5-4):

$$T = F \times MA$$

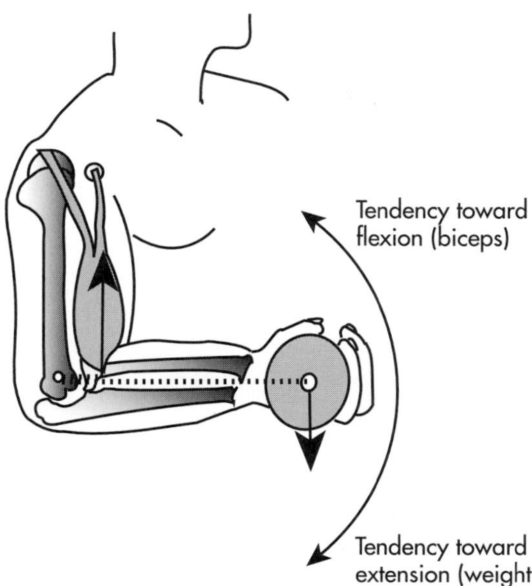

FIGURE **5-4**
The factors in creating a tendency toward elbow flexion are the force of contraction in the biceps and its distance from the axis. The factors in creating a tendency toward elbow extension are the weight of the object held in the hand and its distance from the axis at the elbow.

The moment arm is affected by the exact place on the lever or bony segment on which the force acts, the **point of application.** On a skeletal segment the point of application is synonymous with the muscle's insertion.

Equilibrium of Torques

Successful movement against resistance involves overcoming the resistance and depends on upsetting the balance of tendencies in one direction versus the other. Forces tend to move objects. Only when the tendency toward flexion created by the biceps is greater than the tendency toward elbow extension created by a weight held in the hand does rotary motion (flexion) occur in the direction of the biceps.

When the weight is too heavy or we want to hold the weight still, we exert effort and no movement occurs. The effort creates a tendency toward flexion; however, this tendency is balanced by an equal and opposite tendency toward extension created by the weight of the object. The two tendencies are balanced. Because the balance describes equal tendencies for rotation, equilibrium of rotary tendencies, or **equilibrium of torques,** exists.

We constantly are confronted with equilibrium of torques. ***Donna Nelson,*** our food server, provides a clear example. Donna uses the equilibrium of up and down forces to hold the tray and the equilibrium of torques to balance the tray as she removes food items. She positions items on the tray based on their relative weights. Heavier food items go near the center, where her hand elevates the tray. Lighter items surround the center.

Figure 5-5 shows Donna's tray in rotary equilibrium. For the purpose of our discussion, assume the tray rotates clockwise or counterclockwise in the plane of the

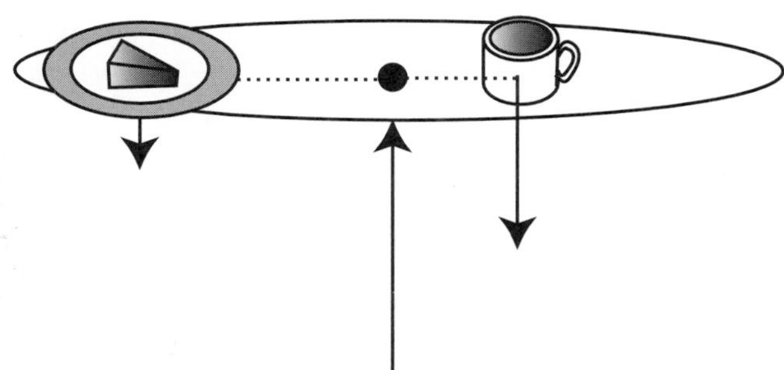

FIGURE **5-5**
Donna's tray is in rotary equilibrium. The force vectors are drawn to scale and indicate the greater force of the full mug of coffee. Notice also the greater distance, or moment arm, between the axis and the dessert. This longer moment arm gives the lighter-weight dessert an advantage equal to the heavier coffee mug.

page. The axis of rotation is at her hand, and items on the tray to the right and left of her hand exert opposite tendencies toward rotation because of their weight and distance from her hand. If the coffee mug is removed, so is its tendency to rotate the tray counterclockwise. The result is a tendency toward counterclockwise rotation because of the weight of the plate of cheesecake. Donna must balance the weight of the cheesecake side of the tray before she removes the coffee cup.

Lever Systems

Because torque involves both force and moment arm, we cannot use a 4.45-kg muscle contraction force to counteract 4.45 kg of resistance. The amount of muscle force needed depends on the muscle's moment arm (distance of the muscle force from the joint axis) and the moment arm of the resistance. The arrangement of the two moment arms on the lever with respect to each other and

TABLE 5-1
Classification of Levers

Levers are classified according to the placement of the axis, resistance force, and force generated by the machine (muscle force) to move the resistance.

	LOCATION OF AXIS	LENGTHS OF MAs	DIRECTION OF FORCES*	DIRECTION OF MOTION
First Class	Between the two forces	Resistance force equal, or one greater than the other	Same	Opposite
Second Class	On one end	Resistance force MA always less	Opposite	Same
Third Class	On one end	Resistance force MA always greater	Opposite	Same

MA, Moment arm.
* Forces in equilibrium

to the axis of motion varies. The three variations represent three classes of levers (Table 5-1).

EVERYDAY LEVERS

We use lever systems every day to make our lives easier. Without these adaptive devices, we could not perform many common functions. A lever allows us to use a handle to extend the moment arm, which changes the mechanical advantage of the forces we exert to overcome resistance.

The seesaw is an example of a first-class lever, in which the mechanical advantages of effort and resistance are more or less balanced on either side of the axis. Other examples are doorknobs, steering wheels, and circular faucet valves. In each case, force is exerted on opposite sides of the center, the location of the axis. When lever extensions are placed on circular doorknobs or faucets, they become second-class levers, the most popular adaptive devices.

Second-class levers lend a mechanical advantage to the force of effort. The amount of force necessary to operate a second-class lever decreases in proportion to the length of the handle. Most bottle openers are designed as second-class levers (Figure 5-6). A wheelbarrow is another example (Figure 5-7).

Second-class levers are common due to the inherent mechanical advantage. A second-class lever allows force of effort to operate on a longer moment arm than that of the resistance force. We choose a wrench with a longer handle to loosen a stubborn nut because this arrangement extends the exertion force moment arm. One disadvantage of the longer moment arm is that it forces the hand to travel a greater distance. Once the nut loosens, we usually grab the handle toward the nut because we no longer need so much leverage.

Third-class levers, which favor the mechanical advantage of resistance, are not as popular as second-class levers, but history provides one infamous example. Medieval warriors who wanted to hurl objects toward castle walls as fast and as high as they could designed the catapult. Flinging objects was their primary concern, and plenty of warriors existed to provide the effort. The third-class lever provided the speed and distance the warriors needed (Figure 5-8).

MUSCULOSKELETAL LEVERS

In the body, most muscles operate on short moment arms because their insertions are close to the joint axis. As a result, muscles typically generate greater forces than the weights of resistance they encounter. Resistance forces, especially those held in the hand, have the mechanical advantage of being an arm's length from the joint axis.

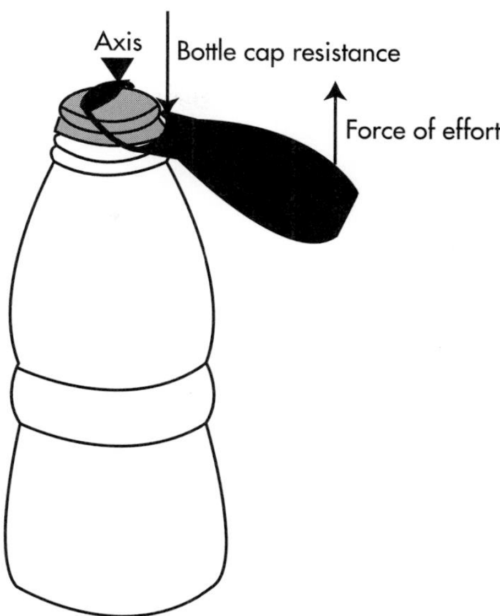

FIGURE **5-6**
A bottle opener is a second-class lever.

At first glance the human body is at a disadvantage and thus inefficient. Actually, a powerful advantage is at work, but it is a less obvious one. Understanding this advantage involves an understanding of leverage and lever systems.

Most bone-joint chains, or kinematic chains, in the body are examples of third-class levers (See Table 5-1). The axis of rotation is located on one end, the resistance force (object being lifted) is near the other end, and the force of muscle contraction is applied between the two, similar to a catapult. In a third-class lever, resistance force always has a greater moment arm than muscle force. Muscle force must be greater than resistance force, however, to compensate for the short moment arm at which the muscle operates. Because third-class levers require so much effort, we often consider them examples of poor mechanical advantage that should be avoided in tools and adaptive devices.

However, third-class levers provide advantages in amount and speed of movement. In our bodies, muscles and bones rotate around joints. In this way, distal parts of extremities can travel greater distances at faster speeds than proximal body parts. Our ability to lift objects is advantageous, but our ability to move them through great distances at fast speeds is even more essential. Third-class levers provide the only way to position an object at the end of a lever.

Another advantage of the third-class lever lies in the nature of muscle contraction. Muscles can shorten only

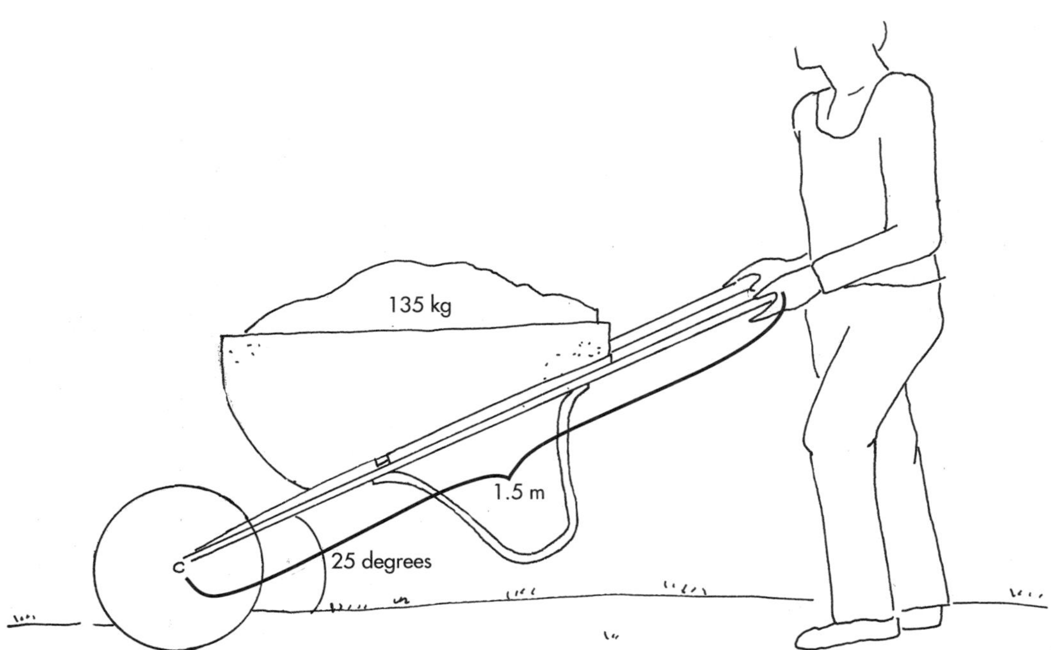

FIGURE **5-7**
This wheelbarrow has handles 1.5 m long from axis to hand placement. Because the upward force is applied by the hands onto the handles, this distance is the moment arm of the force exerted by the body. The load (135 kg) is directed downward and is closer to the axis. The exertion force operates at the longer moment arm.

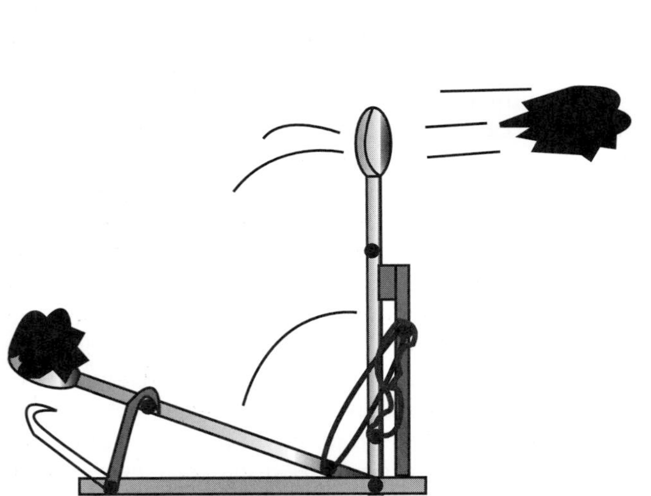

FIGURE **5-8**
The catapult is a third-class lever.

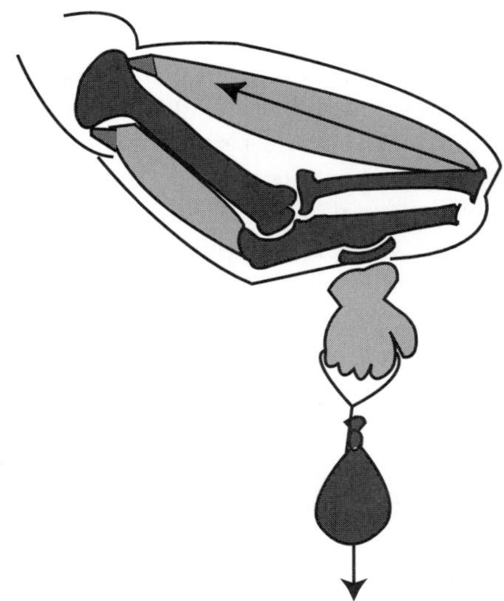

FIGURE **5-9**
If the upper extremity were a second-class lever with the moment arm for the resistance less than that for the muscle force, several problems would result.

BOX 5-1

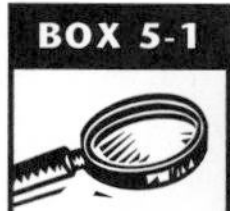

A **CLOSER** LOOK

A Hand in a Different Place

Switching the hand's location from the end to the middle of the forearm poses a number of problems. A few we have not yet considered follow:

1. *Functional reach would be greatly decreased.*
2. *Clothing would have to be redesigned.*
3. *Eating would be interesting. You would have to position your drink at arm's length because your distal forearm would reach beyond the far side of the plate every time your hand scooped food on the near side.*
4. *Shaking hands would be very difficult. You would have to be careful not to poke your acquaintance in the nose with your distal forearm.*
5. *Typing speed would be decreased. You would have to learn touch typing. (With practice, you possibly could use your distal forearms to turn the pages of the book from which you're typing.)*

so much; they have limited excursion capabilities. If muscles operated within second-class lever systems, muscle moment arms would be longer than those of the resistance being moved. As in the case of the wrench handle, the longer the moment arm (handle), the greater the amount of distance through which it must be moved.

Imagine the hand extending from mid forearm and the brachialis inserting on the distal radius. (This would be a second-class lever [See Table 5-1.]) The brachialis would have a mechanical advantage, a longer lever arm, compared with the resistance (Figure 5-9). However, because the distal end of the radius is the farthest point from the axis (elbow joint), it moves through a greater distance at greater speed than the hand. The brachialis attached to this more distal insertion would have to contract through twice the distance than the distance through which the hand would have to move. It also would have to contract faster, and regardless of its speed, the hand would move at half that speed. We already have seen that muscles have the ability to contract only a limited amount of distance. In addition, the force of contraction suffers if the muscle contracts too fast (A Closer Look Box 5-1).

The third-class lever makes more sense in muscle movement. The muscle can contract slowly and through much less excursion to move the hand faster in a greater arc of motion. Because most muscles attach close to the joints they move, moment arms are typically short compared with moment arms for the resistance held in the hand. Muscles must shorten one-fourth or less the length of the distance the hand travels. However, the muscle must generate enough force to make up for its short moment arm (poor mechanical advantage). We easily can increase muscle strength, whereas muscle excursion is fixed.

External and Internal Torques

Two kinds of torque—internal and external—operate on the human body. Forces operating outside the body produce **external torque.** For example, the external torques produced by various food items are Donna's main considerations in balancing her food tray.

Muscles acting on their attachments to bony segments produce **internal torque.** We think of these bony segments as a system of levers. Internal forces of muscle contraction and external forces create tendencies to rotate in one direction or another.

Although Donna may not concentrate on internal torque, it plays just as important a role in the tray's balance as its external counterpart. The full tray exerts a tendency toward shoulder adduction. Donna's shoulder abductors create an equal tendency toward abduction. When the two tendencies are balanced, she successfully holds up the tray.

Differentiating between equal tendencies is important. When forces operate on different moment arms, the magnitude of each opposing force is different, which allows these forces to generate equal and opposite tendencies to rotate. The actual value of the opposing forces and the torque they generate can be determined with a simple formula.

TORQUE VALUE

To determine specific tendencies toward rotation, identify and draw the forces and moment arms involved in each tendency. When Donna holds up her tray, the tendencies at play are shoulder adduction and abduction. The rotating segment is the humerus, and the axis of rotation is the front-to-back axis for abduction/adduction. The force for adduction is the weight of the food tray, and the force for abduction is contraction of the deltoid muscle. (Other shoulder abductors are working, but consider only the deltoid.) The forces of adduction and abduction are both represented as vectors.

The weight of the food tray and its contents are directed straight down from the tray's center of gravity. The weight of the tray times its moment arm (the distance from the vector representing the tray's weight to the axis in the shoulder joint) creates the tendency to-

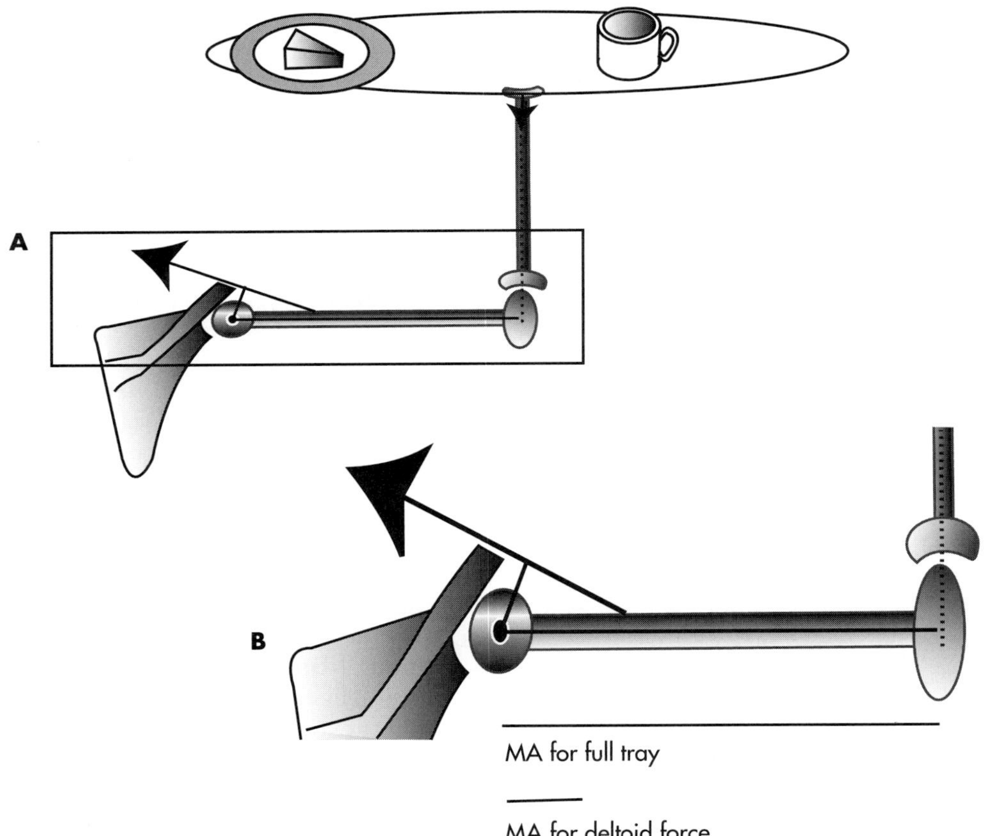

FIGURE **5-10**
A, Equilibrium of abduction/adduction torque at the shoulder. **B,** Notice the greater force the deltoid needs to compensate for its short moment arm *(MA).* The deltoid force has a poorer mechanical advantage (shorter moment arm or shorter lever) and must make up for this shortcoming by producing a greater amount of force than the force of the food tray.

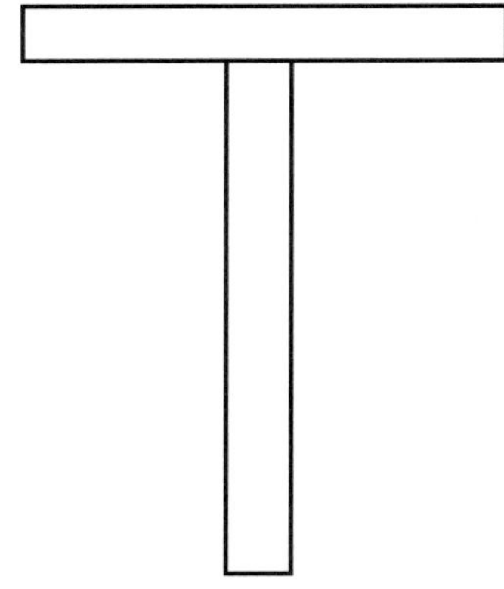

FIGURE **5-11**
A T square helps identify the true (perpendicular) distance from force to axis.

ward adduction. Donna carries a 4.45-kg tray about 26 cm from her shoulder joint. Convert kilograms to newtons, and the torque involved in the tendency toward adduction is the product of the 4.45-kg tray and the 26-cm moment arm, or 1157 N-cm. In other words, multiply force by moment arm.

Because Donna can elevate the tray successfully, we know the 1157 N-cm of adduction tendency is balanced by the abduction effort of the deltoid. This 1157 N-cm of tendency toward abduction involves a different combination of force and moment arm because the deltoid inserts so close to the shoulder axis of abduction/adduction. To generate the 1157 N-cm of tendency to balance the food tray, the deltoid must produce 223 N of force.

Why must the deltoid create 223 N to balance a 44.5-N force of the food tray? The food tray weight (force) is

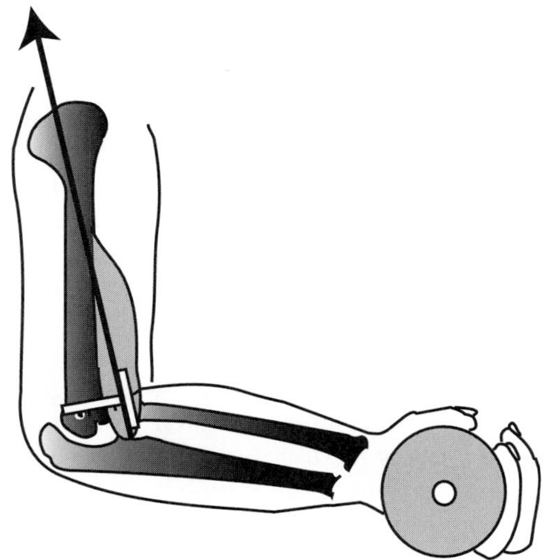

FIGURE **5-12**
The T square is used to determine the distance from the force to the axis.

farther away (26 cm) from the shoulder joint axis and has greater leverage than the deltoid. The deltoid pulls with greater force closer to the axis (5.2 cm) to compensate for its inferior leverage. (Figure 5-10, *A* indicates the different amounts of force with different-length vectors.)

Let us consider how we determine the deltoid force and its moment arm. If we visualize abduction and adduction as a balance between two sets of factors (two force-moment arm sets creating opposite tendencies), we can determine how much force the deltoid muscle must exert to balance the tray. We know the weight of the tray and can measure the moment arms. All that is left is to determine the force the deltoid exerts.

The force of the tray is 44.5 N. Measure the moment arm by measuring the distance from the tray's force vector to the axis. Use a homemade T square made from two cardboard strips attached to each other at 90-degree angles (Figure 5-11). Place one arm of the T square on the force vector (originating where Donna balances the tray with her hand) and slide the T square along the vector in the direction of the axis. Stop when the other arm of the T square intercepts the axis of the shoulder joint and draw a line connecting the axis to the force vector. (Figure 5-12 shows this process for the moment arm of the brachialis at the elbow.) This is the perpendicular distance, the moment arm for the resistance force.

Draw a vector originating from the deltoid's insertion and along its fibers that indicates the direction the deltoid muscle fibers must contract. (Do not draw the arrowhead because the magnitude of this force is not yet known.) Use the sliding T square to measure the distance from the muscle force to the axis and draw this line, the moment arm for the deltoid force.

When both moment arms are represented, measure the length of each and calculate the force of the deltoid. (Your value for the deltoid moment arm may differ slightly from this book's. If so, substitute your value for the 5.2-cm value shown below.)

When Donna holds the food tray, the equation looks like this, and the answer is rounded:

Shoulder adduction tendency = Shoulder abduction tendency

$$44.5 \text{ N} \times 26 \text{ cm} = \underline{\qquad} \text{ N} \times 5.2 \text{ cm}$$

$$1157 \text{ N-cm} = \underline{\qquad} \text{ N} \times 5.2 \text{ cm}$$

$$\frac{1157 \text{ N-cm}}{5.2 \text{ cm}} = 223 \text{ N}$$

The force the deltoid needs to balance the heavier tray is 223 N. Knowing the magnitude of the deltoid force, go back to the line drawn from the deltoid insertion and measure the distance along this vector according to the scale used to draw the tray's force vector. Using a scale of 1 cm = 20 N, measure 11.2 cm from the insertion and draw the arrowhead at that point. Erase any part of the original line extending beyond the arrowhead.

CHANGING FACTORS DURING CONSTANT TORQUE

We have thought about, measured, determined, and drawn the values of the factors (force magnitude and moment arm) that produce a tendency to rotate (torque). We must realize that these factors often change during movement, even though the amount of torque this combination generates remains the same. However, the amount of torque generated in maximal effort changes depending on joint position.

Torque during maximal effort changes as the magnitude of the force and moment arms change. A movement may not feel as strong in one joint position as in another. This can be puzzling because movement does not change the cross section of the muscle, and cross section determines strength. However, movement does change the length of the muscle, and the length of a muscle at the start of its contraction can affect the amount of force the muscle can generate. Movement also often results in changes in the length of the moment arm. The combination of these changes, including muscle length and moment arm, produces different torques at different joint positions.

Changes in moment arm are palpable in the biceps tendon anterior to the elbow. When the forearm is supinated and the elbow flexed to 90 degrees, find the moment arm

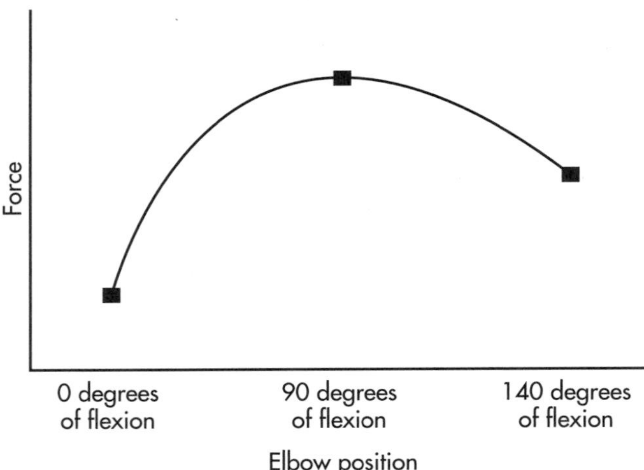

FIGURE **5-13**
The torque generated by the force of contraction of the elbow flexors is shown at different places in the elbow-flexion arc.

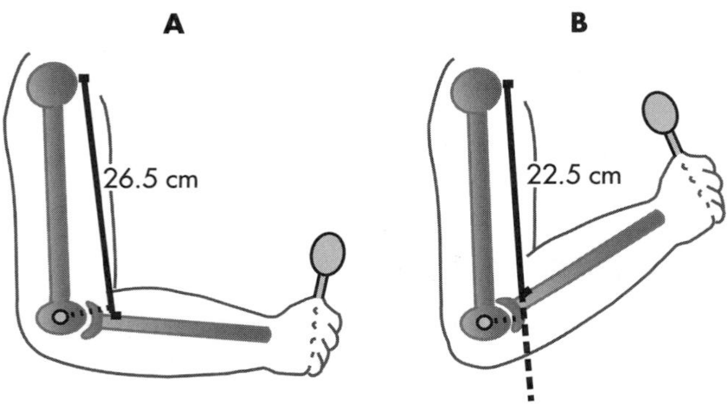

FIGURE **5-14**
Jason's internal torque is affected by changes in length in both the muscle and moment arm. **A,** He begins the movement with the elbow flexed to 90 degrees. **B,** He reaches an elbow position that shortens the moment arm and muscle.

by placing the thumb on the medial epicondyle of the humerus, the approximate location of the side-to-side axis, and the index finger on the biceps tendon. Slowly extend the forearm. The distance between the thumb and fingers decreases, providing a good approximation of the changing moment-arm length for the biceps.

The clearest, least technical way to measure changes in force magnitude (muscle contraction) and moment arm is to perform a series of isometric efforts at different joint positions. Each contraction begins at a different point in the range, and maximal effort is met by matching resistance so that no shortening occurs during the contraction. A maximum isometric torque curve (Figure 5-13) is used to plot the results of this exercise.

Isometric torque curves provide values to illustrate the concept that movement is weaker in one position than in another. For example, ***Jason Black*** has been working on eating independently, but he cannot completely lift a utensil to his mouth. Jason performs best when the table height is adjusted so that his elbow is flexed to 90 degrees as he begins to bring his hand to his mouth. Sitting erect with proper vertebral extension, Jason gets a good start away from the plate but is unable to continue flexion long enough to reach his mouth. He begins the motion at the strongest point in the torque-curve range. However, continued flexion brings his elbow to a position in which less torque is produced. (The changing moment arm and muscle length are shown in Figure 5-14.)

Is the problem too short a moment arm or too short a muscle? In elbow flexion, both occur beyond 90 degrees. In joints in which the moment arm shortens but the muscle lengthens, the improved muscle length compensates for the shorter moment arm and torque remains more constant.

Summary

We are accustomed to associating force with movement and thus more force with faster movement or greater strength. Rotary movement expands our thinking and helps us realize that the amount of force is only part of movement. Placement of force with respect to the axis of motion also plays a key role. Together, magnitude and placement result in a tendency to set bony segments and external objects into circular motion. (Circular motions and the tendencies of different muscles to cause them are addressed in Chapters 6 and 8.)

Applications

APPLICATION **5-1**

Effort Needed to Open and Close a Valve

Find a sink on which lever faucet handles have replaced round handles. With the faucet securely off, try to turn on the water, holding the handle at its end. Turn it off and try again, holding the handle closer to the screw connecting the handle to the valve. Is there a difference in how easily the valve opens? Identify the axis of rotation and the moment arm.

APPLICATION **5-2**

External Torque Produced by a Barbell

In Chapter 4, we considered activities in ***Spiros Prasso's*** work treatment program. Continuing to build his upper-extremity strength, Spiros lifts a 5-kg barbell from a seated position (Figure 5-15). His forearm measures 35 cm from the elbow-joint axis to the palmar crease where the barbell rests. How much external torque does the barbell

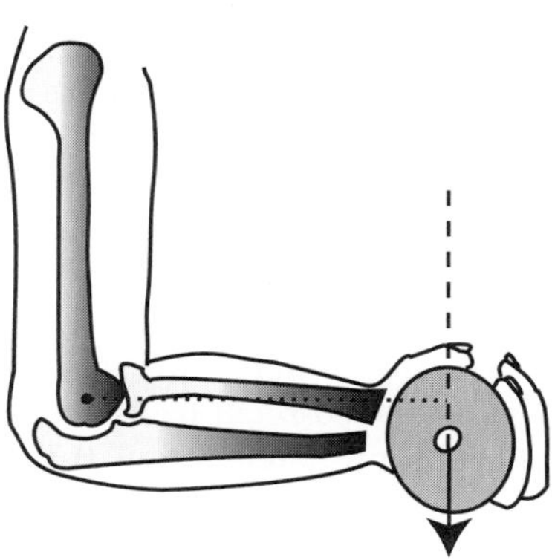

FIGURE **5-15**
External torque is the tendency of the weight to produce elbow extension.

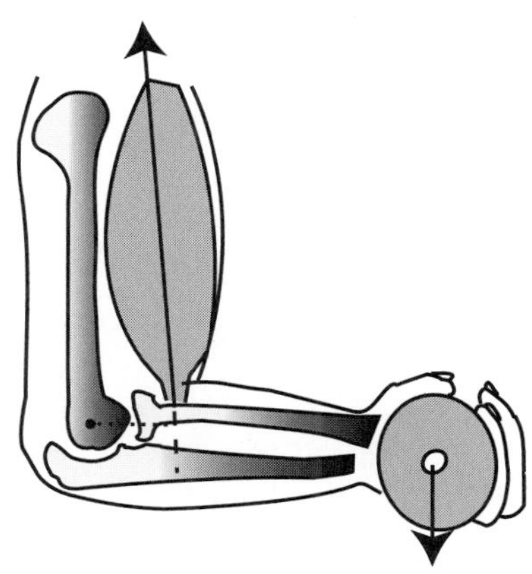

FIGURE **5-16**
Internal torque is the tendency of the biceps to produce elbow flexion.

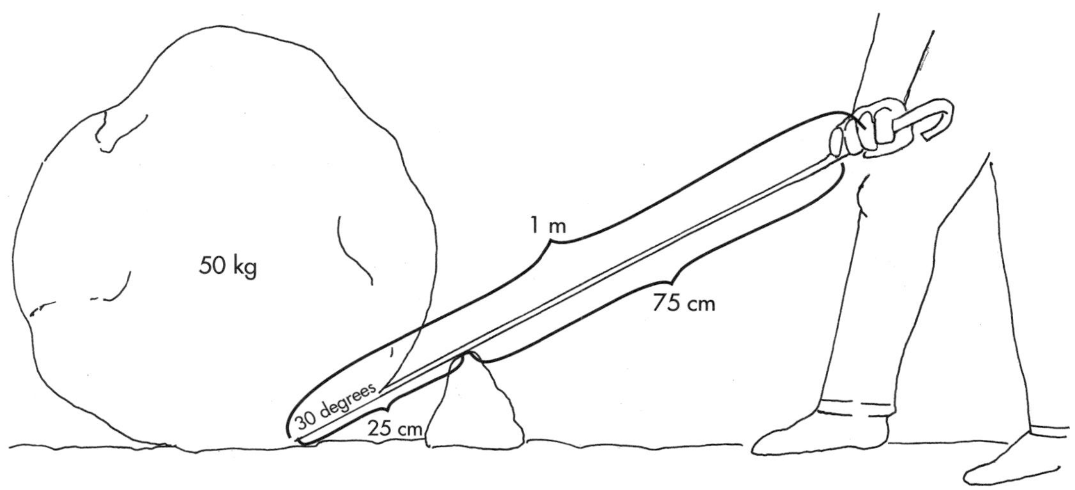

FIGURE **5-17**
A 1-m crowbar is placed so that its axis is 25 cm from a 50-kg rock and 75 cm from the end of the handle. The crowbar is angled 30 degrees from the ground. Converting centimeters to meters and kilograms to newtons, how much effort is needed to lift the rock?

produce when the elbow is flexed to 30, 60, 90, and 120 degrees? Is the external torque the same throughout the range of motion? If not, how does it change and why?

APPLICATION **5-3**
Force Produced by the Biceps

In Figure 5-16, Spiros supports the same 5-kg barbell from a seated position. Let us say the only functioning elbow flexor is the biceps brachii. It inserts 8.5 cm from the elbow's side-to-side axis for flexion. The torque produced by the biceps matches the amount of torque at each joint position in the previous application because the biceps supports the barbell. The moment arms for the biceps at the different joint positions are as follows: 6 cm at 30 degrees, 8 cm at 60 degrees, 8.5 cm at 90 degrees, and 6 cm at 120 degrees of flexion. How much force is produced at 30, 60, 90, and 120 degrees of flexion to support the barbell in an isometric contraction? Is the amount of biceps force the same in each contraction? If not, how does it change and why?

APPLICATION **5-4**
Effort Needed to Lift a Rock with a Crowbar

In Figure 5-17, Spiros uses a 1-m crowbar to lift a 50-kg rock in his work-hardening program. The crowbar is placed over a small rock set 25 cm from the end of the crowbar, which is placed under the rock. The crowbar is set at a 30-degree angle from the ground. What kind of

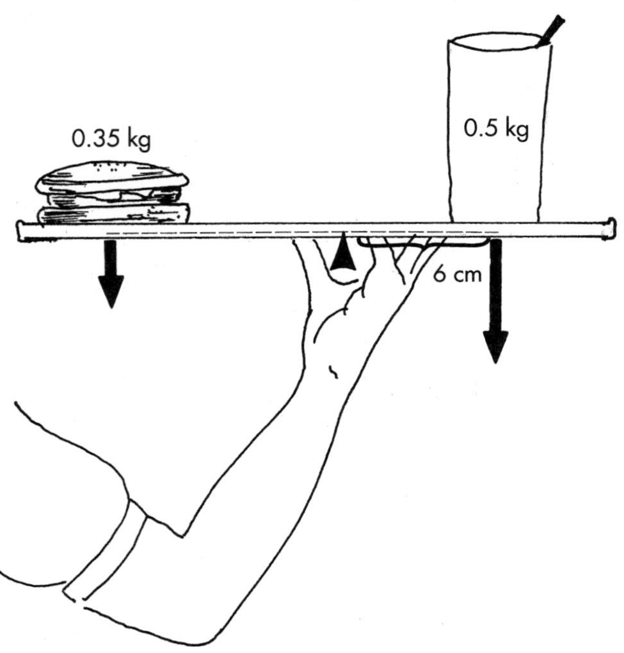

FIGURE **5-18**
To balance this tray of food on one hand, the torque produced by the drink must equal the torque produced by the sandwich.

lever is this? Converting centimeters to meters and kilograms to newtons, how much effort must be applied to the crowbar to lift the rock? What is the advantage of using the crowbar?

APPLICATION **5-5**

Balance Needed to Hold a Tray of Food

In Figure 5-18, Donna carefully places each item a certain distance from the center of the tray. If a soft drink weighing 0.5 kg is placed 6 cm from the center of the tray, how far must a sandwich weighing 0.35 kg be placed from the center of the tray?

See Appendix C for solutions to Applications.

RELATED READINGS

Hall SJ: *Basic biomechanics,* ed 2, New York, 1995, McGraw-Hill.

Luttgens K, Hamilton N: *Kinesiology: scientific basis of human motion,* ed 9, Madison, Wis, 1997, Brown & Benchmark.

Nordin M, Frankel VH: *Basic biomechanics of the musculoskeletal system,* ed 2, Philadelphia, 1989, Lea & Febiger.

Wiktorin CH, Nordin M: *Introduction to problem solving in biomechanics,* Philadelphia, 1986, Lea & Febiger.

Basic Concepts Applied to Musculoskeletal Regions

SECTION **OUTLINE**

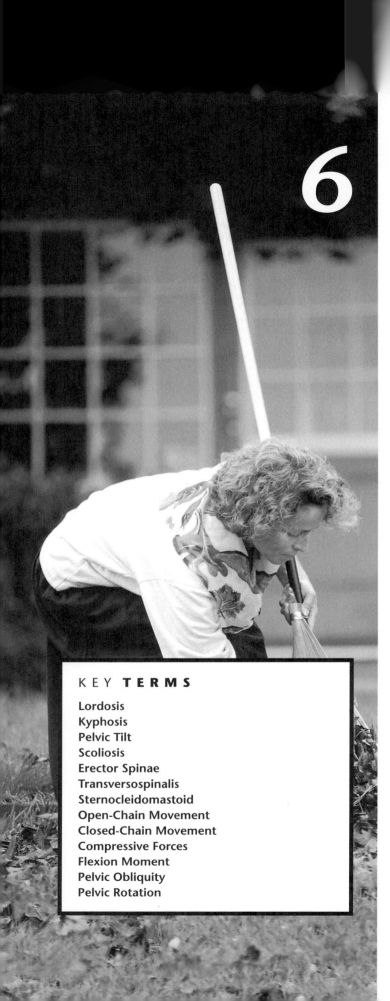

6 The Head and Torso

CHAPTER **OUTLINE**

BACKGROUND

Pathological Curves

Lumbar curve

Scoliosis

TORSO MOVEMENTS

Bilateral and Unilateral Contractions

Erector spinae

Transversospinalis

Sternocleidomastoid

Flexor (abdominal)

Open- and Closed-Chain Movements

Trunk Positioning

Stabilization

Forces Acting on the Head and Torso

Neck

Erector spinae

L5 disk

Seating and Positioning

Stabilization principles

Common restraint systems

SUMMARY

KEY **TERMS**

Lordosis
Kyphosis
Pelvic Tilt
Scoliosis
Erector Spinae
Transversospinalis
Sternocleidomastoid
Open-Chain Movement
Closed-Chain Movement
Compressive Forces
Flexion Moment
Pelvic Obliquity
Pelvic Rotation

The head and trunk house all the organs that support life. Because these organs are composed of delicate tissues, the head and trunk must protect these structures. The skull, spine, rib cage, and pelvis are rigid bodies that protect delicate organs. Skin, tendons, ligaments, cartilage, and fascia provide additional protection.

Although the fragile structures enclosed are most secure when the body is not moving, the bony structures of the head and torso must move many times in many amazing ways each day. Sometimes these movements reposition the trunk. In many cases the head, vertebrae, and pelvis accompany upper- and lower-extremity movement. The torso provides a stable base for use of the extremities and adds to their movements.

Background

The skull is composed of 23 bones connected primarily by fibrous, suture-type joints. The jaw joins the skull with a synovial joint called the *temporomandibular joint,* allowing individuals the freedom to eat and communicate. Most of the head's muscle mass is dedicated to performing these essential activities. Numerous small muscles controlling eye movement, eyelid blinking, facial expression, and attenuation of the hearing mechanism make subtle but important contributions to an individual's ability to interact with the environment.[1]

Excluding the first two, all the vertebral bodies attach to each other via symphyses, cartilaginous joints containing intervertebral disks. Each disk is made up of cartilaginous tissue attached to the vertebral bodies at their top and bottom edges. In the disk's center is a jellylike substance known as the *nucleus pulposus.* The structure of the vertebrae and the intervening disks form a strong, flexible column capable of absorbing a great deal of shock.

Additional intervertebral articulations involve small synovial facet joints that allow the vertebral arches (spinous and transverse processes) to move—one on the other—in small amounts. All articulations allow one vertebra to move on the other in three planes, although the amount of movement per plane differs from one region to the next.

Three curves occur in the sagittal plane. They are independent of muscle function but are altered when muscles contract to move the column. The 7 cervical vertebrae form an anterior convex curve (Figure 6-1).

The 12 units of the thoracic spine form a posterior convex curve (Figure 6-2). The thoracic vertebrae are unique because each body has articulating surfaces directed laterally to receive the ribs. Each rib connects with these surfaces on the upper and lower edges of adjacent vertebrae. The rib cage is composed of seven pairs of true ribs that attach directly onto the sternum. Five pairs of false ribs are connected to the thoracic spine only and have indirect anterior connections. The rib cage protects the heart and lungs with a bony enclosure that limits movement of the thoracic spine in both flexion and extension.

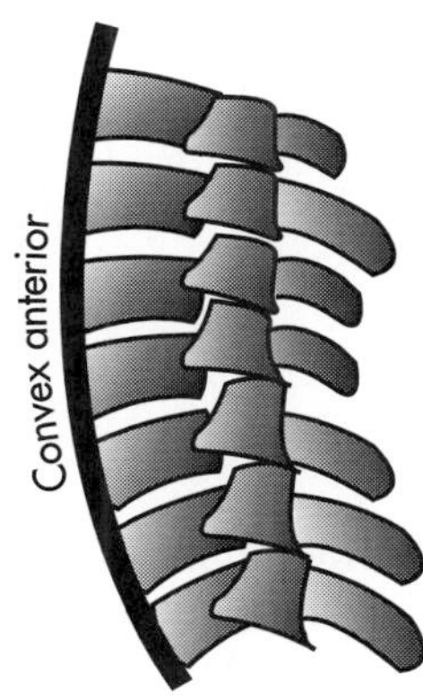

FIGURE **6-1**
The cervical curve. Curves are named in a variety of ways. The clearest language consistently names only the orientation of the convexity, as shown here.

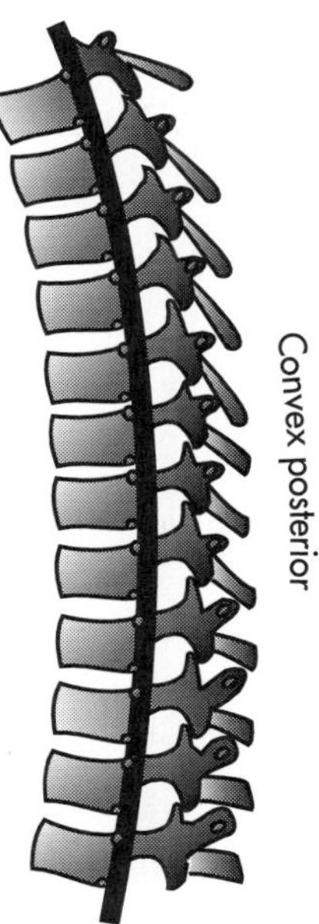

FIGURE **6-2**
The thoracic curve is the reverse of the cervical and lumbar curves.

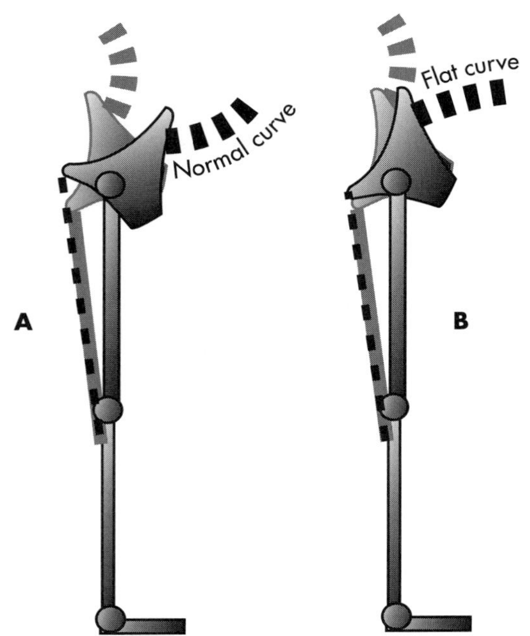

FIGURE **6-3**
A, Normal-length hamstrings allow full flexion of the trunk and pelvis. **B,** Short hamstrings become stretched early as the trunk flexes onto the thigh. As they are stretched to their limits, hamstrings prevent further movement of the pelvis. Continued efforts to bend all must occur in the vertebral column and are exaggerated in the lumbar area.

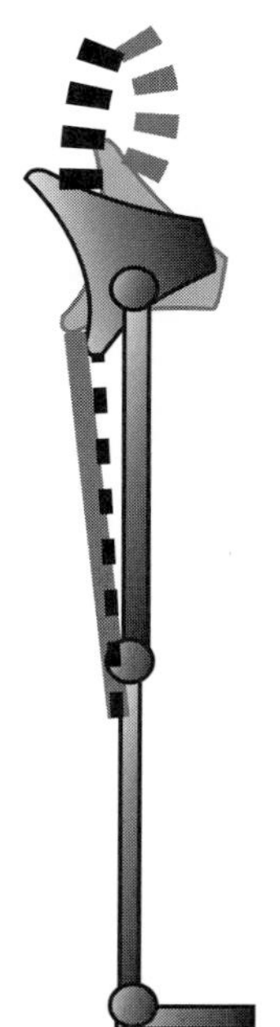

FIGURE **6-4**
Posterior pelvic tilt and a resting posture of reversed lumbar curve secondary to short hamstring length. Note that the pelvic position is described according to the direction of movement of the anterior superior iliac spine.

The low back is made up of 5 lumbar vertebrae forming an anterior convex curve like that in the cervical region. The lumbar curve shapes as a child learns to stand upright, sit, and walk. It serves to keep the head's center of gravity in line with the pelvis. Pelvic position greatly influences the shape of the lumbar curve via the articulation of the fused sacral vertebrae with the fifth lumbar vertebra (L5).

The lumbar region joins the 5 fused sacral vertebrae, referred to as the *sacrum,* at the lumbosacral joint. The sacrum also articulates with the ilia of the pelvis at the sacroiliac joint. Because of this connection, pelvic position and vertebral curves are related.

PATHOLOGICAL CURVES

The normal curves just described can become exaggerated for several reasons, including poor posture and abnormal pelvic position. The cervical and lumbar curves may become exaggerated **(lordosis),** flattened, or even reversed. (In Figure 6-3 the lumbar curve is flattened posteriorly *[B]* and the normal lumbar curve is convex anteriorly *[A].*) The thoracic curve typically increases as upright posture decreases. An exaggeration of the thoracic curve or any posterior convex curve is referred to as **kyphosis.** Because the thoracic region is linked to regions above and below it, kyphotic posture may be associated with cervical lordosis and flattened or reversed lumbar curve, in which the lower back rounds out.

An exaggerated anterior **pelvic tilt** can cause lordosis of the lumbar curve commonly called "sway back." Likewise, a posterior pelvic tilt may cause a flattened or re-

BOX 6-1

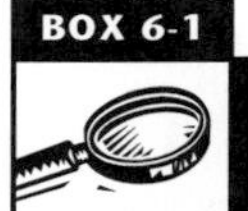

A **CLOSER** LOOK

Posterior Pelvic Tilt and Reversed Lumbar Curve

Comedians often use body postures to create characters. "Grimley," played by Martin Short on Saturday Night Live, *was a perfect example of an individual with extremely short hamstrings. Grimley had severe posterior pelvic tilt and reversed lumbar curve, which gave the lower half of the character's vertebral column a completely rounded-out appearance. Short hamstrings also affected his gait, which caused him to walk with a short swing and partially flexed knees. Remember that the hamstrings are hip extensors and knee flexors.*

versed lumbar curve. Sometimes the pelvic position develops in response to a change in the lumbar curve. Either way, pelvic position and lumbar curve are intimately related.

Lumbar curve

When hip flexors or extensors are not stretched regularly, they may assume shorter resting lengths. Many of us have short hamstrings. We notice this as we extend our knees and attempt to touch our toes. First the torso flexes onto the lower extremities at the hip. Then the back begins to flex and round out until hip flexion reaches its extreme. At this point we usually experience tightness in the posterior thighs as the hamstrings stretch to their farthest points (passive insufficiency). As these hip extensors tighten, they pull inferiorly on the ischial tuberosity (origin) and limit hip flexion by stopping pelvic motion (Figure 6-3,*B*).

Extremely short hamstrings can exert this same pull on the pelvis with even less hip flexion, as in walking. The short hip extensors cause the pelvis to assume a tilted position (posterior pelvic tilt). The pelvis pulls the lower lumbar vertebrae with it in a posterior direction, which can reduce, flatten, and even reverse the lumbar curve (Figure 6-4 and A Closer Look Box 6-1).

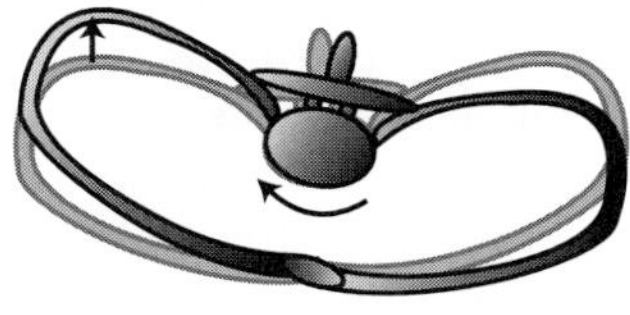

FIGURE **6-5**
In a view from above, a rib pair turns with a vertebra to which it is attached.

Scoliosis

The curves previously described occur in the sagittal plane and therefore are visible from a side view only. Curves in the sagittal plane are normally occurring curves, even though they may become the more extreme in pathological conditions.

Scoliosis describes a curve in the frontal plane visible from an anterior view. Scoliosis is always a pathological condition. Extreme cases involve two or more curves in opposite directions that give the appearance of an S. Scoliosis is unique in not only its orientation in the frontal plane but also its rotation of the vertebral bodies.

When scoliosis occurs in the thoracic region, the ribs that attach to vertebrae exhibit movement in the horizontal plane. Because the ribs attach to the vertebral bodies and each body rotates, each pair of ribs turns like a steering wheel (Figure 6-5). This motion forms a raised area, or hump, posteriorly as the posterior aspect of the moving ribs pushes on superficial soft tissue. The posterior ridge occurs on the side of the convexity of the scoliotic curve; therefore a scoliosis that is convex on the right side is associated with a hump on the right side. (The three pathological curves are summarized and compared with normal alignment in Figure 6-6.)

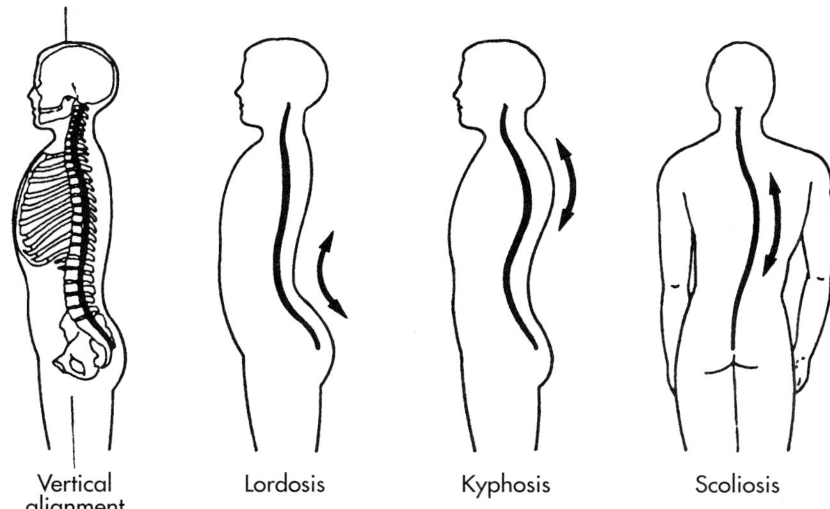

FIGURE **6-6**
Normal alignment versus three pathological curves. (Modified from Hall SJ: *Basic biomechanics,* ed 2, New York, 1995, McGraw-Hill.)

Torso Movements

Many deep muscles of the back attach to the skull, vertebrae, ribs, and pelvis. These deep muscles maintain the strength and integrity of the spinal column and allow for posture, movement, and maintenance of position. Movements of the vertebral column occur in all three planes of motion: extension and forward flexion in the sagittal plane, lateral flexion to either side in the frontal plane, and rotation to either side in the horizontal plane.

BILATERAL AND UNILATERAL CONTRACTIONS

The head must have a wide range of motion to position sensory organs such as the eyes, ears, nose, and mouth for optimal gathering of information. For this reason the cervical vertebrae form the most mobile section of the spine and allow movement in all three planes.

The first cervical vertebra is called the *atlas.* The atlas is a ringlike structure that attaches to the skull via bilateral synovial joints, which primarily allow flexion and extension of the skull onto the neck.

The second cervical vertebra is called the *axis.* It has a toothlike protuberance, the dens (odontoid process) onto which the atlas fits and rotates. The head rotates on the neck at this joint, but the entire cervical region can rotate as the head shakes "no."

Muscle contractions in three major groups of muscles—the erector spinae, transversospinalis, and flexors (four pairs of abdominal muscles)—produce cervical, thoracic, and lumbar movements. The first two groups are segmental. They originate deep in the back in lower segments and insert onto higher segments. The muscles are paired, right and left, and named according to the segments of insertion. For example, the longissimus thoracis and longissimus cervicis are sections of the erector spinae group. As a rule, more superficially placed fibers span a number of vertebrae and deeper fibers span fewer segments.

Erector spinae

Because our interest is in movement, not strictly anatomy, we can differentiate the two groups of deep back muscles by the directions of their fibers. The **erector spinae** muscles mostly run parallel to the vertebral column and consist of three major divisions: the spinalis, running spine to spine; the longissimus, running largely from transverse process to transverse process; and the iliocostalis, running from rib to rib.

Let us review some fundamentals about muscle action on joints. If a muscle force pulls through the axis of motion, no tendency for rotation and no movement occur. We say no "moment" occurs for the movement because although force exists, no moment arm exists and therefore no tendency (torque). If the force of contraction pulls at some distance away from the axis, torque exists; movement then can occur because the muscle contracts.

All three divisions of the erector spinae are posterior to the side-to-side axes for flexion and extension and can extend the vertebral column. Except for the spinalis division, this group lies to the left and right of the front-to-back axes and also can flex laterally (Figure 6-7).

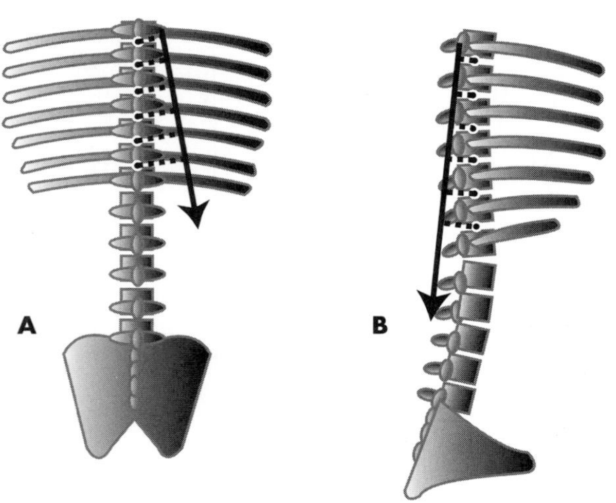

FIGURE **6-7**
The relationship of the erector spinae muscles to the side-to-side **(A)** and front-to-back **(B)** axes. Notice that a moment arm can be drawn from force to axis, quantifying the distance from the axis at which the force pulls. Different views (posterior for lateral flexion and side for extension) are necessary to view movement in different planes.

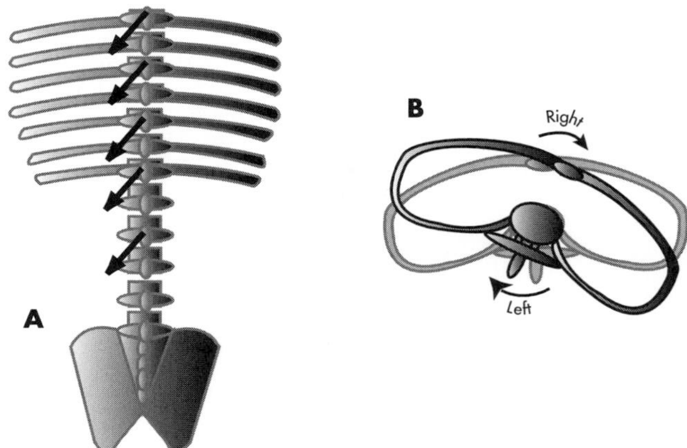

FIGURE **6-8**
A, The transversospinalis group rotates the vertebrae by pulling the medial insertion (spinous process) toward the lateral origin (transverse process). **B,** One point of confusion in the terminology is that when the trunk "turns right" (anterior facing right), the spinous process moves left.

With all these options, why does only one movement occur when three are possible? Contraction of the left erector spinae laterally flexes the column to the left (the same side); contraction of the right erector spinae laterally flexes the column to the right. These statements describe unilateral contractions. A bilateral contraction of the erector spinae (left and right sides) cancels the lateral flexion effects (equilibrium of tendencies in opposite directions). The net effect of bilateral contraction is extension. Each vertebral muscle has the potential for action at multiple axes, so unilateral and bilateral functions must be differentiated.

Transversospinalis

The **transversospinalis** group is primarily responsible for rotation of the vertebral column. This group, segmented and paired like the erector spinae group, contains fibers not parallel to the column. Generally, as concentric contractions occur, the group's laterally placed origins on transverse processes of more inferior segments pull insertions on spinous processes laterally. These contractions serve mainly to rotate the vertebrae, which turn one side of the trunk to the opposite side. For example, the left transversospinalis rotates the trunk so that it turns to face right (Figure 6-8).

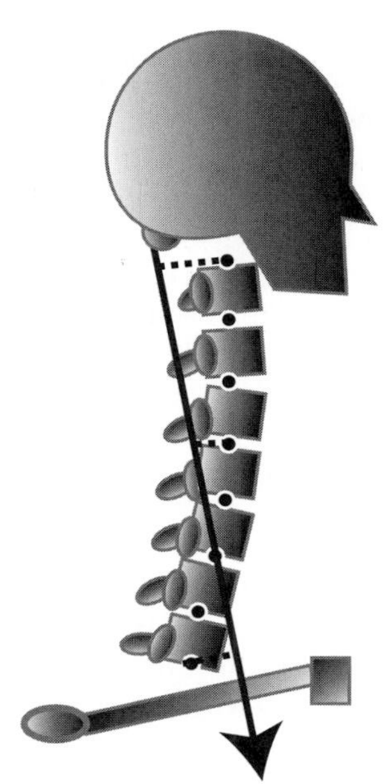

FIGURE **6-9**
Relationship of the sternocleidomastoid muscle to various head and neck side-to-side axes.

Sternocleidomastoid

Head movements often accompany those of the vertebral column, so head and neck movements deserve special consideration. The **sternocleidomastoid** is the most prominent of the anterior neck muscles that attach to the head. Each side of this paired muscle originates from the sternum and proximal clavicle anteriorly and inserts posteriorly on the mastoid process of the skull. The sternocleidomastoid is typically misunderstood as a head extensor and neck flexor. To clearly understand its function, we must observe how the force of this muscle acts on various axes of flexion and extension in the head and neck (Figure 6-9).

At its insertion on the mastoid process the sternocleidomastoid lies posterior and inferior to side-to-side axes of the sagittal plane. It extends the head on the neck and hyperextends the neck. Near its origin on the sternum, the force of contraction runs anterior to the side-to-side axis at the base of the neck and can flex the head and neck onto the trunk. All these functions involve bilateral contractions.

A clear understanding of the sternocleidomastoid helps us realize its inadequacy when it functions without ample support from the other neck muscles. Bilateral contraction of the sternocleidomastoid muscle alone results in extension of the head, hyperextension and virtual collapse of the cervical region, and flexion of the head and neck onto the trunk (Figure 6-10). This lack of chin

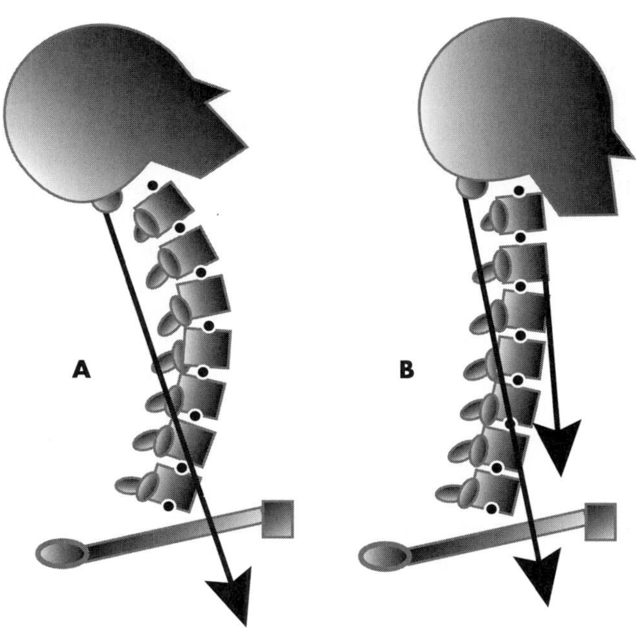

FIGURE **6-10**
A, Appearance of the head and neck when the sternocleidomastoid acts alone. **B,** The same muscle acts in conjunction with a deep cervical flexor, the longus colli, to prevent hyperextension of cervical vertebrae.

tuck and failure to elongate the neck often is seen in individuals with cerebral palsy and interferes with mouth closure and chewing.

Normally the sternocleidomastoid contracts along with a deep cervical flexor, the longus colli, which prevents hyperextension in the cervical vertebrae. These two muscles, together with vertebral extensors, help individuals gaze forward, elongate the neck, and tuck the chin. Specifically, the sternocleidomastoid partially extends the head on the neck while the longus colli prevents cervical hyperextension, and the highest segments of the erector spinae group partially extend the head and neck onto the trunk.

Flexor (abdominal)

The four paired abdominal muscles help the trunk flex and rotate. They also protect the internal contents of the abdominal and pelvic cavities.

The rectus abdominis flexes the trunk as its superior attachment on the sternum is pulled inferiorly toward its attachment on the pelvis. Overstretching of the rectus abdominis creates less of an upward force on the pubic symphysis, which can cause anterior pelvic tilt and lumbar lordosis.

The fibers of the external abdominis oblique follow an angle similar to the fingers of the hands placed in front trouser pockets. Each side of the external abdominis oblique attaches inferiorly and medially to the pelvis and usually pulls its more superior lateral insertion to the right or left in unilateral contractions. For example, the right external oblique rotates the trunk anteriorly and leftward. Like the transversospinalis, the external abdominis oblique rotates the trunk to the opposite side of the muscle's location. Some lateral flexion to the same side also occurs because of the muscle's lateral relationship to the front-to-back axis of the frontal plane. Finally, this paired muscle has an anterior relationship to the side-to-side axis of the sagittal plane; a bilateral contraction cancels all rotational and lateral flexion and flexes the trunk forward.

One layer deeper, the fibers of the internal abdominis oblique run opposite those of the external oblique. Unilateral contraction of the internal oblique pulls the medial attachment on the lower ribs toward the more lateral attachment on the pelvis, rotating the muscle to the same side. That is, the right internal oblique rotates the trunk anterior to the right with some lateral flexion to the same side. Bilateral contraction flexes the trunk.

The innermost layer is the transversus abdominis, and its fibers run horizontally. This layer primarily supports the internal contents; it also helps the trunk laterally flex and rotate.

Posteriorly, two major muscles—the quadratus lumborum and the iliopsoas—protect the abdominal contents. The quadratus lies next to the spine from the lower ribs to the iliac crest of the pelvis. Its fibers are mostly vertical, laterally flexing the vertebral column to the same side in a unilateral contraction. The iliopsoas is composed of two smaller muscles—the psoas major, which originates on the lumbar spine, and the iliacus, which originates on the pelvis. These two muscles join in a tendon attaching to the lesser trochanter of the femur. The iliopsoas flexes the thighs at the hips. When the insertion at the femur is stabilized, the iliopsoas flexes its more proximal attachment and pulls the pelvis forward into flexion over the thigh. The iliopsoas, through its effect on pelvic tilt, maintains the normal lumbar curve.

OPEN- AND CLOSED-CHAIN MOVEMENTS

The upper extremity is a chain of segments connected at joints. When the free distal end of the extremity moves, it is an **open-chain movement.** Open-chain movements involve stabilization of the origin, concentric contraction, and movement of the insertion. This combination yields motion at the distal end of the extremity. Many functional movements involving lifting of objects or movement of the hands in various personal hygiene and home-management tasks are open-chain movements.

The phrase *open chain* helps differentiate specific movements. Muscles know only to shorten, not which attachments to move; however, proximal attachments (origins) typically are stabilized by links to the trunk. Because of proximal stabilization, a concentric contraction moves the distal segments in relation to more proximal segments in the trunk. For example, the forearm flexes onto the arm through open-chain elbow flexion, whereas the upper extremity flexes in relation to the trunk through open-chain shoulder flexion.

Many movements do not follow this scheme and are described differently. In a push-up or pull-up, the hand, the distal end of the chain, is stabilized and the trunk moves in relation to the upper extremity. In a sit-up, the trunk flexes over the hip onto the thigh. A deep-knee bend brings the anterior leg to the dorsum of the foot in dorsiflexion, but the toes do not move away from the floor. In each case the insertion is stabilized and the origin moves. These are **closed-chain movements.**

The distinguishing feature between closed- and open-chain movements is the function of the distal end of the chain. In open-chain movements, muscles contract across joints to move segments with distal ends that move freely in space. The same muscles contract across the same joints to produce closed-chain movements when distal ends are stationary.

The trunk produces many closed-chain versions of shoulder and hip movements. Lifting a suitcase involves open-chain shoulder extension and elbow flexion, whereas

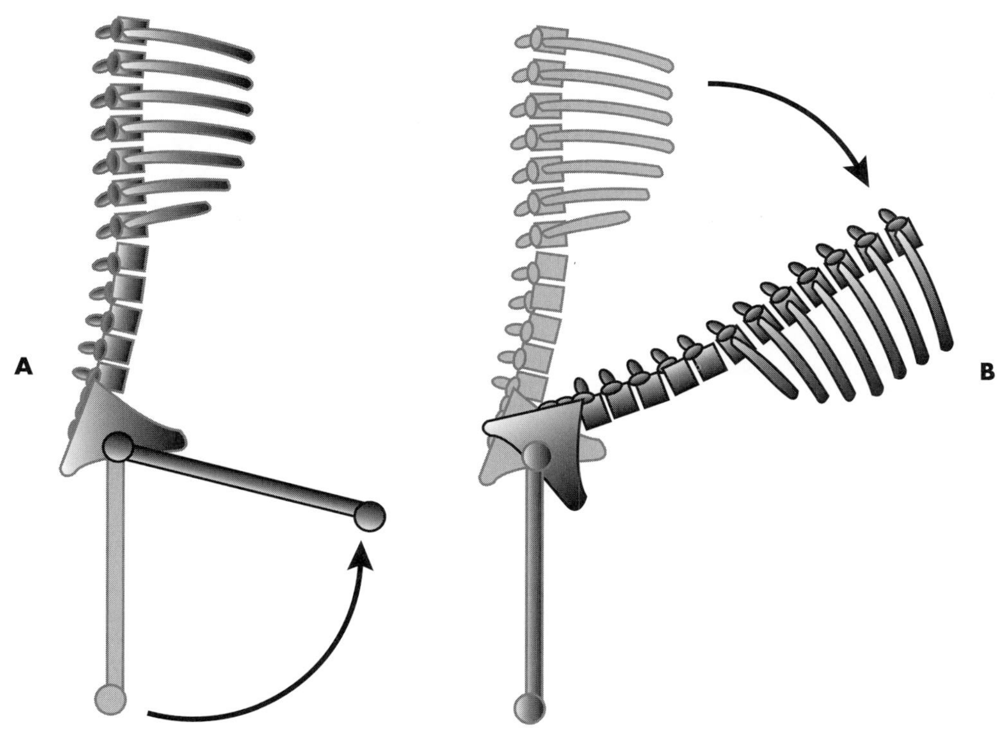

FIGURE **6-11**
Open- **(A)** versus closed-chain **(B)** hip flexion.

pulling the body up to the hand on a bar involves closed-chain shoulder extension and elbow flexion. Kicking the foot up in front of the body is open-chain hip flexion, whereas bending the trunk over to touch the toes is closed-chain hip flexion (Figure 6-11). Walking yields the most commonly experienced closed-chain movements. The foot is planted, and the trunk moves over it in closed-chain hip extension. This alternates with open-chain hip flexion as the leg swings forward to take another step.

TRUNK POSITIONING

Effective use of the extremities requires a stable base. In many cases this base (the trunk) not only provides stability but contributes to movement. In forward reach the trunk remains upright. As the body reaches farther forward, vertebral flexion accompanies scapular protraction, shoulder flexion, and elbow extension. In side reach the trunk flexes laterally. As the body reaches across the chest with the right arm to grab an object on the left, the trunk rotates. Upright posture and the three major vertebral movements accompany a multitude of upper-extremity movements.

Stabilization

Any examination of trunk movements associated with extremity functions leads to a focus on the scapula and pelvis. Movements of the arm at the shoulder and the thigh at the hip involve activation of muscles inserting on the humerus or femur. Movements of insertions require stabilization of origins; this stabilization involves activation of muscles originating in the trunk and inserting on the scapula or pelvis.

While lying in a supine position to perform straight-leg raises, the abdominals tighten. Why do the abdominals contract when the hips simply flex to raise the lower extremities slightly into the air? Remember, muscles shorten and move whichever attachment moves easiest. Hip flexors originating from the pelvis and crossing the hip to insert on the femur can tilt the pelvis forward more easily than they can raise the entire lower extremity against the pull of gravity. If the pelvis (origin) were not stabilized, the hip flexors would tilt the pelvis and have little contractility left to flex the hip and raise the lower extremity (Figure 6-12).

Thus the rectus abdominis guarantees a stable pelvis by pulling upward on its attachment to the pubic symphysis. Because the hip flexors are unable to move their origins, they shorten and move their insertions, achieving the desired leg raise by flexing the hip.

A similar sequence occurs when the upper extremities abduct. Both glenohumeral abductors originate largely from the scapula and insert onto the humerus. As they shorten, the scapula, which weighs less than the

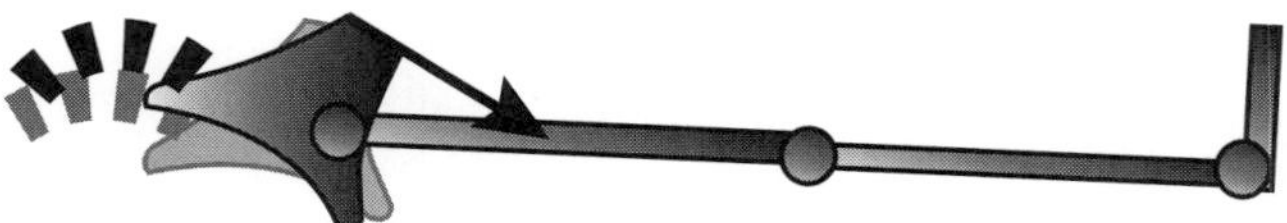

FIGURE **6-12**
Movement of the pelvis when hip flexor origins are not stabilized.

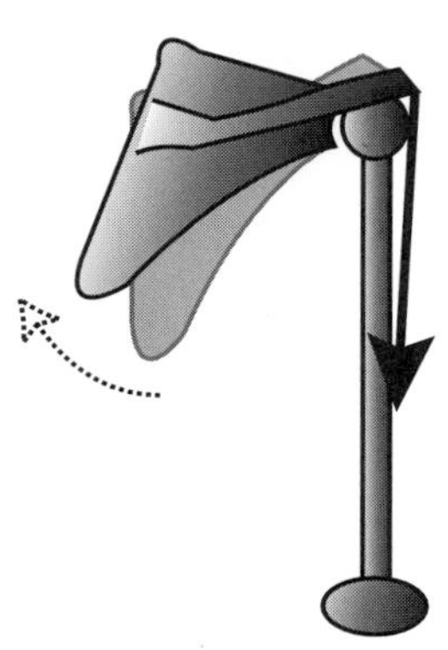

FIGURE **6-13**
Movement of the scapula when arm abductors act on their origins because the upward scapular rotators are not stabilized.

upper extremity, moves first. If the scapula were not stabilized, the abductors would waste their excursion rotating the scapula downward instead of abducting the arm (Figure 6-13). In the normal pattern, contraction of the upward scapular rotators prevents movement at the origins of the arm abductors. These upward rotators are superficial trunk muscles that originate on the trunk and insert onto the scapula. Stabilizing trunk muscles are essential for extremity movements.

FORCES ACTING ON THE HEAD AND TORSO

Clinical observation of the head and vertebral column involves the realization that we live, play, and work under gravity's constant influence. Muscle contractions that maintain upright posture inevitably cause **compressive forces** to act on the vertebral bodies and disks. We must account for these forces in activity analysis.

Neck

The owner of a small company contracted with an OT practitioner after several computer operators complained of neck pain and upper-back tightness during normal working days. All operators used identical equipment and spent approximately 6 hours at their computer terminals. The most seriously affected operator, ***Oliver Xiong,*** is about 2 m tall and weighs 65 kg. ***Nancy Grant,***

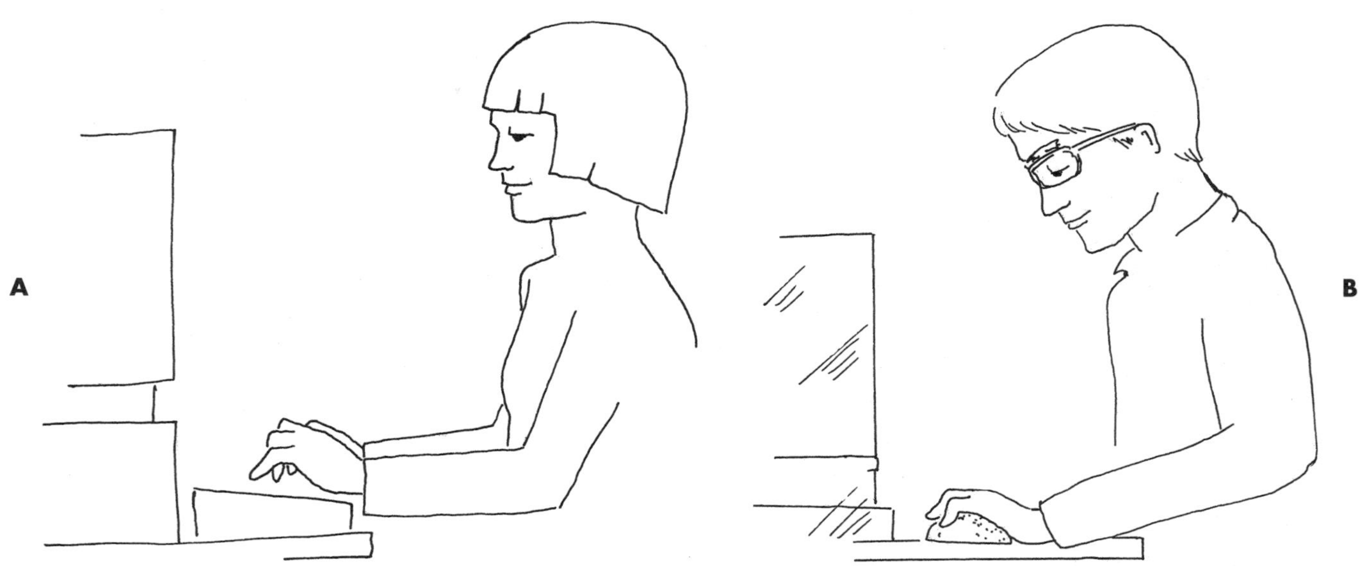

FIGURE **6-14**
A, Nancy, a computer operator, sits with her head erect. **B,** Oliver, her co-worker, sits with his head held at a 30-degree angle.

another operator, is less seriously affected. She is about 1.6 m tall and weighs 60 kg. The OT practitioner estimates that their heads each weigh about 5 kg (see Appendix B, Table B-1). Figure 6-14 shows these operators at their terminals. Nancy generally sits with her head erect, whereas Oliver generally sits with his head flexed to 30 degrees.

The OT practitioner wants to know the force, or load, on each operator's intervertebral disks and how it changes in different positions. First, the force of muscle contraction in the spinal extensors must be determined because contraction of these muscles to extend the cervical region produces substantial compression (linear force) and extension (rotary force).

Although the cervical region contains a number of side-to-side axes, the OT practitioner focuses on the axis of motion at cervical vertebra 5 (C5), about 3 cm above the palpable spine of C7. The head's center of gravity is the portion of the temple closest to the temporomandibular joint. With the head erect, the distance from the axis of motion to the center of gravity of the head is 2 cm. With the head flexed, this same distance is 6 cm. The distance of the erector spinae to the axis of motion is 4 cm when the head is erect and when it is flexed to 30 degrees.

In Figure 6-15 a diagram of Nancy's head shows the opposing forces and their moment arms. Forces are at play in opposite directions, which normally causes tendencies toward rotation in opposite directions. Because little or no movement is present, equilibrium exists. The torques (tendencies) in opposite directions are equal; thus torque of flexion equals torque of extension. The sum of all torques *(T)* equals zero ($\Sigma T = 0$).

Calculate the force of the erector spinae muscles by using the formula for equilibrium of torques, which considers the force *(F)* and moment arms *(MA)* in opposite directions. To indicate opposite directions, assign one torque a positive sign and the opposite a negative sign:

$$\begin{aligned} \Sigma T &= 0 \\ \text{Torque}_{\text{extensors}} + (-\text{Torque}_{\text{gravity}}) &= 0 \\ (F_{\text{extensors}} \times MA_{\text{extensors}}) + (-F_{\text{gravity}} \times MA_{\text{gravity}}) &= 0 \end{aligned}$$

In this equation, $F_{extensors}$ and $F_{gravity}$ are the forces created by the erector spinae and gravity. Moment arms (distance or force from the axis) for the extensors and gravity are $MA_{extensors}$ and $MA_{gravity}$. Remember to convert centimeters to meters and kilograms to newtons:

$$\begin{aligned} F_{\text{extensors}} \times 0.04\ \text{m} - (50\ \text{N} \times 0.02\ \text{m}) &= 0 \\ F_{\text{extensors}} \times 0.04\ \text{m} &= 50\ \text{N} \times 0.02\ \text{m} \\ F_{\text{extensors}} &= \frac{1\ \text{Nm}}{0.04\ \text{m}} \\ F_{\text{extensors}} &= 25\ \text{N} \end{aligned}$$

Disk compression involves a linear force in which both gravity and the erector spinae muscles pull downward, so the reaction force on the disk must be an equal upward force. Forces up equal forces down, or the sum of all forces equals zero ($\Sigma F = 0$). Converting kilograms to newtons, calculate the reaction force on the C5 disk by using the formula for equilibrium of forces. Downward forces are assigned negative signs:

$$\begin{aligned} \Sigma F = 0 &= F_{\text{reaction}} + (-25\ \text{N}) + (-50\ \text{N}) \\ F_{\text{reaction}} &= 25\ \text{N} + 50\ \text{N} \\ F_{\text{reaction}} &= 75\ \text{N} \end{aligned}$$

When Oliver's head is flexed to 30 degrees, the compressive forces are greater due to the increased torque produced by gravity acting on the head and a stronger contraction in the erector spinae to maintain neck extension (Figure 6-16). Converting centimeters to meters and kilograms to newtons, calculate the force of the erector spinae, using gravity's larger moment arm:

$$\begin{aligned} \Sigma T &= 0 \\ \text{Torque}_{\text{extensors}} + (-\text{Torque}_{\text{gravity}}) &= 0 \\ (F_{\text{extensors}} \times MA_{\text{extensors}}) + (-F_{\text{gravity}} \times MA_{\text{gravity}}) &= 0 \\ (F_{\text{extensors}} \times 0.04\ \text{m}) - (50\ \text{N} \times 0.06\ \text{m}) &= 0 \\ (F_{\text{extensors}} \times 0.04\ \text{m}) &= 50\ \text{N} \times 0.06\ \text{m} \\ F_{\text{extensors}} &= \frac{3\ \text{Nm}}{0.04\ \text{m}} \\ F_{\text{extensors}} &= 75\ \text{N} \end{aligned}$$

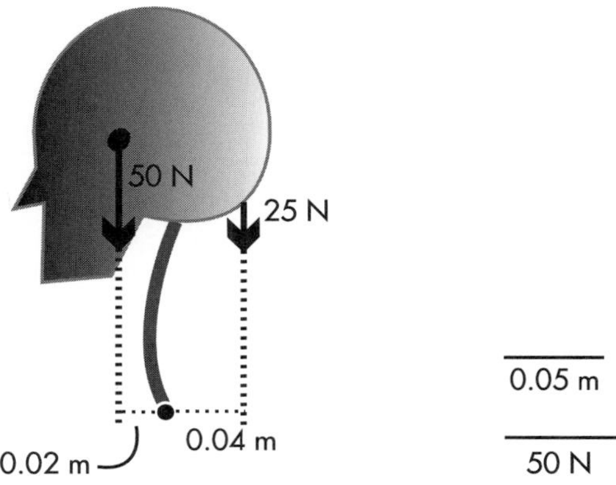

FIGURE **6-15**
With the head erect, the force the erector spinae muscles need to maintain erect posture is 25 N. The reaction force on the C5 disk is 75 N upward the sum of the two forces directed downward. (Centimeters are converted to meters and kilograms to newtons.)

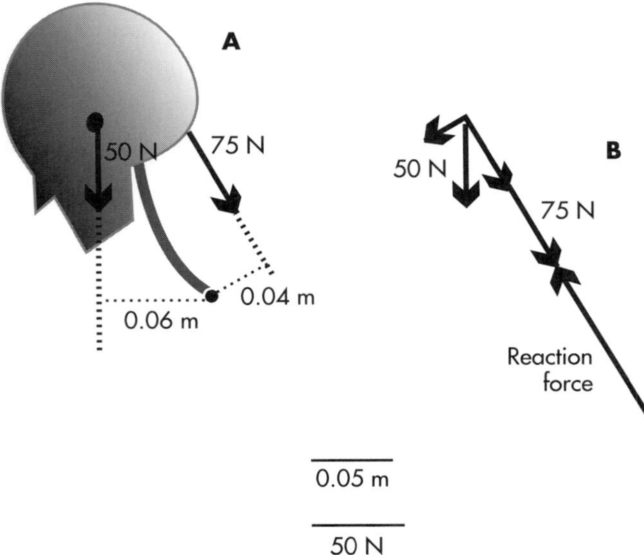

FIGURE **6-16**
When the head is at a 30-degree angle, the force the erector spinae muscles must exert to maintain this posture is 75 N **(A)** and the reaction force increases accordingly. With the head at 30 degrees, most of the weight exerts a compression effect on the vertebral column; compression from the stronger erector spinae contraction is greater. The reaction force exerted toward the head equals the sum of the two forces directed toward the shoulders **(B).**

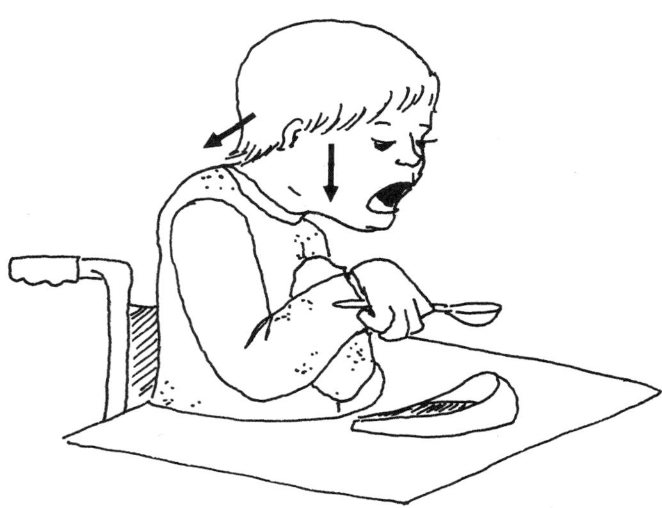

FIGURE **6-17**
When Jason eats with his head angled forward, this requires more endurance than his head can sustain.

Although not all the head's weight in this position compresses the spine, the reaction force is greater at 30-degrees flexion than in the upright position. More than half the weight of the head compresses the spine, and the contraction force of the head and neck extensors more than doubles (see Figure 6-16, *B*).

Thus the more the head is maintained in a flexed position, the greater the effect of gravity and the greater the strength of contraction of the erector spinae to balance the head. This causes the cervical spine to compress even more.

An OT practitioner must make a number of determinations to draw this scenario. In establishing the class of lever, the practitioner must determine the relationships of the forces of effort and resistance to the axis of motion. In this case the axis of motion lies between the two forces, creating a first-class lever. Spinal muscles must exert greater effort when the head moves from alignment with the spinal axis of motion. This effort is in direct proportion to the distance of the head's center of gravity from the spinal axis of motion. The effort force rises quickly with a minimal amount of motion.

Nancy needs minimal effort to keep her head erect, but Oliver, who holds his head flexed to 30 degrees, needs three times as much effort. This produces about 50% more compressive force on the corresponding disk. Oliver pulls his head erect frequently during his 6-hour shift at the computer terminal and suffers muscle fatigue and soreness. Placing the video display terminal higher encourages an erect rather than flexed posture and relieves some muscle fatigue. Oliver, Nancy, and the other computer operators also should take frequent breaks and slowly stretch their neck muscles to relieve the forces of neck flexion.

OT practitioners know that posture is an important consideration in the analysis of fatigue and discomfort in activity. If the head is not in alignment, activity is more difficult, causing the individual to become fatigued more easily. Figure 6-17 shows ***Jason Black,*** a student with cerebral palsy, trying to eat in the school cafeteria. He has difficulty lifting the utensil to his mouth. To compensate for his upper-extremity difficulties, Jason flexes his head forward to meet the spoon. This solves one problem but creates another. The greater degree of flexion requires more effort to support his head than Jason would need with better posture. The added fatigue and discomfort he experiences cause him to stop before he has satisfied his hunger.

Erector spinae

Spiros Prasso's job requires he lift 25-cm and 46-cm boxes to shoulder height (Figure 6-18). All boxes weigh 18 kg. While the upper extremities lift the boxes, the erector spinae maintain back extension. OT practitioners work-

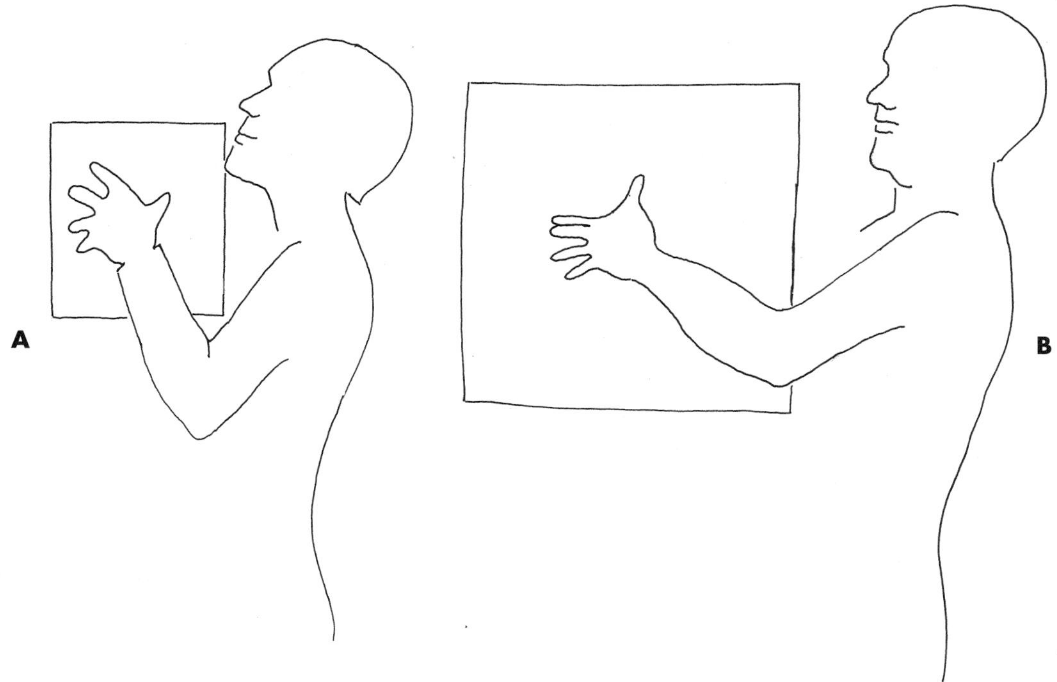

FIGURE **6-18**
A, Spiros holds the 25-cm box 20 cm from the axis of motion at the L5 disk. **B,** He holds the 46-cm box 40 cm from the axis of motion at the L5 disk.

ing with Spiros must know the force that the erector spinae muscles need to lift each box and the reaction force (load) on the L5 disk in each case. How can the practitioners adapt the work environment when the loads on the disk are greater than desired?

An OT assistant visiting Spiros' job site uses the following information to determine the forces involved:

1. The force of the erector spinae group operates 5 cm from the axis of motion at the L5 disk.
2. Spiros weighs 70 kg, so the assistant estimates that his upper-body weight is about 40 kg.
3. His body position as he lifts (head extended and trunk inclined backward) forms a center of gravity 2 cm dorsal to the axis of motion in the L5 disk.
4. When he holds the 25-cm box, its center of gravity is 20 cm from his axis of motion.
5. He holds the 46-cm box with its center of gravity 40 cm from his axis of motion.

Notice that the weight of the upper trunk falls dorsal to the axis of motion and acts as an extensor at the L5 disk. This decreases the amount of effort the erector spinae need to lift the boxes.

Figure 6-19 is a diagram of the relevant forces and moment arms. With the formula for equilibrium of torques, calculate the tendency toward extension created by the erector spinae muscles. The weight of the box (180 N) creates a tendency toward flexion; the weight of the upper trunk (400 N) and the erector spinae force create the tendency toward extension. Remember to convert centimeters to meters and kilograms to newtons:

$$0 = (F_{box} \times MA_{box}) + (-F_{body\ weight} \times MA_{body\ weight}) + (-F_{extensors} \times MA_{extensors})$$

$$0 = (180\text{ N} \times 0.2\text{ m}) + (-400\text{ N} \times 0.02\text{ m}) + (-F_{extensors} \times 0.05\text{ m})$$

$$0 = 36\text{ Nm} - 8\text{ Nm} + (-F_{extensors} \times 0.05\text{ m})$$

$$F_{extensors} = \frac{28\text{ Nm}}{0.05\text{ m}}$$

$$F_{extensors} = 560\text{ N}$$

Calculate the reaction force on the L5 disk using the force equilibrium condition $\Sigma F = 0$. Because the force of gravity on the box, body, and erector spinae muscles pulls downward, the reaction force on the disk must push upward with equal force:

$$0 = F_{reaction} + (-180\text{ N}) + (-400\text{ N}) + (-560\text{ N})$$

$$F_{reaction} = 180\text{ N} + 400\text{ N} + 560\text{ N}$$

$$F_{reaction} = 1140\text{ N}$$

Figure 6-20 shows the forces and moment arms involved in lifting the larger box. Converting centimeters

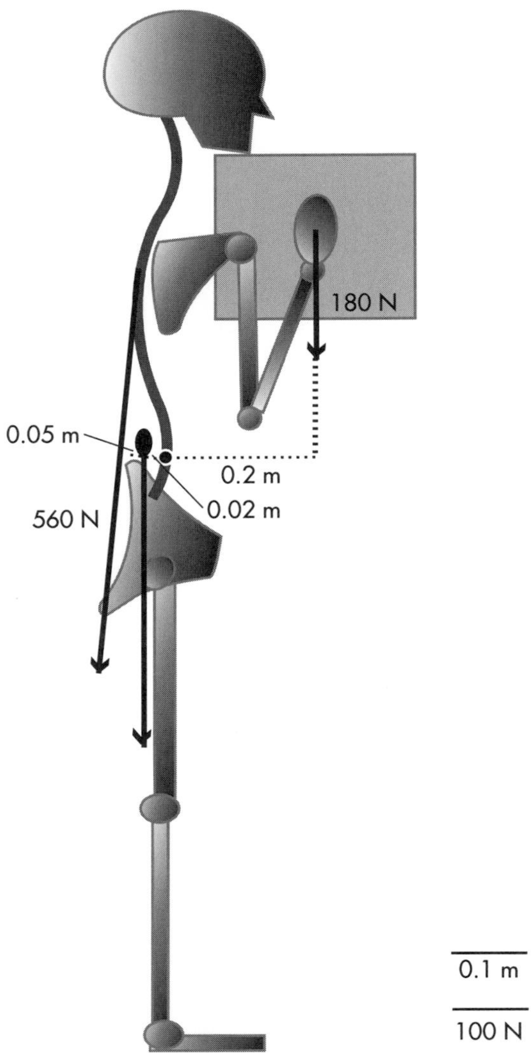

FIGURE **6-19**
A force of 560 N is necessary to hold a 25-cm box 20 cm from the axis of motion at the L5 disk. Carrying the box in this position causes an upward reaction force of 1140 N on the L5 disk.

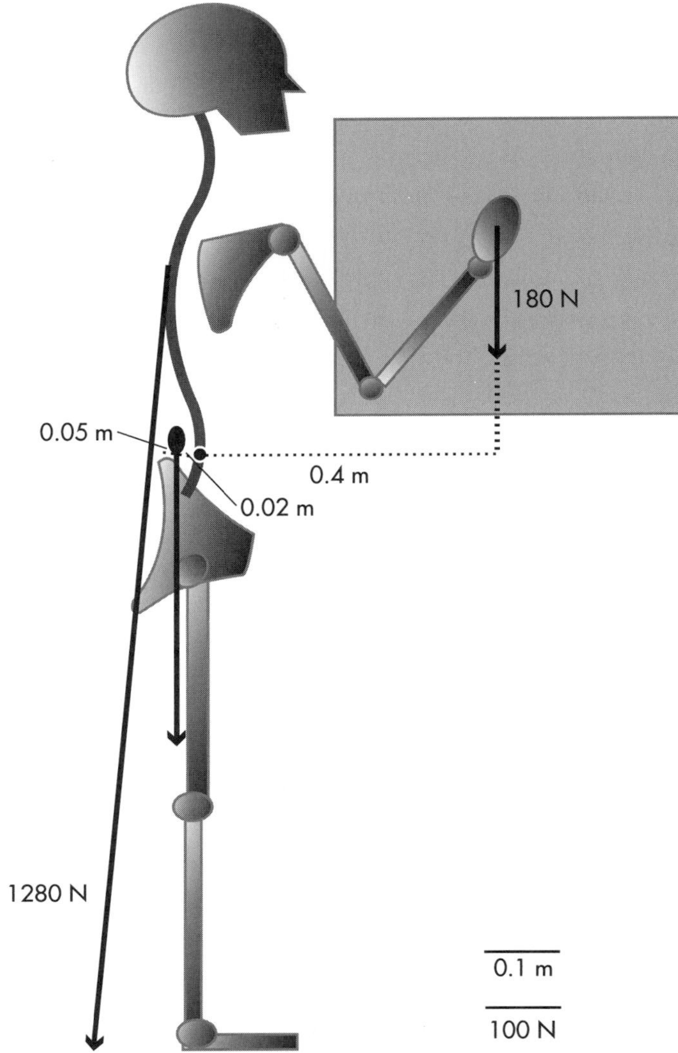

FIGURE **6-20**
A force of 1280 N is required to hold a 46-cm box 40 cm from the axis of motion at the L5 disk. Carrying the box in this position causes an upward reaction force of 1860 N on the L5 disk.

to meters and kilograms to newtons, calculate the force of the erector spinae and the reaction force:

$$0 = (180\ \text{N} \times 0.4\ \text{m}) + (-400\ \text{N} \times 0.02\ \text{m}) + (-F_{\text{extensors}} \times 0.05\ \text{m})$$

$$0 = 72\ \text{Nm} + (-8\ \text{Nm}) + (-F_{\text{extensors}} \times 0.05\ \text{m})$$

$$F_{\text{extensors}} = \frac{64\ \text{Nm}}{0.05\ \text{m}}$$

$$F_{\text{extensors}} = 1280\ \text{N}$$

Calculate the reaction force:

$$F_{\text{reaction}} + (-180\ \text{N}) + (-400\ \text{N}) + (-1280\ \text{N}) = 0$$

$$F_{\text{reaction}} = 180\ \text{N} + 400\ \text{N} + 1280\ \text{N}$$

$$F_{\text{reaction}} = 1860\ \text{N}$$

As the size of the box increases, its center of gravity moves farther from the axis of motion in the L5 disk and its moment arm increases. The longer moment arm means the weight creates a greater tendency toward vertebral flexion, or a greater **flexion moment.** To balance this tendency, Spiros uses twice as much force to lift the larger box, even though it weighs the same as the smaller box. The larger box creates a larger disk load.

Using the smallest possible box reduces the magnitude of the moment arm of the box and decreases the amount of effort required to lift the box. Figure 6-21 shows that a long, narrow box can decrease the effort the erector spinae must exert but increase the amount of effort the shoulder muscles must exert.

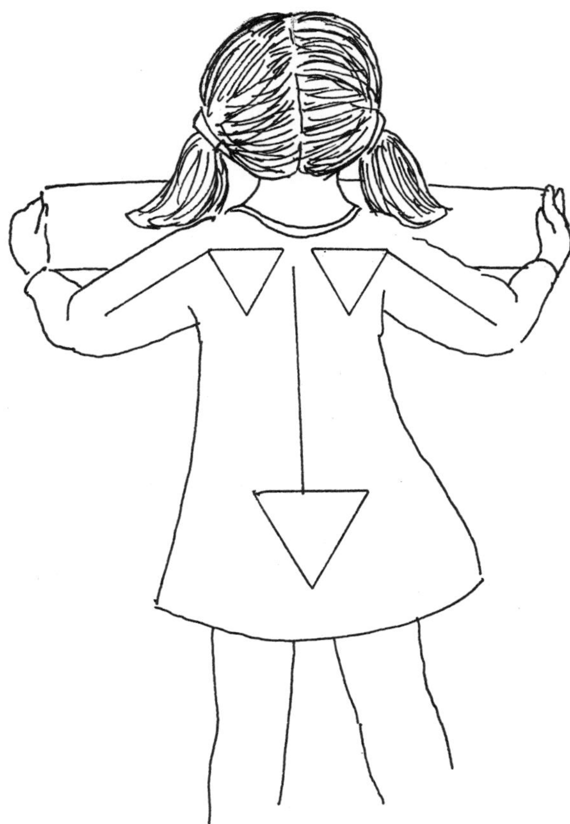

FIGURE **6-21**
Carrying a long, narrow box may decrease loads on the vertebrae but increases loads on the shoulders.

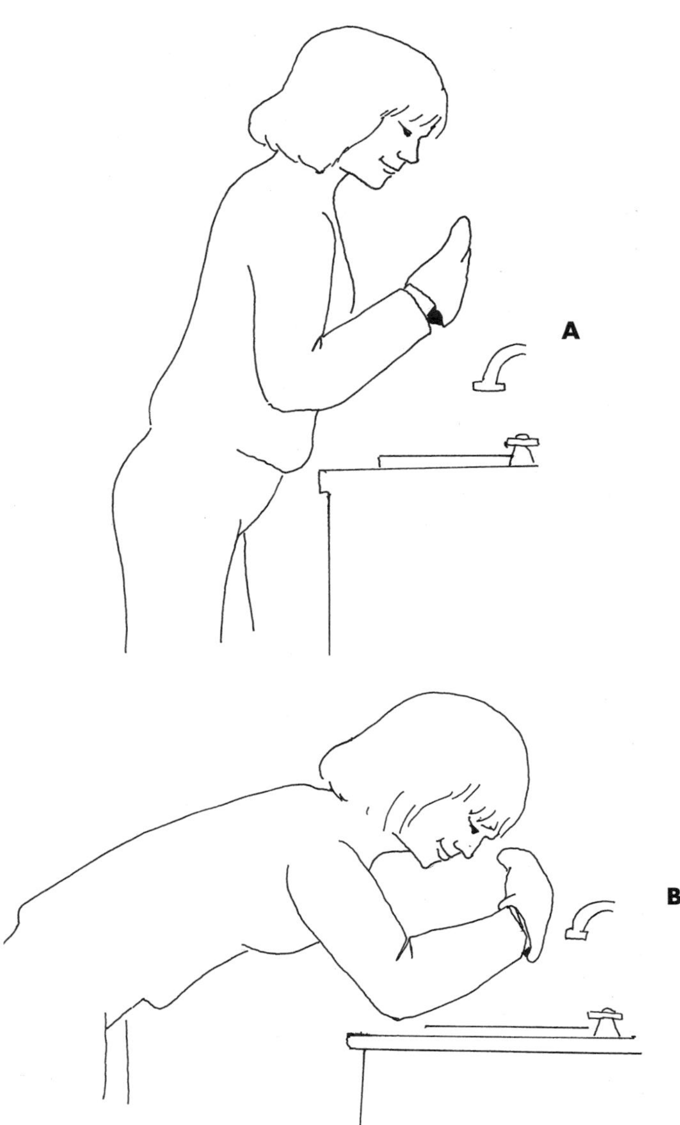

FIGURE **6-22**
A, When Nancy stands at the sink, the L5 vertebra forms a 30-degree angle to the floor. Her elbows are 20 cm from the axis of motion at the L5 disk. **B,** When she bends over the sink, the L5 vertebra forms a 70-degree angle to the floor. Her elbows are 52 cm from the axis of motion at the L5 disk.

As Spiros' muscles become fatigued, he compensates by using rapid, jerking motions to shift the load's center of gravity as close to his axis of motion as possible. He arches his back, shifting his body's center of gravity farther back to lengthen its moment arm. The OT practitioners note that this works because it intensifies the effect of his body weight as an extensor. However, they remind him that hyperextension increases the load on the smaller facet joints of the vertebrae and creates stress on ligaments along the anterior portion of the vertebrae. Because no safe way exists to compensate for the large flexion moment the boxes create, the OT practitioners also encourage his employer to package each load so the the load's center of gravity remain close to the body at all times.

L5 disk*

The OT practitioner returns to the computer company where Oliver and Nancy work to present a program on preventing injury with improved body mechanics. During the program, Nancy explains that she often notices back pain when she prepares for bed. Figure 6-22 shows how she leans over a sink to perform personal-hygiene activities. To demonstrate why back pain occurs, the OT practitioner uses a diagram with both arms held in a bilaterally symmetrical posture.

When Nancy stands, the center of gravity for her head and trunk falls 17 cm from the axis of motion in the L5 disk and the center of gravity for her arms falls 20 cm

*See Appendix C for graphic and mathematical solutions to this problem.

from the L5 disk. When Nancy bends, the center of gravity for her head and trunk is 31 cm from the L5 disk and the center of gravity for her arms is 52 cm away from the L5 disk. Nancy weighs 60 kg.

The erector spinae force needed to counteract the force of gravity is 5 cm from the axis of motion in the L5 disk. Remember that a force pulling directly through an axis (zero moment arm) creates no moment, or has no tendency toward extension; thus the force created by contraction produces a linear motion. An extension force acting at a small moment arm creates some extension tendency, but most force moves the segment along a line. The erector spinae have a short moment arm, and their linear movement causes the vertebral bodies to move closer and compress the intervertebral disks.

How much force do the erector spinae need to counteract the weight of the head, trunk, and arms when Nancy stands erect versus when she bends? How much compressive force operates on the L5 disk in each position? How can the OT practitioner adapt this activity to reduce the effort needed by the erector spinae and the load imposed on the L5 disk?

The OT practitioner notes that the weights of the head, trunk, and arms fall anterior to the axis of motion and assigns them positive values while assigning the counteractive force of the erector spinae a negative value (see Appendix B, Table B-1).

Figures 6-23 and 6-24 show forces and moment arms. Calculate the force of the erector spinae using the formula for equilibrium of torques ($\Sigma T = 0$). Nancy's head and trunk together weigh 34 kg and exert force 17 cm from the axis of motion. Her arms weigh 6 kg and have a moment arm of 20 cm. Converting centimeters to meters and kilograms to newtons, calculate the force generated by the erector spinae muscles when she stands upright at the sink:

$$\Sigma T = 0 = (340\ \text{N} \times 0.17\ \text{m}) + (60\ \text{N} \times 0.2\ \text{m}) + (-F_{\text{extensors}} \times 0.05\ \text{m})$$

$$0 = 57.8\ \text{Nm} + 12\ \text{Nm} + (-F_{\text{extensors}} \times 0.05\ \text{m})$$

$$F_{\text{extensors}} = \frac{69.8\ \text{Nm}}{0.05\ \text{m}}$$

$$F_{\text{extensors}} = 1396\ \text{N}$$

When Nancy leans over the sink, the erector spinae must support the increased effect of gravity on her trunk. Notice how everything changes as the moment arms increase:

$$\Sigma T = 0 = (340\ \text{N} \times 0.31\ \text{m}) + (60\ \text{N} \times 0.52\ \text{m}) + (-F_{\text{extensors}} \times 0.05\ \text{m})$$

$$0 = 105.4\ \text{Nm} + 31.2\ \text{Nm} + (-F_{\text{extensors}} \times 0.05\ \text{m})$$

$$F_{\text{extensors}} = \frac{136.6\ \text{Nm}}{0.05\ \text{m}}$$

$$F_{\text{extensors}} = 2732\ \text{N}$$

The erector spinae work twice as hard when Nancy bends over a sink as they do when she stands next to the sink. Remember that the small moment arm for the back extensors results in more linear (compressive) force than extension force. In fact, most compressive forces on the disk are caused by activation of the erector spinae. The compressive forces on the disk caused by the weight of the body are actually less when the body bends than when it stands.

Bending introduces another force, shear, into the equation. Shear force is parallel to the surface on which the force acts. In this case the amount of shear is small—about 13%—and negligible compared with the large amount of compressive force acting on the disk (see Appendix C).

Most sinks are so low that individuals must bend to perform daily tasks like washing the face or brushing the teeth. Figure 6-25 shows how Nancy can reduce the stressful forces on her low back by supporting some of her body's weight with one arm. Figure 6-26 shows another way to reduce stressful forces. By bending the knees and lowering the body, this individual places her face closer to the sink, which requires less lumbar flexion. When the hip joints move to bend the body, the low back is held in extension, so lumbar disks experience less anterior pressure.

SEATING AND POSITIONING

The drastic effect gravity has on the vertebral column is most evident in muscle weakness or imbalance. When we look at an unsupported column, we see how the different vertebral muscles manage the column against the predominant influence of gravity.

Stabilization principles

The pelvis is the foundation of stabilization. All the straps and pads in the world do very little to support a weak vertebral column unless the pelvis is stabilized. The company where Oliver and Nancy work supplies all its employees with $2000 chairs, but as Oliver becomes fatigued and slouches to view his screen, his pelvis slips forward and ruins the vertebral alignment the chair was designed to maintain. OT practitioners who specialize in positioning know that the pelvis is the key to stabilization.

The pelvis helps the body maintain a normal lumbar curve. We learned how anterior pelvic tilt affects the normal lumbar curve and how posterior tilt accompanies reversed lumbar curve. Positioning the pelvis in a slight anterior tilt allows weight to bear on the ischial tuberosities (as it should) and allows the body to maintain a normal lumbar curve (convex anteriorly) if the lumbar spine is mobile (A Closer Look Box 6-2). A lumbar pad or cushion can provide anterior pelvic tilt and maintain lumbar positioning if the cushion is placed where the lumbar curve should be. Placement too high or too low puts pres-

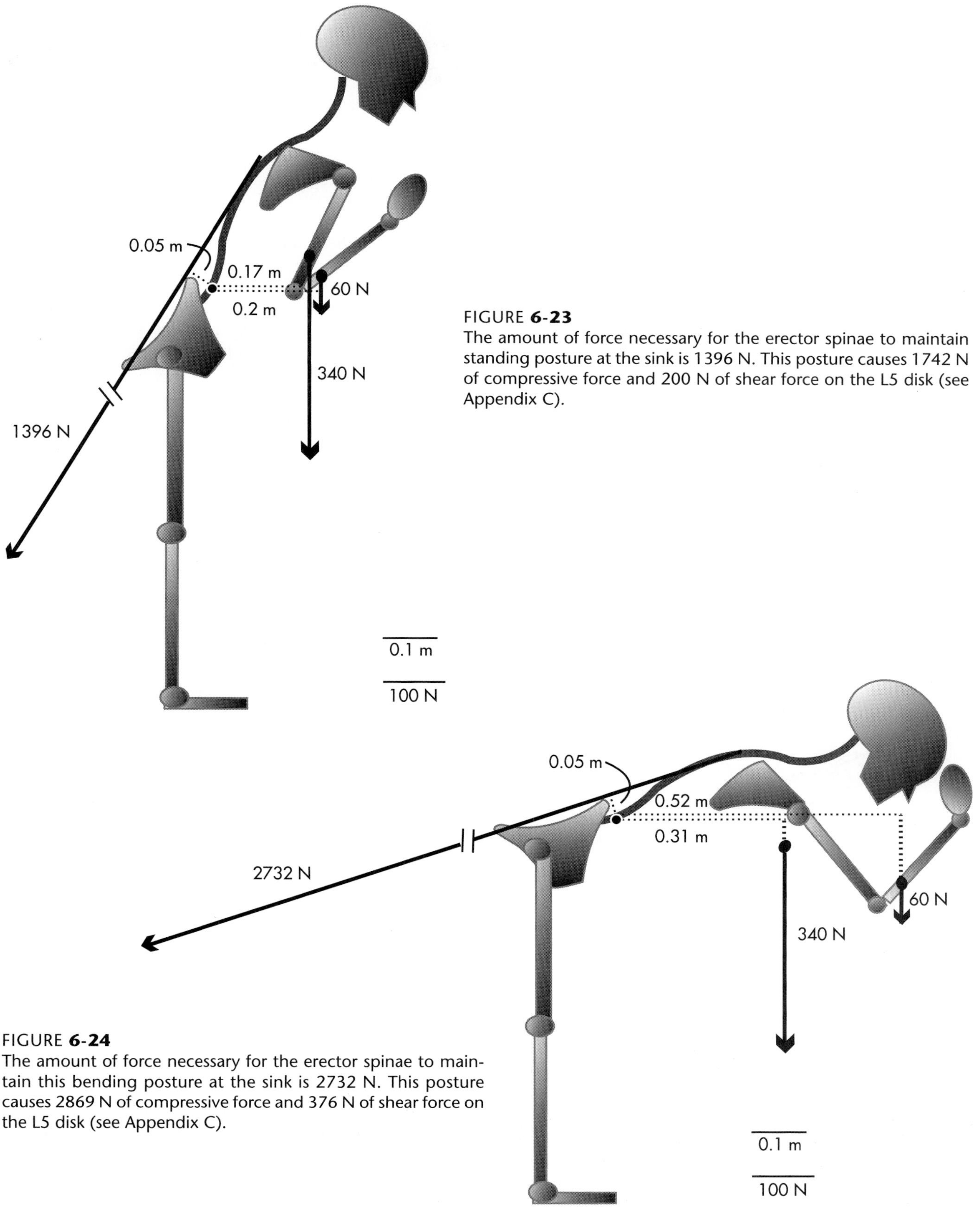

FIGURE **6-23**
The amount of force necessary for the erector spinae to maintain standing posture at the sink is 1396 N. This posture causes 1742 N of compressive force and 200 N of shear force on the L5 disk (see Appendix C).

FIGURE **6-24**
The amount of force necessary for the erector spinae to maintain this bending posture at the sink is 2732 N. This posture causes 2869 N of compressive force and 376 N of shear force on the L5 disk (see Appendix C).

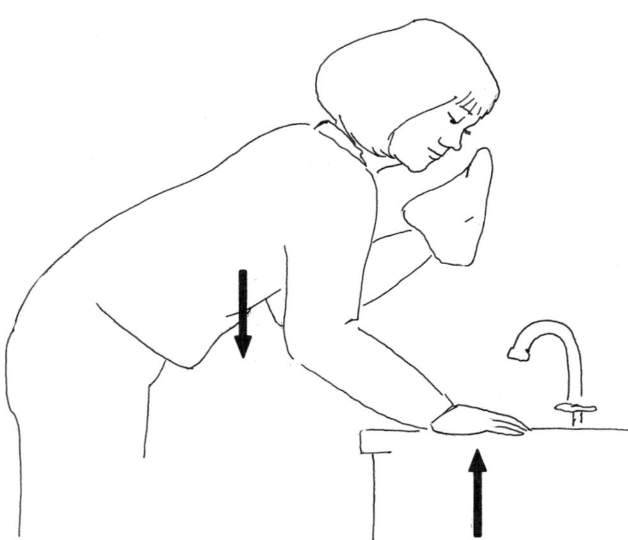

FIGURE **6-25**
Supporting her body weight with one arm on the countertop allows Nancy to share the weight of the upper trunk with the upper-extremity muscles by using less back-extensor force. This means less compressive force is generated. As Nancy raises the washcloth to her face, the need to flex decreases.

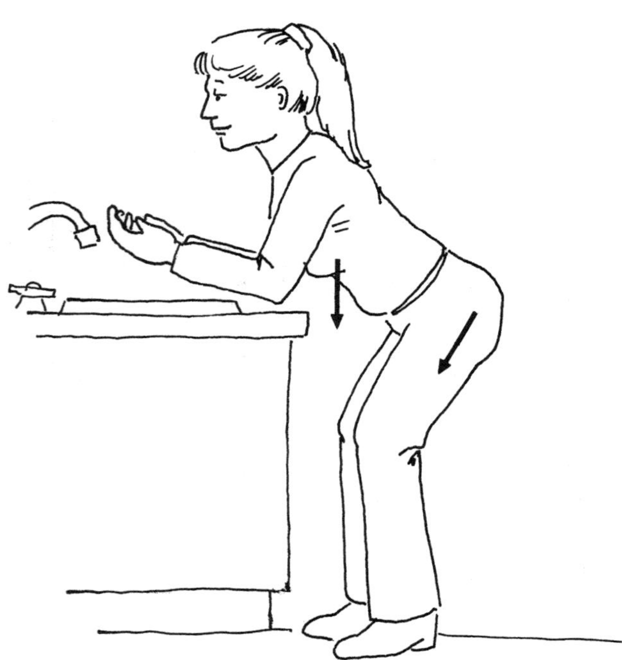

FIGURE **6-26**
Bending at the knees allows this individual to lower her face to the sink without bending her back. The weight of the upper trunk works at a smaller moment arm, and the back extensors produce a smaller contraction force. She keeps the lower portion of her back straight and decreases the forces acting on the lower part of her back as she bends over the sink.

BOX 6-2

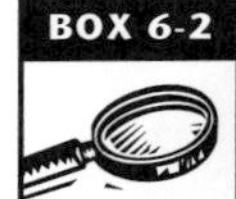

A **CLOSER** LOOK

Evaluations

The OT practitioners who work with Jason know that the first step toward changing his positioning is an evaluation. To begin, they determine the mobility of his spine. Some postures are present for so long in individuals that they become fixed and must be accommodated rather than corrected by external supports. Jason has a fixed reversed lumbar curve (convex posteriorly). A lumbar pad puts undue pressure on the posterior spinous processes and is likely to cause skin breakdown if his pelvis is tightly secured. If the pelvis is not tightly secured, the lumbar pad pushes Jason from the seat instead of reestablishing lumbar lordosis.

The OT practitioners then determine whether Jason's hamstrings are long enough to allow his pelvis to be positioned in anterior tilt. They compare passive range of motion of the hips into flexion with his knees extended versus flexed. The larger the discrepancy in the amount of hip flexion, the more his hamstrings limit movement. Jason's hamstrings are so short that he cannot achieve 90 degrees of hip flexion, even with his knee flexed.

Armed with this information, the OT practitioners begin to develop a seating system that allows Jason greater than 90 degrees of knee flexion with hip flexion at 90 degrees.

sure on the thoracic or sacral vertebrae, respectively. Because both these regions normally protrude posteriorly, an improperly placed lumbar roll serves only to push the individual forward from the chair.

Overtight hamstrings can frustrate attempts at repositioning by prestabilizing the pelvis. The OT assistant experienced this problem when first meeting Jason. The OT assistant attempted to reposition Jason with an anterior pelvic tilt, but his short hamstrings stretched as the pelvis brought his ischial tuberosities (hamstring origin) backward from the hamstring insertions below the knee. Tightness in the hamstrings prevented pelvic movement, and the desired degree of anterior tilt was not possible (see A Closer Look Box 6-2).

The OT assistant also noted that Jason's hamstrings were shorter on the left side than on the right. Jason could not achieve bilateral hip flexion to 90 degrees because his left hip stopped at about 85 degrees. Jason's left posterior thigh hit the sitting surface first as the OT assistant attempted to create a more optimal sitting posture. Because Jason's left hip could not flex farther, his

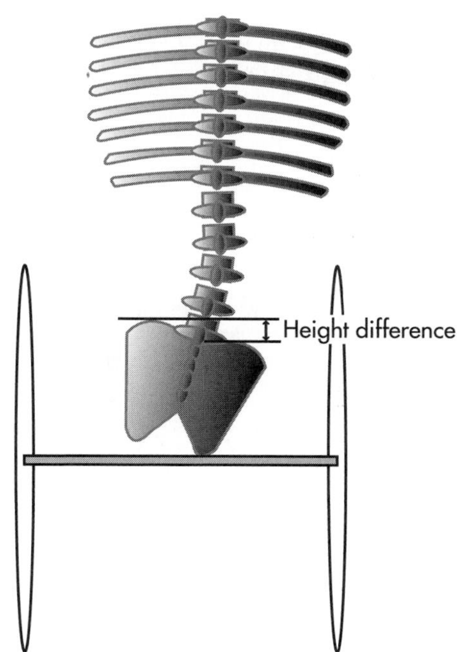

FIGURE **6-27**
When an individual with asymmetrically short hamstrings attempts to sit, pelvic obliquity may result.

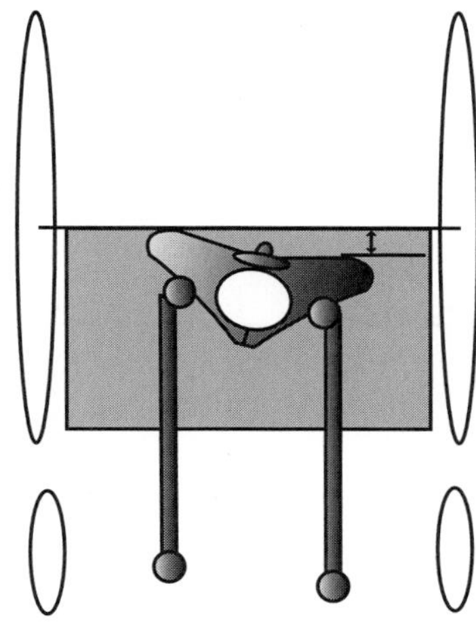

FIGURE **6-28**
Pelvic rotation from a top, or superior, view.

left pelvis moved upward as the right hip flexed into 90 degrees. The OT assistant referred to Jason's position as **pelvic obliquity,** in which his left iliac crest is higher than the right (Figure 6-27).

Often, asymmetrical hamstring length results in another type of pelvic repositioning. Jason could not achieve hip flexion of 90 degrees on his left side. After several minutes of trying to maintain this posture, his pelvis shifted anteriorly instead of upwardly. The OT assistant observed this **pelvic rotation** by looking at him from above and noting that his hips were no longer in the same vertical, or frontal, plane (Figure 6-28).

Seating must address any pelvic positions that occur because of muscle shortness across the hips. Unless the pelvis is accommodated, all other attempts at support are futile. An asymmetrical seat depth or seat height may be a desirable adaptation to the sitting surface. A 45-degree seat belt also can secure the pelvis.

Alignment in superior regions follows pelvic stabilization. Lateral supports medially direct forces in the thoracic region. These lateral supports counter lateral forces of the vertebral segments caused by gravity. Straps hold the trunk to the seat back so that lateral supports can apply pressure to the intended regions. In addition, anterior-posterior and lateral supports provide the stabilization the head requires.

Other vertebral and pelvic issues deal less with orthopedics and more with neurology. For example, a wedge cushion encourages greater than 90 degrees of hip flexion to reduce extensor spasms and improve overall sitting posture. The wedge cushion is an ideal solution to a seating problem when it addresses the area with the least amount of support.

Sometimes increased support is not only unnecessary but also harmful. For example, OT practitioners working with Jason are concerned that his head supports yield muscle contractions that push against the surfaces of the supports. They plan to tilt his wheelchair back so that his head's center of gravity is just behind his pelvis, stabilizing his head on a small rear support. This position allows Jason to use his neck flexors to raise his head upright and neck extensors to maintain the position. When he becomes fatigued, he can relax into a semireclined position that still allows him to view his surroundings. The semireclined position facilitates muscle contractions that allow him to hold his head erect without external supports.

OT practitioners must approach external supports in positioning differently than when they attempt to change alignment and muscle length in splinting. Good positioning accommodates fixed positions and prevents problems in one area, like the pelvis, from negatively affecting vertebral alignment in other regions. Positioning support should prevent further degradation of alignment. Support should be provided only after the OT practitioner decides that an individual cannot position the body alone. External support does not strengthen muscles; it only replaces the need for an individual to maintain good sitting posture. For a deeper understanding of positioning, more study is recommended.

Common restraint systems

Upholstered reclining chairs have a long history in nursing homes. They operate as beltless restraints by increasing gravity's moment arm. Caretakers recline the chair until gravity's moment arm for extension exceeds the ability of the body's trunk flexors to produce enough flexion for the individual to rise from the seat.

Seat belts with buckles or Velcro placed out of reach restrain more active individuals. These seat belts are usually waist straps that are quite uncomfortable; discomfort generally serves as the principal reason individuals attempt to remove the belts. Waist straps attach to the wheelchair back and have no real effect on positioning. The waist strap's point of contact is the soft abdomen. Tightening the belt produces severe discomfort and can affect breathing. The belt must be somewhat loose to be tolerated, so the pelvis usually slides forward. This action results from the downward pull of gravity and increases when an individual uses a lower extremity to propel the wheelchair, as is common after a stroke.

Nursing staff at Maple Grove Skilled Care Facility requested that the OT department outfit ***Quentin Keller*** with a lap tray to help him improve his positioning. No matter what they said, he tried to unbuckle his seat belt or slide under it. To make matters worse, he had seriously abraded the skin on his sacrum by sliding down in his chair, placing him at risk for developing a pressure sore. The nurses hoped the lap tray would bypass regulations about restraints and put to rest their worries that Quentin would fall. Leaning on a tray, they thought, may remove some pressure from his sacrum.

The OT practitioners found Quentin using his right leg to drag himself down the hall in an old wheelchair. They noticed that the posterior tilt he assumed when pulling himself down the hall had caused him to develop a kyphotic thoracic curve. OT staff brought Quentin into their clinic for measurements and, by the end of the week, outfitted him with a more effective 45-degree belt.

The angled belt attaches at the junction of the seat and the back to form a 45-degree angle with the sitting surface. It anchors the pelvis deep into the corner of the chair. The belt allows Quentin to assume a stable sitting position. He experiences no discomfort, so he does not try to remove it. Because the belt anchors him more securely in the chair, Quentin can propel himself more easily and the abrasions on the sacrum can heal, as his body sits more erect in his chair. The OT practitioners explain that the lap tray would only have compounded Quentin's problems by stabilizing the trunk at an even higher position and making forward pelvic slide even easier.

The waist belt and lap tray each fail to do what the 45-degree belt does best—anchor Quentin's pelvis into the corner of the chair. Because the 45-degree belt is lower than the waist belt and lap tray and does not compress abdominal and pelvic organs, it can be tightened enough to be effective without being uncomfortable. It puts gentle but firm pressure on the pelvis, which slides forward under less effective devices. When the belt is effective and comfortable, it removes Quentin's original motivation to remove the belt and the clasp can be placed within his reach. Thus the belt is no longer a restraint. The end result is comfortable, good posture without a restraint. When a 45-degree belt secures the pelvis, the lap tray becomes a tabletop alternative, not a restraint.

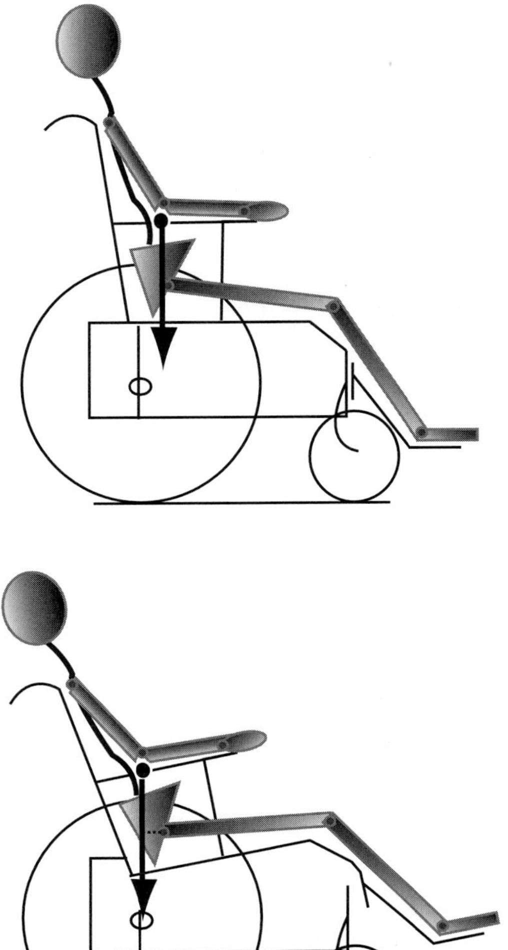

FIGURE **6-29**
Slight backward tilting of the chair promotes a tendency toward closed-chain hip extension, counteracting the effect of momentum when the chair is stopped suddenly.

A wedge cushion also anchors an individual without using a belt. A wedge places the hips in more than 90 degrees of flexion and produces the same effect as if the individual were sitting on a sofa. On sofas and overstuffed chairs the hips are flexed beyond 90 degrees. The hip and knee extensors, both necessary when the individual stands, are placed in weak positions in their range, making them less effective from this position. (Remember isometric torque curves?) The wedge can be effective, but it produces increased hip flexion and raises the feet. The OT practitioner must elevate the footrests to support the weight of the lower leg; otherwise, too much pressure is placed on the posterior thighs, causing another problem.

Many people use chest belts to restrain the body's forward momentum when the wheelchair is stopped suddenly. ***Bernice Richards,*** who works as a singer in a cocktail lounge, uses an electric wheelchair. She has trunk instability secondary to C5 quadriplegia and was outfitted with a chest belt but feels that the belt obscures her sequined tops.

Bernice and her OT practitioner discussed various options and decided to tilt her chair backward. The angle of the chair back places Bernice's upper body center of gravity behind the hip axis for flexion and extension. In this position the upper body produces a tendency toward closed-chain hip extension. This counteracts the forward momentum toward closed-chain hip flexion she experiences when her chair is stopped suddenly and decreases the need for a chest restraint (Figure 6-29).

Summary

The bony and soft-tissue structures of the head, neck, and trunk provide a stable but flexible shell to protect vital organs, a stable base for movement of the extremities, and a mobile base from which to extend the upper extremities. Despite its design, the back should not be used to lift the trunk from a forward-flexed position. The vertebral extensors, with their short moment arms, produce more compression than extension force. Maintaining upright posture requires little extensor force and causes minimal compression of the intervertebral disks. In contrast, lifting with the back uses a great deal of extensor force and introduces enough compression to damage disks.

Biomechanics can explain and provide solutions for many common problems associated with body positioning. Basic principles in this chapter serve as a basis for two of the most common problems an OT practitioner encounters:

1. Providing external support from the pelvis upward along the vertebral column when internal stability fails because muscles are too weak
2. Assessing restraints from the perspective of positioning principles and considering failure and discomfort from restraints as results of poor positioning

Applications

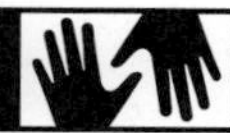

APPLICATION 6-1
Upper-Extremity Reach

Identify how the trunk participates in the following reach patterns. Determine the active groups of trunk muscles in each case:

1. Reach forward with both hands as far as you can without flexing the hips past 90 degrees.
2. Reach to one side or the other as far as you can. (Shoulder abduction should be about 90 degrees.)
3. Reach straight up as far as you can.
4. Reach as far as you can to the left side by bringing your right arm in front of your shoulders.

APPLICATION 6-2
Open- and Closed-Chain Hip Movements

Sit with your legs crossed in front of you and hips flexed to at least 90 degrees. Compare this with long sitting. (To achieve long sitting, lie in a supine position and sit up so that your hips are flexed to 90 degrees and your knees fully extended with your feet in front.) Is long sitting a different feeling? Compare hip flexion movements for crossed-legged sitting with long sitting. What happens in long sitting when you reach forward to touch your toes?

APPLICATION 6-3
Stance

Dr. Paul Zimmerman, a dermatologist with a busy private practice, needs help adapting his office environment to minimize his back pain. He is most uncomfortable bending over his examination table. He has begun doing some office-based surgery and must hold this position for an hour or more in some procedures. Placing one foot on a step stool relieves the doctor's back pain and makes it possible for him to complete surgical procedures with minimal discomfort. Why?

See Appendix C for solutions to Applications.

REFERENCE

1. Williams PL, Bannister LH: *Gray's anatomy: the anatomical basis of medicine and surgery,* ed 38, New York, 1995, Churchill Livingstone.

RELATED READINGS

Hall SJ: *Basic biomechanics,* ed 2, New York, 1995, McGraw-Hill.
Jacobs J, Bettencourt CM: *Ergonomics for therapists,* Newton, Mass, 1995, Butterworth-Heinemann.

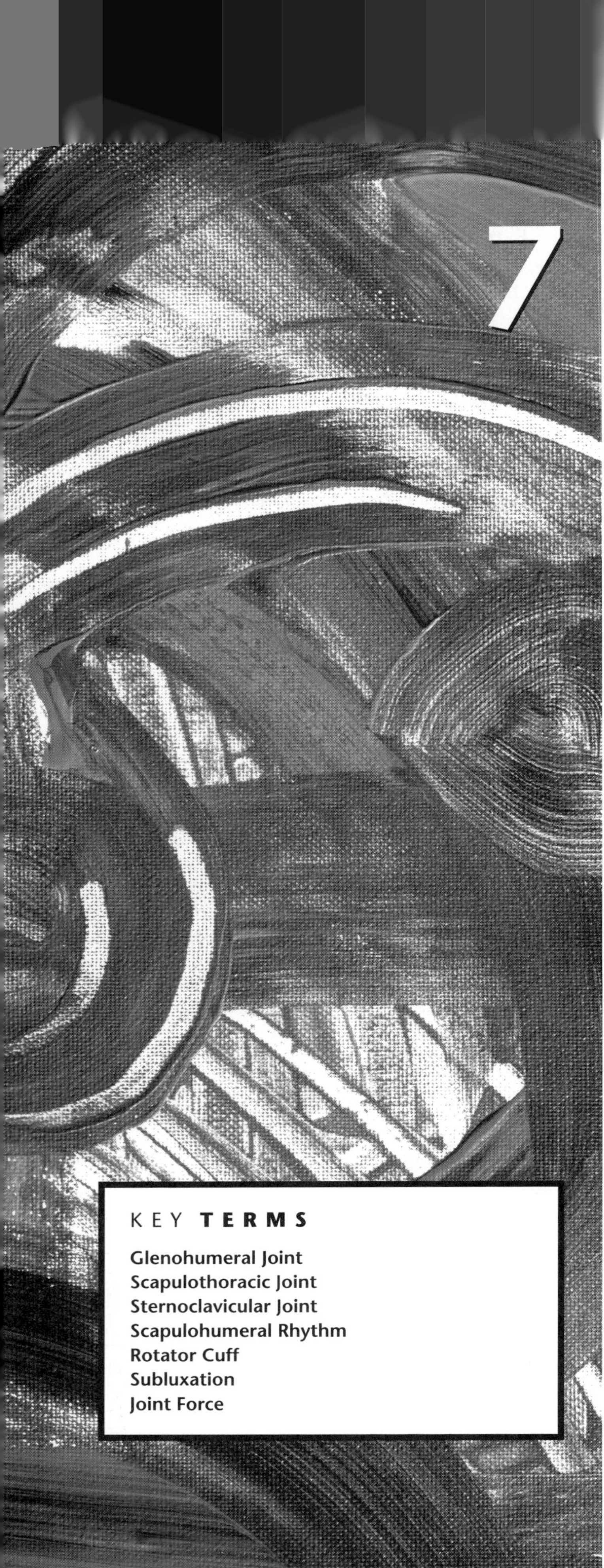

7 The Proximal Upper Extremity

CHAPTER OUTLINE

KEY TERMS

Glenohumeral Joint
Scapulothoracic Joint
Sternoclavicular Joint
Scapulohumeral Rhythm
Rotator Cuff
Subluxation
Joint Force

T ***hrough the ages,*** individuals have used tools to adapt to their environments. Most of us associate tool use with hand use. This chapter focuses on reaching, the important proximal counterpart of tool use. Any meaningful manipulation of materials by the fingers and thumbs depends on stabilization and arm movement.

Shoulder motion can position the hand the length of the arm in a 360-degree arc. With the elbow extended, we can touch, adjust, hold, and manipulate objects at the edge of that arc and flex the elbow to reach within the extremes of the arc. Various combinations of shoulder and elbow movements place the hand at multiple points in space. Each multiple joint in the upper extremity has a designated amount of freedom of movement. Steindler[6] described the ability to place the hand in a variety of places as a joint chain displaying degrees of freedom.

The Shoulder Complex

We often refer to shoulder movement as if it occurs in a single joint. Early lessons in anatomy highlight the shoulder's classification as a ball-and-socket joint that moves in three planes. This emphasis on glenohumeral articulation downplays the importance of other joints in the shoulder complex. Acting alone, the **glenohumeral joint,** even in its 3 degrees of freedom, does not allow the hand to reach above the head or in any extreme of forward or backward reach.

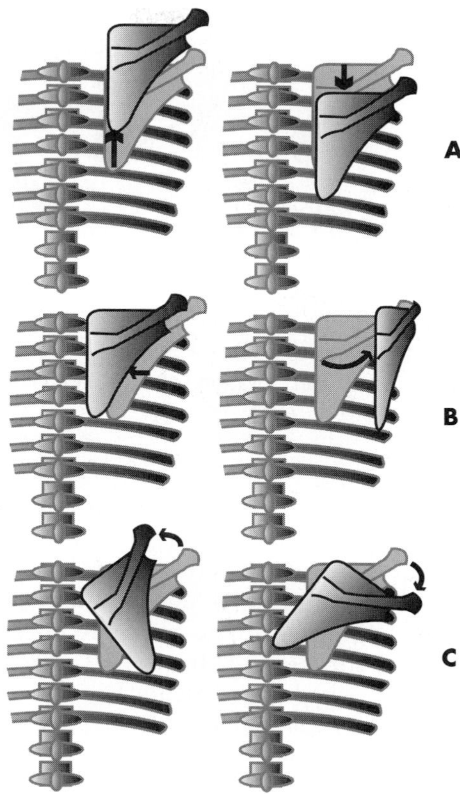

FIGURE **7-1**
The various movements of the scapula include elevation and depression **(A)**, retraction and protraction **(B)**, and upward and downward rotation **(C)**.

ARTICULATIONS

The scapula makes a critical contribution to upper-extremity movement and function. Its articulation with the thorax **(scapulothoracic joint)** allows movement of the scapula in six directions: elevation and depression, protraction and retraction, and upward and downward rotation (Figure 7-1). Scapular movements are integral parts of various upper-extremity reach patterns. Forward reach includes elbow extension, shoulder flexion, and scapular protraction. Placing the hand high above the head requires full elbow extension and shoulder flexion with upward scapular rotation. Reaching the hand behind the back requires just the opposite—downward scapular rotation, full glenohumeral internal rotation and extension, and elbow flexion.

The relationship between the clavicle and the scapula makes this freedom of movement possible. The upper extremity's bony attachment to the axial skeleton occurs solely at the **sternoclavicular joint,** a small, freely movable synovial joint. The clavicle articulates with the scapula at the acromioclavicular joint. Thus when the scapula moves, so does the clavicle. However, clavicular motions do not have official names. Generally, frontal-plane movement occurs with scapular-plane elevation and depression and upward and downward rotation, whereas horizontal-plane movement occurs with scapular protraction and retraction.

Movement or restriction of one segment allows movement or restriction of another. Therefore if the sternoclavicular joint restricts clavicular movement, scapular movement decreases. In this way, decreased scapular movement limits upper-extremity use.

MUSCLES

Reviewing anatomy to locate muscle attachments and innervations may help reduce confusion over which muscles move the scapula and which move the humerus at the glenohumeral joint. Kinesiology involves determin-

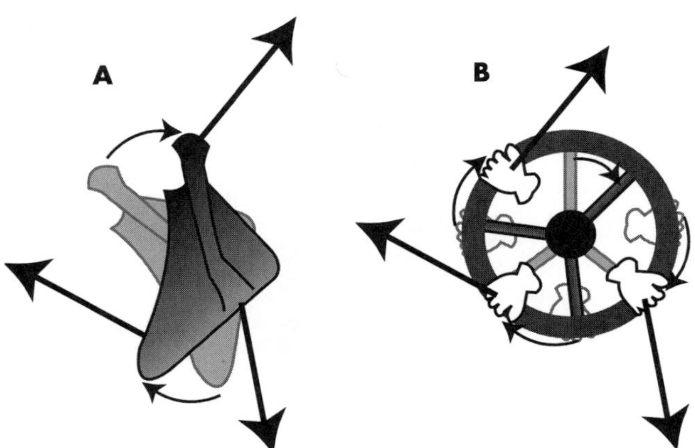

FIGURE **7-2**
The scapula and upward rotation **(A)** compared with the turning of a steering wheel **(B)**.

ing which muscles do what and why. Instead of memorizing or rememorizing functions, try to develop a three-dimensional image of the entire shoulder region.

The upper trapezius and levator scapulae, which originate on the spine and run downward to insert onto the scapula, elevate the scapula by shortening to pull their insertions up toward their origins. Gravity's pull is the force most responsible for scapular depression, the opposite movement. Scapular depression to raise the trunk to transfer from a wheelchair or bear weight on crutches is against resistance. Performing such tasks requires concentric contractions of the lower trapezius, latissimus dorsi, and pectoralis major muscles, which originate below and reach up to insert onto the scapula. The latter two scapular depressors move the scapula mostly through their strong attachments to and downward pulls on the humerus.

The upper and lower trapezius and lower fibers of the serratus anterior originate in very different places, but imagining the insertions of these muscles moving toward their origins clarifies how they produce upward scapular rotation. Their effect on the scapula is similar to three hands on three different points of a steering wheel. A hand on the right pulls down, another on the bottom pulls left, a hand on the left pushes up, turning the wheel right, or clockwise. Upward rotation of the left scapula is a similar movement. The lower trapezius inserts near the root of the scapular spine and pulls down, the lower serratus pulls the inferior angle lateral, and the upper trapezius pulls the acromion up (Figure 7-2 and A Closer Look Box 7-1).

Downward scapular rotation, like scapular depression, is mostly a result of gravity. The rhomboids (major and minor) rotate the scapula downward against resistance.

BOX 7-1

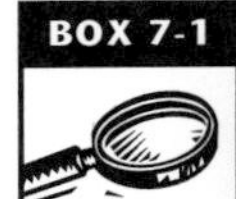

A **CLOSER** LOOK

Scapular Rotation

The terminology for scapular rotation differs depending on the part of the scapula the eye follows. Because the glenoid articulates with the humerus and in a sense points the way for the hand, references to scapular movement follow glenoid movement. The glenoid faces upward to allow positioning of the hand above the head, so this movement is referred to as upward scapular rotation. During this movement, the inferior angle moves laterally. The term lateral scapular rotation *originated from this perspective. Although the description is correct, it does not depict in which direction the distal upper extremity moves.*

The same is true for scapular protraction and retraction versus scapular abduction and adduction. In protraction the glenoid moves around the side of the thorax to face forward, holding the hand in front of the trunk. The vertebral border of the scapula moves from the midline. Emphasis on the movement of the vertebral border leads to a view of protraction as scapular abduction. The opposite movement, retraction, adducts the vertebral border back toward the midline.

Scapular protraction and retraction follow the contour of the thorax while bringing the scapula forward the backward (see A Closer Look Box 7-1). The insertion of the serratus anterior enables the scapula's costal surface to remain fully adjacent to the convexity of the thorax throughout the arc of movement. The serratus originates on the vertebral border of the scapula and winds under it and around the thorax to attach onto the same border. The serratus would pull the scapula forward regardless of where on the scapula it inserted, but protraction would not look the same if it inserted onto the scapula's lateral border. As the scapula pulled forward and rocked against the rib cage, the vertebral border would protrude posteriorly, known as "winging" (Figure 7-3, *A*). Insertion onto the vertebral border pushes the scapula anteriorly from its most posterior part instead of pulling its anterior edge anteriorly. No winging occurs as long as the serratus anterior is intact (see Figure 7-3, *B*).

Retraction, the opposite of protraction, is to some extent due to recoil in the tissues that are stretched during protraction. Because protraction and retraction both occur in the transverse plane, gravity does not affect them. When retraction occurs against resistance or requires

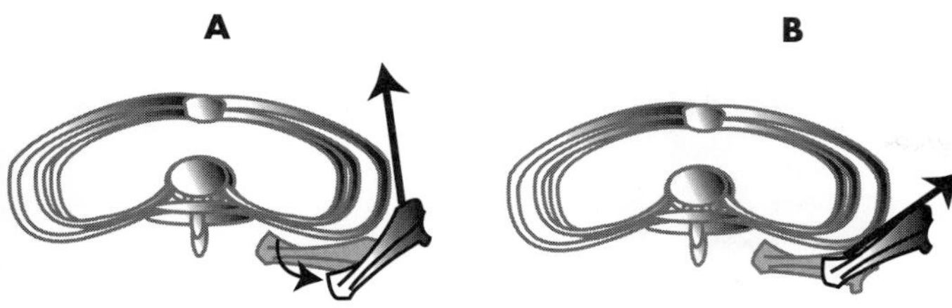

FIGURE **7-3**
A, Scapular protraction and winging would occur if the insertion of the serratus anterior were on the scapula's lateral border. **B,** Its actual insertion on the vertebral border holds the scapula close to the thoracic wall during protraction.

more force than recoil produces, the middle fibers of the trapezius move in a pure motion or combine with the rhomboids to retract and rotate downward.

Closed-chain scapular depression

Closed-chain movements involve stabilization of the distal part of the moving chain to prevent its movement. In Chapter 4, we used a pull-up to demonstrate how shortening of the muscles results in trunk movement when the hand grasps an immovable bar. Elbow flexors shorten, flexing the humerus onto the forearm at the elbow. As the humerus moves, the trunk rises toward the bar, creating closed-chain elbow flexion.

Elevating the trunk for transfer from a wheelchair or onto a table or mat is an example of closed-chain scapular depression. In open-chain depression, the scapula moves downward in relation to the trunk because scapular depressors like the latissimus dorsi and sternal pectoralis major originate lower on the trunk than their insertions on the humerus. When the hand is free in space, concentric contractions cause the humerus to move downward. Because the humerus is attached to the scapula at the glenohumeral joint, the scapula moves downward (depression) in relation to the trunk. Closed-chain movement occurs when the hand is stabilized on the mat or chair seat. Because the hand cannot move downward, as the depressors shorten, the trunk moves upward toward the scapula (Figure 7-4). Understanding the role of the scapular depressors ensures that strengthening activities for such transfers exercise the correct muscles.

Scapular stabilization

Stabilization of the scapula relies on isometric contractions of muscles; the concentric contractions of these muscles produce scapular movement. Two basic concepts in kinesiology explain the need for scapular stabilization. First, when a muscle contracts, it shortens; whether the origin or insertion moves depends on which moves easier. Second, as Newton discovered, the acceleration of an object is related to its mass. The scapula is less massive than the entire upper extremity. Therefore when glenohumeral muscles contract, they move the scapula unless other factors intervene.

All muscles that move the humerus at the glenohumeral joint first require scapular stabilization. Most, except for the pectoralis major and latissimus dorsi, originate on the scapula and insert onto the humerus. Without scapular stabilization, glenohumeral muscles that originate on the scapula would waste their excursion and move the wrong segment.

Shoulder abduction, or flexion, moves the hand against gravity through elevation of the upper extremity and involves both scapular and glenohumeral movement. The scapula must be stabilized before any scapular or glenohumeral movement occurs. The supraspinatus and deltoid muscles together contract to abduct the glenohumeral joint, but their tendency to move the least massive segment rotates the scapula downward. Isometric contractions of the upward scapular rotators produce scapular stabilization, preventing downward rotation (Figure 7-5).

Elevation via abduction

With the scapula stabilized, glenohumeral muscles can contract and abduct. Both the supraspinatus and deltoid muscles can abduct, but the supraspinatus is more pure in its action. The deltoid originates above the glenoid; this attachment and the relatively short moment arm for abduction gives much of the deltoid's force a linear effect, directed parallel to the glenoid. Early in abduction, isolated concentric contraction of the deltoid compresses the structures between the humeral head and the acromion more than it abducts the humerus.

Three factors prevent undesirable elevation of the humerus in abduction. First, the supraspinatus originates medial to the glenoid rather than above, producing a linear effect directed into the glenoid fossa. Early activation of the supraspinatus results in pure abduction without elevation. Second, the combined pull of the infraspinatus, teres minor, and subscapularis directly opposes the elevation effect of the deltoid[1] (Figure 7-6). These smaller muscles pull mostly through the abduction axis and can exert a downward linear pull on the humerus without interfering with abduction. Third, as abduction progresses, the linear component of the deltoid force is directed into the glenoid like that of the supraspinatus early in abduction. This enables continued abduction without humeral elevation.

Only with scapular stabilization, balance of the upward and downward forces affecting the humerus, continued glenohumeral abduction, and upward scapular rotation can an individual raise the hand above the head.

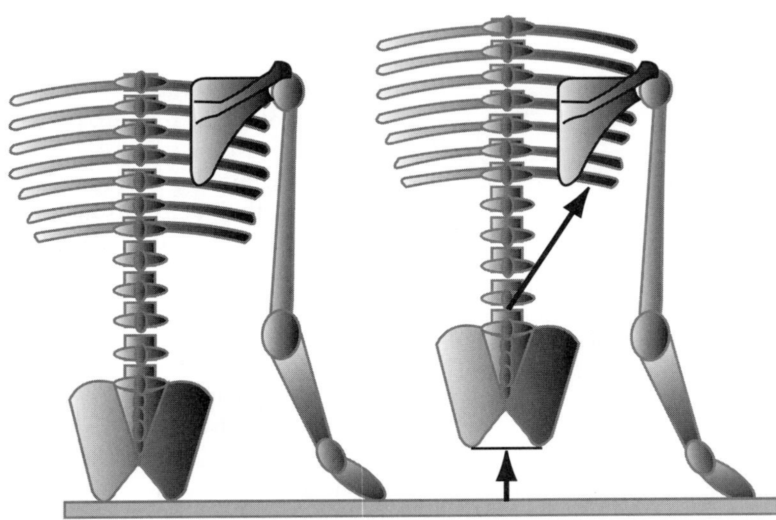

FIGURE **7-4**
Closed-chain scapular depression results in trunk elevation in a transfer from a wheelchair.

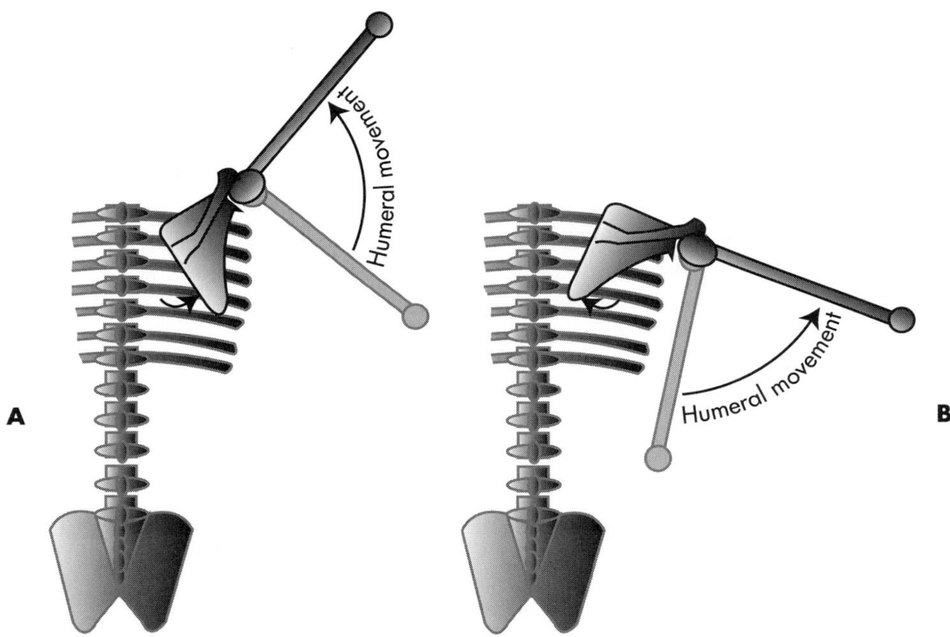

FIGURE **7-5**
Glenohumeral movement with **(A)** and without **(B)** scapular stabilization. Notice that the amount of humeral movement is the same in each case.

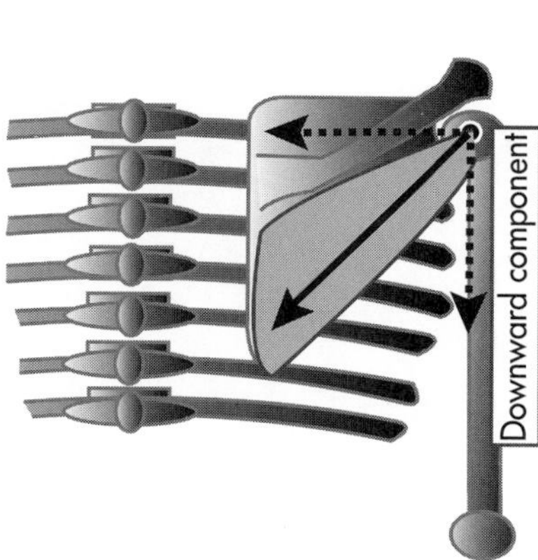

FIGURE **7-6**
The infraspinatus, teres minor, and subscapularis (not visible from this view) pull the humerus downward and inward. The downward component of the force balances the elevating effect of the deltoid early in abduction.

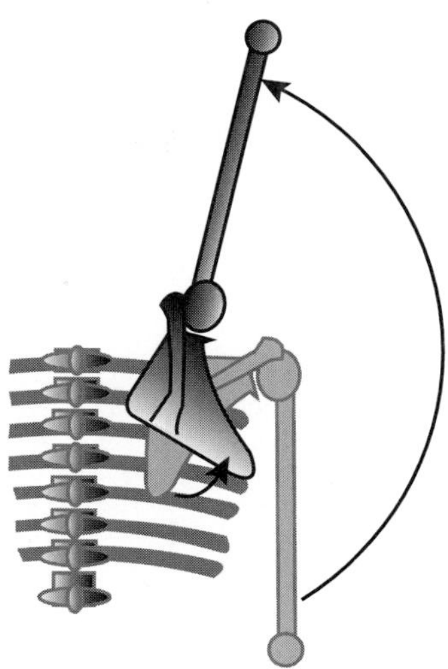

FIGURE **7-7**
Elevation of the upper extremity through abduction requires both a glenohumeral and a scapular contribution.

Scapulohumeral rhythm describes the simultaneous glenohumeral and scapular movements.

Scapulohumeral rhythm
Upper-extremity abduction involves a combination of upward scapular rotation and glenohumeral abduction (Figure 7-7). Various studies have detailed the ratio of scapular to glenohumeral movement. Glenohumeral abduction occurs alone for the first 30 to 40 degrees, followed by a steady contribution of upward scapular rotation. Scapular and glenohumeral movements occur simultaneously but unequally. Glenohumeral motion produces no more than 120 degrees of abduction while upward scapular rotation contributes another 60 degrees. Upward scapular rotation is an essential component in elevation of the upper extremity because 120 degrees of motion cannot place the hand above the head.[5]

Rotator cuff
Four muscles—the subscapularis, supraspinatus, infraspinatus, and teres minor—comprise the **rotator cuff.** We already have described their actions in different functions. This collective name arises out of the appearance and function of these muscles as a circular cuff securing the humeral head close to the glenoid fossa. The glenohumeral ligaments and rotator cuff muscles help stabilize the joint. The rotator cuff is most active when the hand holds objects that produce a downward force on the upper extremity.[1]

Although they stabilize the glenohumeral joint together, individual groupings of rotator cuff muscles demonstrate functional diversity, including two antagonistic, or opposing, actions. The supraspinatus primarily functions as a glenohumeral abductor, whereas the infraspinatus, teres minor, and subscapularis, with their common downward effect on the humerus, balance the upward pull of the deltoid on the humerus early in abduction. The infraspinatus and teres minor externally rotate the humerus because of their locations posterior to the rotation axis. The anteriorly located subscapularis acts as an antagonist, internally rotating the humerus.

Glenohumeral subluxation
After a cerebral vascular accident (CVA), or stroke, the glenohumeral joint commonly becomes partially dislocated **(subluxation).** Although severe spasticity may affect parts of the upper extremity, some glenohumeral muscles are rendered relatively inactive. Because of this shift in muscle balance and slight realignment of the scapula, which causes the glenoid to lose its upward orientation, the normal mechanism securing the humeral head into the glenoid fails.

Normal glenohumeral joint stability involves a certain orientation of the glenoid and the superior joint structures—the joint capsule, supraspinatus, and posterior deltoid. The glenoid faces slightly upward because its inferior edge protrudes more laterally than its superior edge. As the pull of gravity moves the humeral head inferiorly along the glenoid, the humeral head moves laterally as it moves downward. This movement stretches the superior joint structures, and their recoil prevents the humeral head from moving farther downward (Figure 7-8).

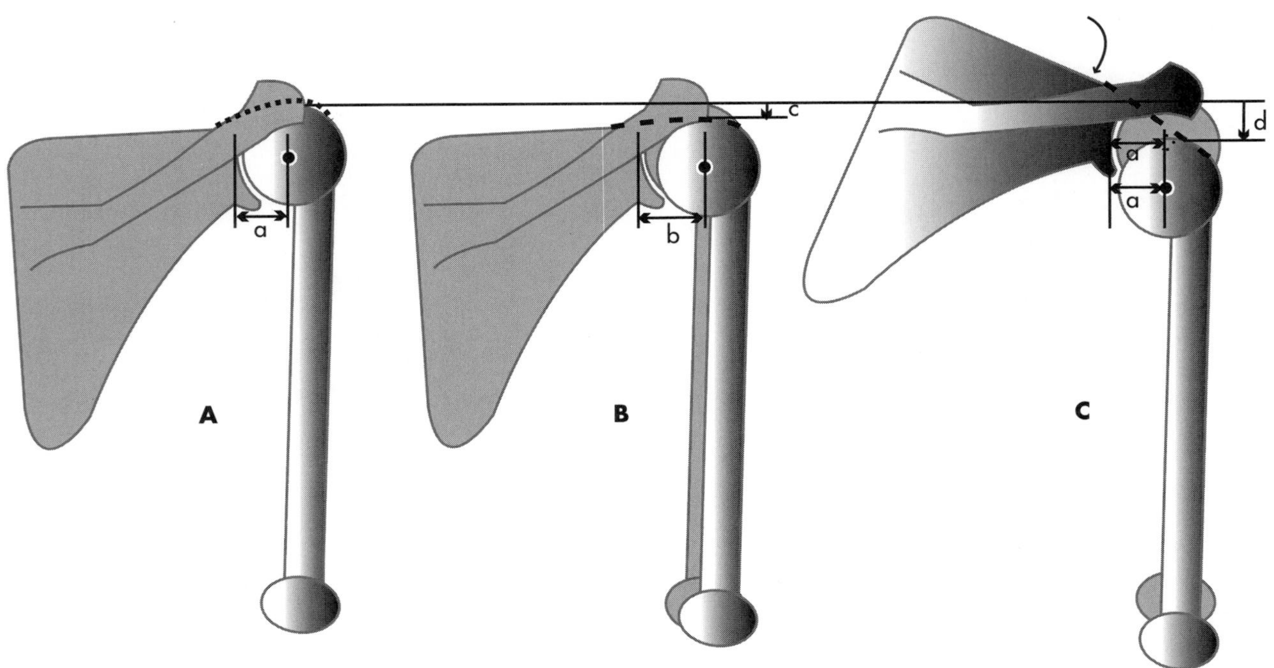

FIGURE **7-8**
A, The humeral head is most medially located when centered in the glenoid; distance *a* is minimal. **B,** Downward movement of the humerus due to gravity is accompanied by lateral tracking of the humeral head as it follows the lateral curvature of the glenoid *(b)*. This increased distance between the glenoid and the head (*a* to *b*) stretches the surrounding soft tissue, which recoils and prevents further downward motion. Thus distance *c* is held to a minimum. **C,** The scapula is more downwardly rotated, and the inferior glenoid has moved out from under the humeral head. Movement down no longer produces lateral tracking. (Distance *a* is the same before and after the humerus drops.) Without lateral movement, the supportive tissues do not tighten and the humerus can move downward a greater distance, resulting in subluxation *(d)*.

When the hand holds a weight, the supraspinatus contracts to provide increased support. The supraspinatus may contract to support the upper extremity even when the hand does not hold a weight.[1] The correlation of subluxation with flaccid paralysis of the supraspinatus after a CVA verifies the role of the supraspinatus in the prevention of subluxation[3] (A Closer Look Box 7-2).

Muscle functions and axes

As we learn more about kinesiology, we realize that understanding a muscle's relationship to the axis or axes it crosses is more important than simply remembering muscle functions. However, a review of anatomy can refresh our minds about the attachments of muscles and their spatial relationships with other structures. Knowing a muscle's location often tells us what tasks it performs in functional activity.

The paired movements of glenohumeral abduction and adduction occur around a front-to-back axis. All muscles situated lateral or superior to this axis abduct this joint. Imagine a string tied to the insertion and pulled parallel to the muscle fibers toward the origin. As long as it maintains the same relationship to the axis, the string produces the same movement as the muscle. Try pulling the string toward a different origin, pulling on the opposite side of the axis; the opposite motion occurs (Figure 7-9).

The middle deltoid and supraspinatus lie superior, or lateral, to the glenohumeral joint; therefore they are glenohumeral abductors. The long head of the biceps shares this lateral relationship to the abduction axis only if the upper extremity is externally rotated. Thus positioning the upper extremity in external rotation allows the long head of the biceps to function as a glenohumeral abductor (Figure 7-10). The pectoralis major (sternal fibers), teres major, and latissimus dorsi have inferior relationships to this axis. They are adductors against resistance. (Remember that gravity is the most constant glenohumeral adductor.)

BOX 7-2

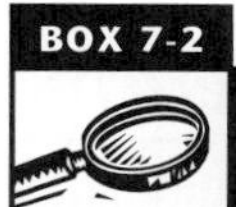

A **CLOSER** LOOK

Glenohumeral Subluxation

Efforts to reduce subluxation have consumed the time and energy of practitioners. Stimulation of the deltoid is an attractive technique because it immediately reduces glenohumeral subluxation by elevating the adducted, relaxed upper extremity. In many cases the target of stimulation is the easily located middle deltoid. Isolation and stimulation of this muscle quickly elevates the humeral head and reduces subluxation—but only as long as the muscle is stimulated. The deltoid will probably not elevate the humeral head on its own.

Basmajian and DeLuca[1] convincingly established that the middle deltoid is "inactive even with heavy pulls on the arm. Other muscles running vertically from the scapula to the humerus, particularly the biceps and long head of the triceps, were conspicuously inactive as well." The two researchers[1] demonstrated that only the supraspinatus and the posterior fibers of the deltoid were active in the prevention of subluxation. Because the middle deltoid does not function normally to hold the humeral head into the glenoid, external stimulation of these fibers is unlikely to reduce subluxation over time. Stimulation may facilitate voluntary control or strengthen the deltoid but does not lead to increased subluxation over time.

OT practitioners who stimulate the middle deltoid to reduce subluxation misinterpret research. Stimulation of the posterior deltoid and the supraspinatus, however, is effective in the reduction of subluxation.[4] Stimulation of these muscles is consistent with Basmajian and DeLuca's findings[1] and preferable to stimulation of the middle deltoid.

Basmajian and DeLuca[1] also explained that the superior joint structures—the joint capsule, supraspinatus, and posterior deltoid—and angulation of the glenoid all help prevent subluxation. If gravity's pull on the upper extremity forces the scapula to rotate downward and the glenoid to lose its orientation, the superior structures lose their effectiveness. In this way, downward movement of the humeral head does not create lateral movement and the superior structures are not stretched. OT practitioners may prevent subluxation successfully by improving an individual's scapular positioning and treating the upward scapular rotators.

Concern over subluxation often centers on the pain the individual is believed to experience. Two separate studies have demonstrated very little association between shoulder subluxation and pain after CVA.[2,7] In fact, more poststroke shoulder pain may be attributed to limited external rotation than to subluxation.[7] Effective treatment strategies for the reduction of shoulder pain and the prevention of stretching in the shoulder capsule include support of the affected upper extremity and use of natural means like lap trays and arm rests to help individuals maintain that support.

Muscles producing glenohumeral flexion, extension, and internal and external rotation depend on their relationships to the axes of movement the same way glenohumeral abductors and adductors do. The pectoralis major, coracobrachialis, biceps long head, and anterior deltoid flex because they pull forward on their insertions anterior to the side-to-side axis. The latissimus dorsi, teres major, and posterior deltoid extend because they pull posteriorly with posterior and inferior relationships to the axis. The pectoralis major, teres major, latissimus dorsi, anterior deltoid, and subscapularis are all internal rotators because they share a medial pull and an anterior relationship to the up-to-down axis for humeral rotation. On the opposite, posterior side of the axis, the infraspinatus, teres minor, and posterior deltoid externally rotate the humerus. Because the supraspinatus pulls through the up-to-down axis and is neither anterior nor posterior to it, it does not rotate, even though it is part of the rotator cuff muscle group.

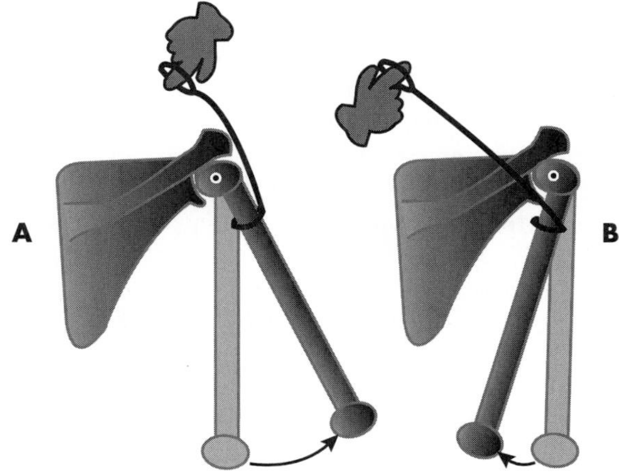

FIGURE **7-9**
A, Pulling a string tied to the deltoid insertion toward the origin, as long as the lateral relationship to the shoulder axis is maintained, produces abduction. **B,** Pulling the string toward a different origin medial to the axis results in adduction.

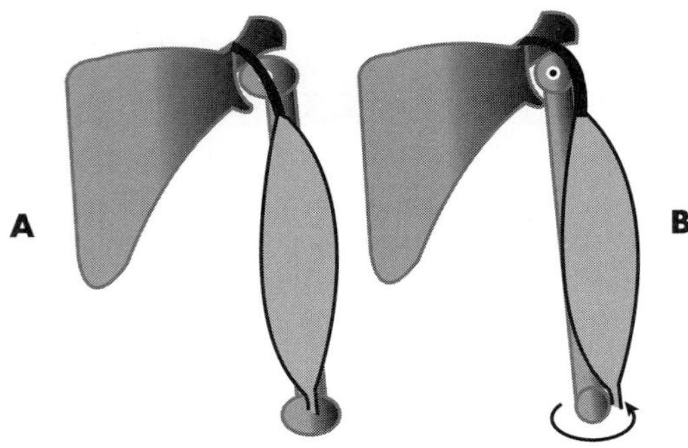

FIGURE **7-10**
A, The humerus is in a neutral position. **B,** The humerus is externally rotated, and the biceps long head acts as a glenohumeral abductor.

BOX 7-3

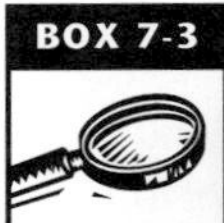

A **CLOSER** LOOK

Drawing of Muscle Function

A drawing of muscle function should include the view from which it is drawn. Always conceptualize the motion you draw occurring in a plane along the surface of the paper. Imagine looking down the axis of motion; therefore for flexion you would look down the side-to-side axis. The axis dictates what view you draw: side-to-side, side view; front-to-back, front (or back) view; and up-to-down, horizontal view (from the top). Remember that the axis of motion always sticks into the plane with a 90-degree orientation, so it appears as a dot on the page located in the center of the convex segment of the joint. For glenohumeral flexion, draw a side view and draw the side-to-side axis as a dot in the center of the humeral head.

Draw muscle force as a vector. In a typical open-chain motion in which the insertion moves, place your pencil on the insertion point and draw a straight line following the direction of muscle fibers toward the origin. If the fibers turn around a bony protuberance, do not follow the fibers but continue to draw the arrow straight, as if it were the tangent of a circle. Remember to make a scale and draw the arrow long enough to indicate the strength of the contraction. The arrowhead indicates the direction of the contraction and thus the movement.

Imagine that strings tied to these insertions are pulled toward the muscle's origins. As long as they match the correct relationships to the axis, a tug on the string produces the same function as the muscle produces (A Closer Look Box 7-3).

The Elbow Complex and Forearm

The elbow joint usually is presented as a hinge joint. However, considering the elbow as a complex of joints more accurately reflects its ability to allow flexion, extension, and radial rotation for supination and pronation. The ulna and radius articulate with the humerus to form a combination of joints.

ARTICULATIONS

Articulation between the humerus and ulna comprises the medial portion of the elbow complex. This ulnotrochlear hinge has one degree of freedom and allows movement (flexion and extension) in only one plane around one side-to-side axis. Laterally, the radius articulates with the humerus to form a shallow ball-and-socket radiocapitular joint. The attachment of the radius to the ulna through the interosseus membrane prevents abduction and adduction of the radius. Thus movement is not allowed at three axes. Flexion and extension and rotation are allowed.

The two more distal joints of the forearm, the proximal and distal radioulnar joints, are uniaxial joints allowing radial rotation for pronation and supination. Proximally the radius spins around an axis at its center. Distally it spins in a larger arc around an axis not in the center but closer to its ulnar edge. The shape of the radius and the manner in which its two ends attach to the ulna account for the different movements of the proximal and distal ends of the radius (Figure 7-11 and A Closer Look Box 7-4).

The radius curves slightly lateral from proximal to distal. A line drawn from the center of the proximal radius runs along the ulnar edge of the distal radius. This line forms the axis for pronation and supination (see Figure 7-11, *B*). Ulnar attachments of the distal and proximal radius complete the design and guarantee the different movement arcs of these two ends.

Proximally, the radius is held close to the ulna by the annular ligament and allowed to spin within the ligament. Distally, the ulnar edge of the radius is held closely adjacent to the ulna by the articular disk. This attachment causes the distal radius to spin around the ulna. (Notice that the radius is attached to the distal ulna on the articulated human skeleton by way of a pin or screw through the center of the ulna.) These different centers of rotation allow the radius to cross over the ulna in pronation so that it brings the hand from palm up to palm down.

FLEXION AND EXTENSION

Elbow flexion occurs when muscle forces are directed proximally, anterior to the side-to-side flexion and extension axis. The biceps, brachialis, and brachioradialis are the largest muscle masses with this relationship. Mus-

BOX 7-4

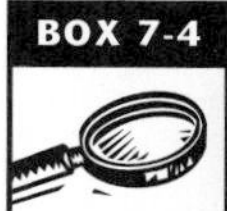

A CLOSER LOOK

A Straight Radius

If the radius were straight like the humerus and had similar proximal and distal attachments, it would rotate around an axis within itself both proximally and distally, spelling disaster for pronation and supination of the hand. The hand would have to completely dislocate from the ulna to pronate and turn the palm down (see Figure 7-11, A). However, its curved design bends the radius away from its long axis (see Figure 7-11, B). This and the different proximal and distal attachments allow the radius to rotate around itself proximally and around the ulna distally. The ulna and the ulnar aspect of the wrist and hand remain connected as the radius brings the hand around the ulna.

cles like the extensor carpi radialis longus and pronator teres, by virtue of their anterior locations and origins on the humeral epicondyles, may assist in elbow flexion. Their attachments close to the flexion axis produce short moment arms for flexion and explain their minimal function in this movement. The triceps has a posterior relationship to the side-to-side elbow axis and serves the major elbow extensor.

Inhibition of the biceps

Flexion of the forearm in forearm supination involves strong activation of the biceps, which both supinates and flexes. When the elbow flexes with the forearm in pronation, the biceps is nearly inactive and elbow flexion occurs mainly through activation of the brachialis.

An electromyographic (EMG) recording of the biceps demonstrates this activation pattern. Flexing the forearm in supination produces a clear signal that indicates activity in the biceps. A constant signal from the biceps when the elbow is supinated and flexed to about 90 degrees indicates an isometric contraction. The signal from the biceps decreases as the forearm pronates, even though the elbow remains flexed to 90 degrees.

The EMG signal changes as different muscles are activated to perform combinations. When the biceps shortens in a concentric contraction, its force creates tendencies toward elbow flexion and forearm supination. (The biceps has a moment arm for elbow flexion and forearm supination, which activate the biceps.) Without the biceps, two muscles—the brachialis is at the elbow and the supinator at the forearm—must be activated.

If the task requires elbow flexion with forearm pronation, the biceps can flex the elbow but the pronator must contract to cancel the supination effect of the biceps on the forearm. Using the biceps in this situation involves activation of two muscles when only one is necessary. The brachialis allows elbow flexion without the tendency toward supination because it inserts only on the ulna and has no pronation or supination effect. Once the forearm is pronated, the brachialis alone flexes the elbow, rendering the pronator unnecessary.

When ***Mary Smith*** arrived at Maple Grove Skilled Care Facility, she held her right arm flexed tightly against her body. She refused to let any nurses or aides move her arm through passive range of motion, so the nursing supervisor contacted the OT department. The OT assistant who

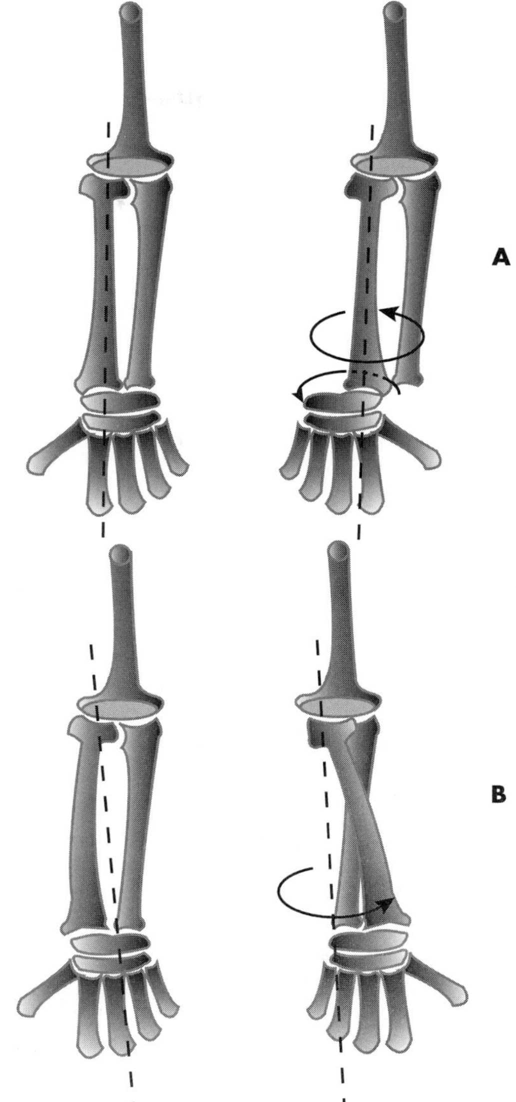

FIGURE **7-11**
Supination and pronation with a straight radius **(A)** would be a disaster. The slightly curved radius **(B)** allows the movement.

went to see Mary explained that putting her arm through range of motion probably would help her not to feel so stiff and sore all the time. The OT assistant promised to try some new techniques that would make range of motion less painful than it had been in the past.

First, the OT assistant gave Mary's right arm a gentle rubdown to gain Mary's trust and then slowly pronated her forearm to inhibit the biceps. The OT assistant explained to Mary that in the past, medical practitioners may have attempted to extend her elbow with her palm up in supination, a position associated with increased activity in the biceps. By pronating the forearm first, the OT assistant inactivated the biceps and made elbow extension easier and more comfortable. The OT assistant continued to explain that elbow extension in pronation stretches the tight biceps tendon even further because both of the biceps' antagonistic movements—extension and pronation—occur simultaneously. After Mary and the Maple Grove nursing staff learned this technique, daily range of motion became easier and more beneficial for everyone.

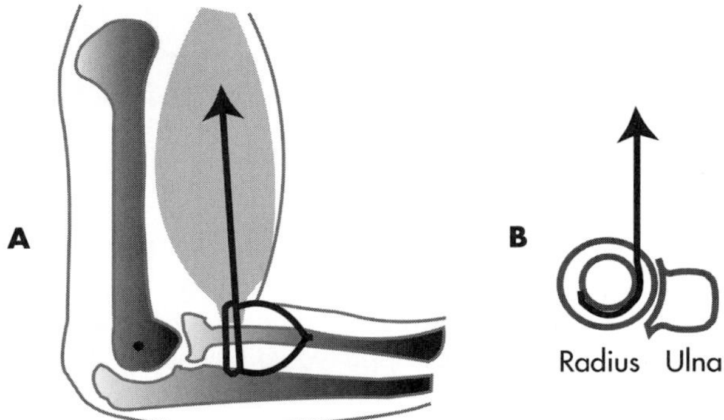

FIGURE **7-12**
The biceps spins the radius like a top to produce the rotation necessary for forearm supination. A side view **(A)** and a cross-sectional view **(B)** of the radius and ulna.

PRONATION AND SUPINATION

Pronation and supination arise from forces that pull the radius across the forearm toward the ulna. Anterior forces (pronator teres and pronator quadratus) produce pronation; posterior forces (supinator) result in supination. The strongest supinator, the biceps, wraps around the radius when the forearm is pronated like a string wraps around a top. Contraction of the biceps spins the top (the radius), producing supination (Figure 7-12). (Flexing the elbow to midposition clarifies this relationship and displays the most effective action.)

The brachioradialis can function as both a pronator and a supinator. Like the muscles previously described, the brachioradialis directs a force that pulls the radius toward the ulna. As the forearm pronates, the brachioradialis' force is dorsal to the axis for pronation and supination and supinates the forearm to midposition. At mid-position it loses this relationship, and its role as a supinator stops. When the forearm is fully supinated, the brachioradialis directs a force on the volar (flexor) side of the axis and causes pronation to midposition (Figure 7-13). The direction of pull and its relationship to the axis help explain the brachioradialis' contradictory functions.

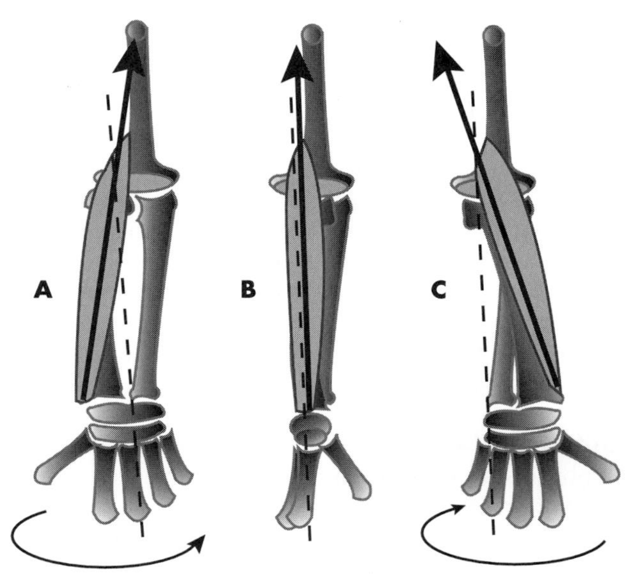

FIGURE **7-13**
The brachioradialis changes its relationship with the pronation and supination axis as it moves the forearm. In this view, intersection of the axis *(dotted line)* by the force vector means the muscle produces movement. **A,** The forearm is supinated, and the brachioradialis pronates. **B,** The forearm is in a neutral position, and the brachioradialis has no effect. **C,** The forearm is pronated, and the brachioradialis supinates.

Isolation of the supinator

The biceps is larger and stronger than the supinator but is not always active. Quieting the biceps and performing supination with only the supinator helps determine function in the radial nerve. Because supination can be performed with the biceps or supinator, two nerves—the musculocutaneous and radial—are involved. If an individual can supinate using only the supinator, an injured radial nerve has regenerated and reconnected.

Eduardo Ybarra visited the hand-therapy clinic after cutting his forearm with a saw. The OT practitioner evaluating him needed to know whether innervation to the supinator had been affected. The OT practitioner knew that performing supination rapidly or with the flexed elbow supporting the weight of the forearm would activate the biceps. Isolating the supinator, the OT practitioner posi-

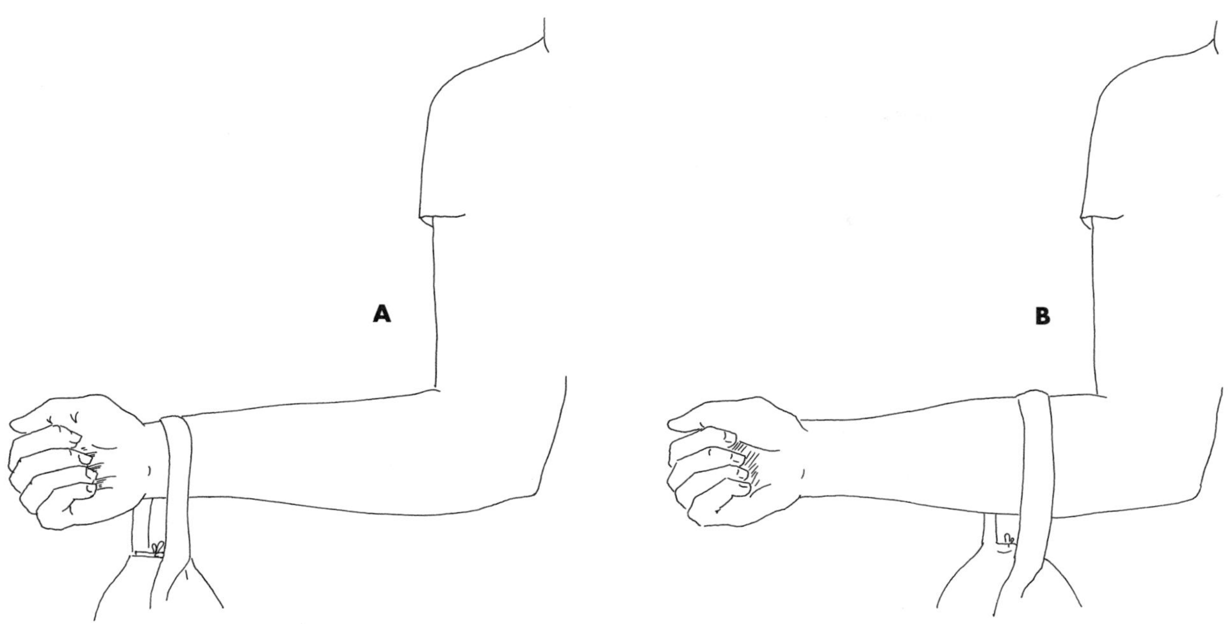

FIGURE **7-14**
Linda places her 5-kg handbag at the wrist **(A)** and near the elbow **(B).**

tioned the forearm in a supported, flexed, and pronated position. The practitioner palpated the biceps tendon in the cubital fossa and instructed Eduardo to turn his palm up slowly. Under normal conditions, the supinator activates alone in this position. If radial nerve function does not return, the supinator remains inactive and the biceps is activated. The OT practitioner did not feel any action in the biceps tendon and concluded that Eduardo's radial nerve was functioning distally at least as far as his supinator.

Function and Adaptation

Ergonomics concerns itself with not only which muscles are active in movement but also how the activity changes under different conditions. Elbow flexors produce an upward force that supports the flexed elbow when the hand holds a weight, but at the same time this muscle force compresses the joint. The biceps force pulls the ulna upward against the humerus **(joint force).**

CARRYING A HANDBAG

Linda Valdez was recently diagnosed with rheumatoid arthritis, and the OT practitioners caring for her are concerned about the large handbag she carries. The handbag puts a hefty load on her elbow flexors. The reaction forces produced by her biceps may damage the fragile elbow joint when she carries this handbag.

In Figure 7-14, Linda, who weighs 60 kg, places a 5-kg handbag at her wrist, 20 cm from the center of rotation at the elbow joint *(A)*. Her elbow is flexed to 90 degrees, and her forearm is supinated. The force produced by the biceps muscle has a moment arm of 4 cm and a line of application parallel to the long axis of the humerus. Linda carries the same purse closer to her elbow, 10 cm from the center of rotation at the elbow joint *(B)*.

The resistance forces produced by Linda's handbag operate with two very different moment arms. How large a force must Linda's biceps muscle generate to counteract the torque produced by the weight of the handbag? From an ergonomic standpoint, how does moving the handbag closer to or farther from the joint affect the forces acting on her elbow joint? How large is the reaction force *(R)* at the ulnotrochlear joint?

To find the weight of Linda's forearm, multiply her total body weight by the percentage of body weight taken up by the forearm and hand (see Appendix B). Remember to convert centimeters to meters:

$$60 \text{ kg} \times 0.02 = 1.2 \text{ kg}$$

Draw the force of gravity affecting the forearm by locating its center of gravity in Appendix B:

$0.43 \times 20 \text{ cm} = 8.6 \text{ cm}$
(from the elbow to the center of gravity in the forearm)

The force of the biceps under each condition requires the equation for equilibrium of torques in opposite di-

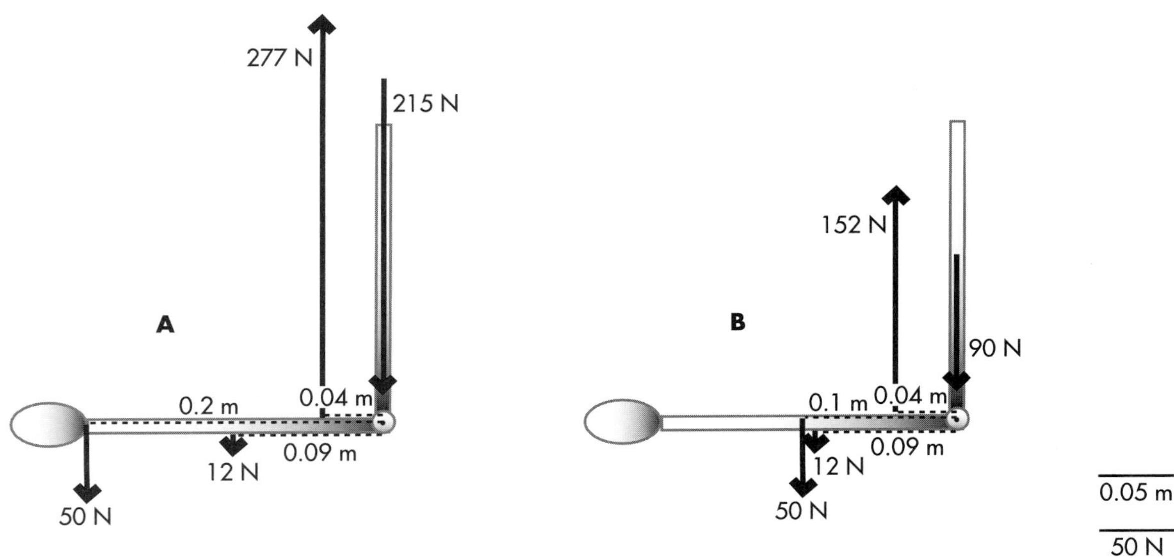

FIGURE **7-15**
A, The biceps must produce 277 N of force when Linda holds her 5-kg handbag at the wrist.
B, A force of only 152 N is needed when she places it closer to her elbow.

rections. Remember to convert centimeters to meters and kilograms to newtons:

$$(50\text{ N} \times 0.2\text{ m}) + (12\text{ N} \times 0.09\text{ m}) = \text{B} \times 0.04\text{ m}$$
$$10\text{ Nm} + 1.08\text{ Nm} = \text{B} \times 0.04\text{ m}$$
$$11.08\text{ Nm} = \text{B} \times 0.04\text{ m}$$
$$\text{B} = 277\text{ N}$$
$$(50\text{ N} \times 0.1\text{ m}) + (12\text{ N} \times 0.09\text{ m}) = \text{B} \times 0.04\text{ m}$$
$$5\text{ Nm} + 1.08\text{ Nm} = \text{B} \times 0.04\text{ m}$$
$$6.08\text{ Nm} = \text{B} \times 0.04\text{ m}$$
$$\text{B} = 152\text{ N}$$

Linda's biceps must contract with greater force as she places the handbag closer to her wrist (Figure 7-15). The upward biceps forces pull up the ulna against the trochlea of the humerus and create compression. The matching downward force (reaction force or joint force) is directed through the humerus and exerted onto the matching surface of the ulna at the joint. A lack of movement up or down creates a state of linear equilibrium. (Remember Newton's law about action and reaction.) Converting centimeters to meters and kilograms to newtons, determine the downward reaction force. Use the formula for equilibrium of upward and downward forces:

$$277\text{ N} = \text{R} + 50\text{ N} + 12\text{ N}$$
$$\text{R} = 277\text{ N} - 50\text{ N} - 12\text{ N}$$
$$\text{R} = 215\text{ N downward}$$
$$152\text{ N} = \text{R} + 50\text{ N} + 12\text{ N}$$
$$\text{R} = 152\text{ N} - 50\text{ N} - 12\text{ N}$$
$$\text{R} = 90\text{ N downward}$$

Linda's biceps works twice as hard to hold the handbag at her wrist; the reaction force more than doubles. The OT practitioners explain the danger of strong joint reaction forces and their destructive effect on Linda's fragile joints. They show her how to protect her joints by moving even relatively light loads closer to the affected joints.

EXTENDING THE ELBOW

Despite her C5 quadriplegia, ***Bernice Richards*** uses elbow extension to operate the brakes on her automobile hand controls. She also plants her hands on the bed and performs a push-up motion to sit up and don her socks. OT interns question OT staff members, "Elbow extension without elbow extensors? How can it be?"

The staff members point out that these movements involve elbow extension and shoulder flexion. Bernice links elbow extension and shoulder flexion by planting her hand. This stabilizes the chain's distal end so that shoulder flexion causes elbow extension. Because Bernice has muscle strength in her shoulders, she can move both the shoulder and the elbow as long as her hand is stabilized. Once Bernice's hand is free in space, elbow and shoulder motions are independent.

The OT interns know that higher cervical segments innervate the shoulder flexors. They begin to visualize how stabilizing the hand affects the interdependency of upper-extremity segments. The elbow-shoulder link creates elbow extension via the shoulder flexors, laying bare the mystery of elbow extension without elbow extensors.

The OT staff members also note that Bernice externally rotates her humerus at the end of the extension movement when pushing her trunk into a vertical position. This terminal external shoulder rotation produces a few more degrees of shoulder flexion and hyperextends the elbow. Because Bernice has 5 degrees or more of elbow hyperextension, she can hold the terminal elbow position using hyperextension as a lock. The weight of her upper trunk creates a force that resists elbow flexion. It is directed behind the elbow axis when the elbow is hyperextended. Bernice's ligaments prevent further hyperextension, and her elbow remains stable in hyperextension as long as her trunk's weight remains posterior to the axis. OT staff members note that individuals often hyperextend the knees to bear weight with little muscular effort when they feel fatigued. Both motions conserve energy, using ligaments to counter gravity.

Summary

The more deeply we study the shoulder and elbow, the more information we discover. Our hands get where we want them to go because of sternoclavicular joint freedom and scapular movement. The rotator cuff muscles form a cuff but are much more than simple rotators. Scapular muscles sometimes move the trunk. Heavy handbags can create dangerous joint-reaction forces. The elbow sometimes flexes and extends because of muscles that move the shoulder. All these mysteries become clear once we apply a few relatively simple concepts from biomechanics.

Applications

APPLICATION 7-1
Muscle Function Simulations

Use duct tape to attach a string to the deltoid tubercle on the humerus. Pull the string toward the (1) acromion lateral to the front-to-back axis, (2) distal clavicle anterior to the side-to-side axis, (3) midspine of the scapula posterior to the side-to-side axis, and (4) sacrum posterior and inferior to the side-to-side axis.

What happens each time? Which muscle does each new pull represent? In the last case, contrast the rotational effect on the humerus with that of the latissimus. In all cases, why do you have to pull so hard to effect movement?

APPLICATION 7-2
Muscle Function Drawings

Prove to yourself that you can demonstrate muscle function by drawing the force of contraction in its proper relationship to the axis of motion. Draw the humerus, elbow, and ulna. Next, draw a force representing the pull of the brachialis on the ulna that produces flexion. Can you redraw the brachialis force as if the brachialis were surgically reattached to become an elbow extensor?

APPLICATION 7-3
Limited Shoulder Strength

Hospital engineers are designing door handles that all patients in the spinal cord unit can use. They have asked the OT department to help them determine how much force average patients have available to operate a door handle using shoulder flexors and abductors. Figure 7-16 depicts a 60-kg man with C5 quadriplegia and fair muscle grades in shoulder flexion and abduction. Figure 7-17 depicts another man with poor muscle grades who can achieve shoulder flexion to only 70 degrees and abduction to 50 degrees. The door handle the engineers are designing must be operated by a movement midway between shoulder flexion and abduction.

The muscle fibers of the anterior and middle deltoid lie approximately at a 30-degree angle from each other and 2 cm from the axis of motion in the glenohumeral joint. With the arm outstretched, the center of gravity for the entire upper extremity falls approximately at the elbow, about 30 cm from the shoulder joint in an average person.

7-3A. How much force is available to individuals with fair anterior and middle deltoid muscle grades?

7-3B. How much force is available to individuals with poor anterior and middle deltoid muscle grades?

7-3C. How much force is available in fair and poor strength ranges when anterior and middle deltoid fibers are combined in midrange?

Discussion. Is any advantage gained through use of a range midway between shoulder flexion and abduction? How can manual muscle testing and goniometry be used as noninvasive methods in the determination of muscle forces available for daily activities?

APPLICATION 7-4
Loads on Upper-Extremity Joints

Keyboarding with an unsupported upper extremity may cause shoulder, elbow, and wrist fatigue. Although these joint positions are not extreme or awkward, gravity's pull on the forwardly positioned arm creates torques at each joint. ***Nancy Grant,*** a computer operator, weighs 50 kg. Determine the amount of torque gravity creates at her shoulder, elbow, and wrist joints (see Appendix B):

1. The upper extremity is 4.8% of total body weight.
2. The forearm and hand are 2.1% of total body weight.
3. The hand is 0.6% of total body weight.
4. The moment arm for the combined center of gravity extending Nancy's shoulder is 7.7 cm.

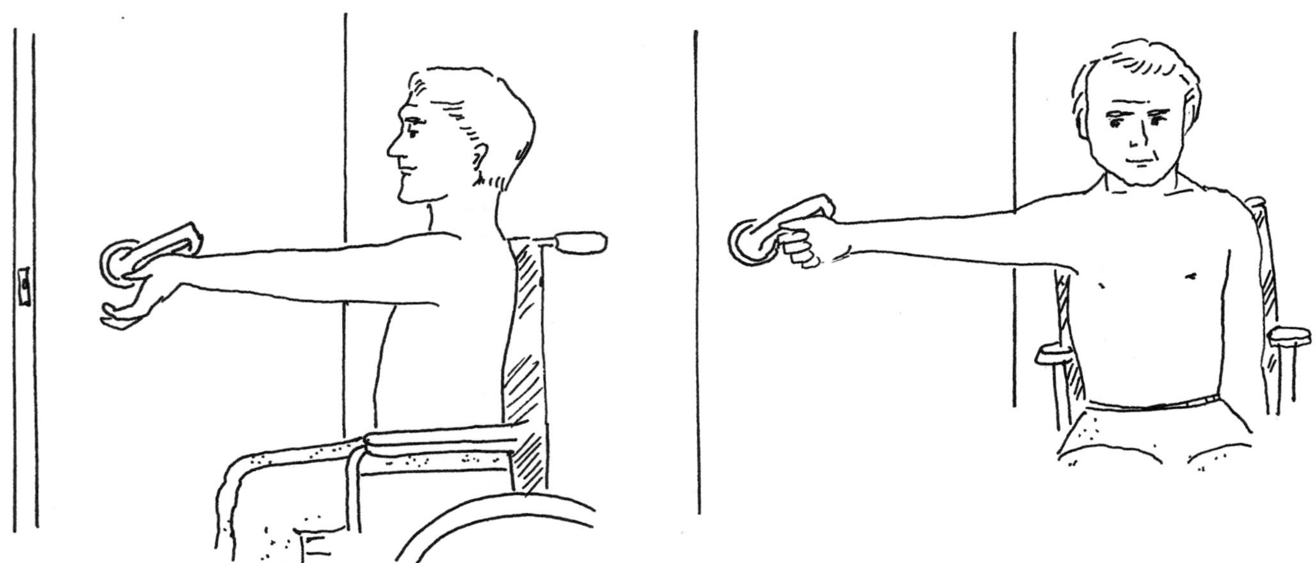

FIGURE **7-16**
The anterior and middle deltoid muscles measure fair strength at 90 degrees of shoulder flexion and abduction, respectively.

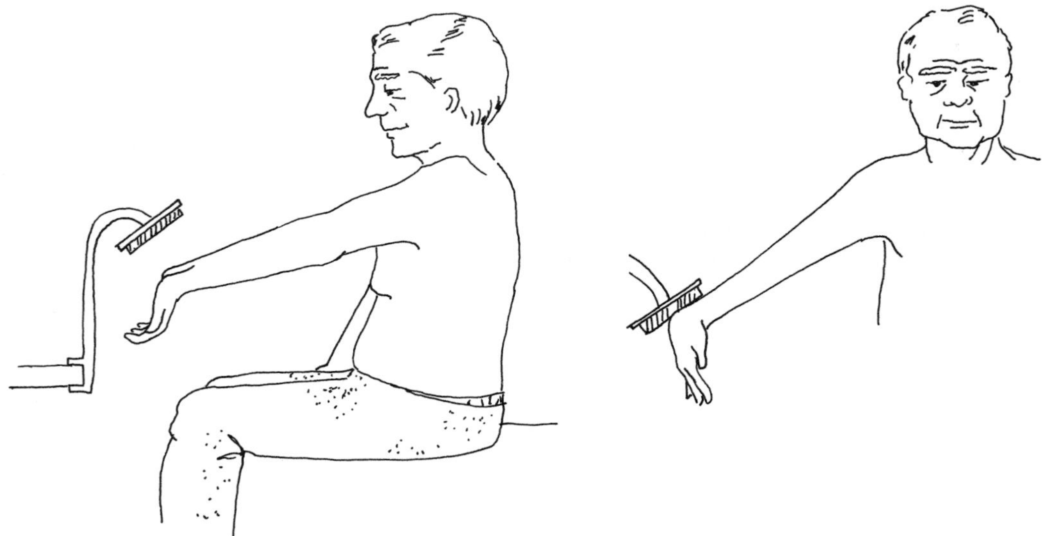

FIGURE **7-17**
Poor muscle grades in the anterior and middle deltoids result in less than 90 degrees of flexion and abduction. In this case, only 70 degrees of shoulder flexion and 50 degrees of abduction are possible.

5. The moment arm for the combined forearm and hand center of gravity extending Nancy's elbow is 6.8 cm.
6. The moment arm for the hand flexing the wrist is 2.3 cm.

Discussion. Interpret the requirements of the shoulder, elbow, and wrist joints in response to the tendencies created by gravity. How can the load on the muscles be reduced?

See Appendix C for solutions to Applications.

REFERENCES

1. Basmajian JV, DeLuca CJ: *Muscles alive: their functions revealed by electromyography,* ed 5, Baltimore, 1985, Williams & Wilkins.
2. Bohannon RW, Andrews AW: Shoulder subluxation and pain in stroke patients, *Am J Occup Ther* 44(6):507-509, 1990.
3. Chaco J, Wolf E: Subluxation of the glenohumeral joint in hemiplegia, *Am J Phys Med* 50:139-143, 1971.
4. Faghri PD and others: The effects of functional electrical stimulation on shoulder subluxation, arm function recovery, and shoulder pain in hemiplegic stroke patients, *Arch Phys Med Rehabil* 75(1):73-79, 1994.
5. Soderberg GL: *Kinesiology: application to pathological motion,* Baltimore, 1986, Williams & Wilkins.
6. Steindler A: *Kinesiology of the human body,* Springfield, Ill, 1973, Charles C Thomas.
7. Zorowitz RD and others: Shoulder pain and subluxation after stroke: correlation or coincidence? *Am J Occup Ther* 50(3):194-201, 1996.

RELATED READINGS

Hall SJ: *Basic biomechanics,* New York, 1995, McGraw-Hill.

Nordin M, Frankel VH: *Basic biomechanics of the musculoskeletal system,* Philadelphia, 1989, Lea & Febiger.

Williams PL, Bannister LH: *Gray's anatomy: the anatomical basis of medicine and surgery,* ed 38, New York, 1995, Churchill Livingstone.

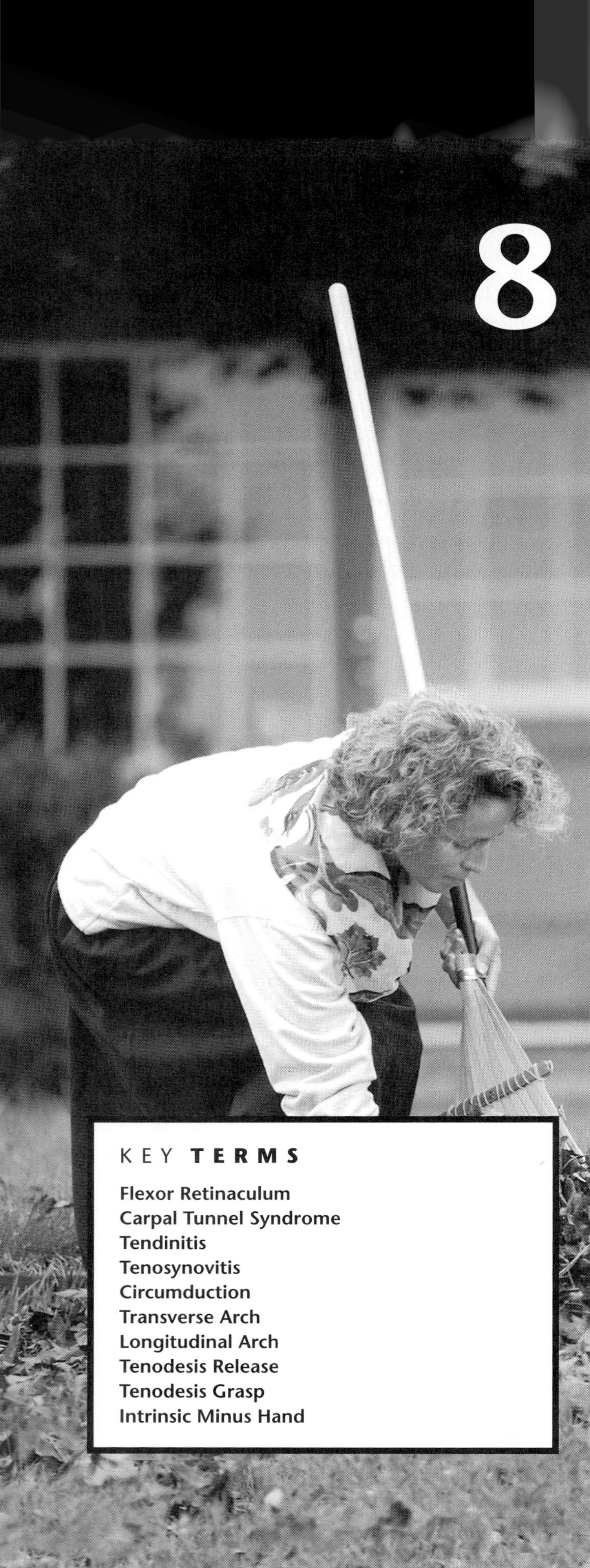

8 The Distal Upper Extremity

KEY TERMS

Flexor Retinaculum
Carpal Tunnel Syndrome
Tendinitis
Tenosynovitis
Circumduction
Transverse Arch
Longitudinal Arch
Tenodesis Release
Tenodesis Grasp
Intrinsic Minus Hand

CHAPTER OUTLINE

C *hapter 7 focused on* the importance of proximal upper-extremity joints, muscles, and movements. Although the hand is not the whole of the upper extremity, in this chapter we see that the hand is worthy of considerable attention. While the shoulder, elbow, and wrist move and position the hand, the hand grasps and manipulates to complete the task.

The same hand that allows us to break boards and cinder blocks in karate can manipulate a needle in microsurgery. The 15 joints in the thumb and fingers allow the hand to adapt to almost any position. A multitude of muscles, each with its own discrete neural control, allows us to perform a range of tasks, from holding a hammer with a power grip to picking up an egg with delicate pressure. We can position our thumb pad opposite the pads of the other fingers precisely enough to grasp one human hair. That same opposition movement locks the entire thumb around a rope tightly enough to support the body's weight.

The Wrist

Much more than a connection of the hand to the arm, the wrist positions the hand so that the long finger flexors and extensors can grasp and release objects. Wrist extensors allow us to grasp objects, and accompanying wrist flexors allow us to release them quickly. Likewise, ulnar deviation at the wrist powers functions such as hammering and throwing.

The wrist joint is composed of 8 carpal bones—joined in a semicircular arrangement around the central capitate bone—framed by the distal radius and ulnar disk. These 10 bones articulate with ligaments that form an arch, the concave surface of which lies at the base of the palm. Its convex surface forms the back of the hand. This osteofibrous structure, which provides a strong and stable attachment for muscles, is the structural foundation for the palm's complex contours.

On the palmar surface the hook of the hamate and pisiform bone on the ulnar side connect through the **flexor retinaculum** (transverse carpal ligament) to the more radially placed scaphoid and trapezium. The concave shape of the combined carpal bones and the fibrous roof provided by the flexor retinaculum form a carpal tunnel. This structure contains a large number of important neurovascular and tendinous structures that pass through to the hand. If these structures remain compressed over long periods of time, the individual can develop **carpal tunnel syndrome** (A Closer Look Box 8-1).

ARTICULATIONS

The wrist is classified as a condyloid joint, which allows movement around two axes. Flexion and extension occur in the sagittal plane around a double side-to-side axis. These movements involve two separate pairs of articulations—the radius and ulnar disk with the proximal row of carpals and the proximal with the distal row of carpals[8] (Figure 8-1).

Abduction and adduction occur in the frontal plane around the anterior-to-posterior axis found in the capitate bone. Frequently, we call wrist abduction *radial deviation* and wrist adduction *ulnar deviation.* **Circumduction** describes a combination of movements. From a neutral position the wrist moves into extension, then in sequence into radial deviation, flexion, and ulnar deviation before it moves back into extension. Because circumduction involves more than one movement, it involves more than one axis, unlike the true rotation in the forearm and arm. When we use paintbrushes and markers to draw circles, we demonstrate everyday examples of circumduction in action.

MUSCLES

Muscles named for their functions at the wrist contain the word *carpi* in their names and originate on or near the distal end of the humerus in association with the humeral epicondyles. The large area of muscle mass in the forearm produces the force the tendons transmit to stabilize the wrist and move the hand. Each muscle that crosses the wrist has a function at the wrist, even if it is named for a movement produced in the hand (finger flexion and extension).

Function depends on a muscle's relationship to the axes of motion, not on its name. Tendons that pass anterior to the wrist's side-to-side axis are wrist flexors, including the flexors carpi radialis and ulnaris and the flexors digitorum superficialis and profundus. Tendons that pass posterior to the side-to-side axis—the extensors carpi radialis longus and brevis, extensor carpi ulnaris, and extensors digitorum, indicis, and digiti minimi—extend the wrist. Although numerous digital muscles affect the wrist, this discussion concentrates first on muscles named for their wrist functions.

The flexors carpi ulnaris and radialis flex the wrist because both are anterior to the side-to-side axis. If they do not function together, movement becomes abnormal. The extensors carpi radialis longus, brevis, and ulnaris lie posterior to the same axis and extend the wrist. The extensors located on the radial and ulnar sides rely on each other to balance the extension.

BOX 8-1

A **CLOSER** LOOK

Carpal Tunnel Syndrome

Wendy Dabdoub *noticed tingling (paresthesia) in her thumb, her index finger, and occasionally in her ring finger (median nerve distribution). She associated this discomfort with her job. Wendy packs fruit for shipment, a job that involves repetitive, simultaneous wrist and finger flexion against resistance; her complaint is common among individuals with similar duties. If it is held too long or assumed and released too frequently against resistance, any extreme or awkward wrist position can lead to carpal tunnel syndrome.*

Carpal tunnel syndrome has a variety of causes, including medical conditions associated with tissue swelling and orthopedic problems. ***Linda Valdez,*** *who has rheumatoid arthritis, is at risk for developing carpal tunnel syndrome, as is* ***Henry Isaacs,*** *who fractured his wrist in a fall at Maple Grove Skilled Care Facility. These risks are fairly obvious, but unless we take a closer look at Wendy's workplace, we cannot determine the cause of her condition.*

In Wendy's case the problem stems from both direct pressure on the median nerve and overuse of the tendons of the flexor digitorum superficialis and profundus. Finger flexion in a position of wrist flexion puts direct pressure on the median nerve between the flexor retinaculum and the flexor tendons. As wrist and finger flexor tendons squeeze the median nerve against the tight flexor retinaculum, wrist trauma results. (We will discuss this in more detail in the section on bowstringing.)

Repeated finger flexion and extension with a flexed wrist forces the finger flexor tendons to travel back and forth on the edge of the flexor retinaculum. This friction inflames the tendons ***(tendinitis)*** *and their sheaths* ***(tenosynovitis),*** *which causes swelling in the wrist.*

The carpal tunnel is a closed passage top to bottom and side to side. Structures passing through lie close together with little room to spare. Thus swollen tissues take up more room, squeezing the tunnel's contents. The cramped space puts direct pressure on the median nerve, which decreases blood flow to this nerve (ischemia). Paresthesia (the "pins-and-needles" sensation) on the radial half of the hand, the area of skin supplied by cutaneous branches of the median nerve, is often the first sign of trouble. If pressure continues, nerve damage affects both the cutaneous and motor fibers of the median nerve. Malfunction of motor fibers or altered sensory feedback may weaken grasp, a secondary symptom. Prolonged, poorly managed carpal tunnel syndrome causes atrophy of the hand's thenar muscles.

Removing the damaging influence (overuse) is the most reasonable treatment in Wendy's case. Cutting the flexor retinaculum (carpal tunnel release surgery) to cure overuse, although it creates more room in the passage, ignores the real cause of the problem. Returning to the harmful practices responsible for the tendinitis and swelling usually leads to recurrence. Job-site analysis and appropriate recommendations are likely to generate more lasting solutions.

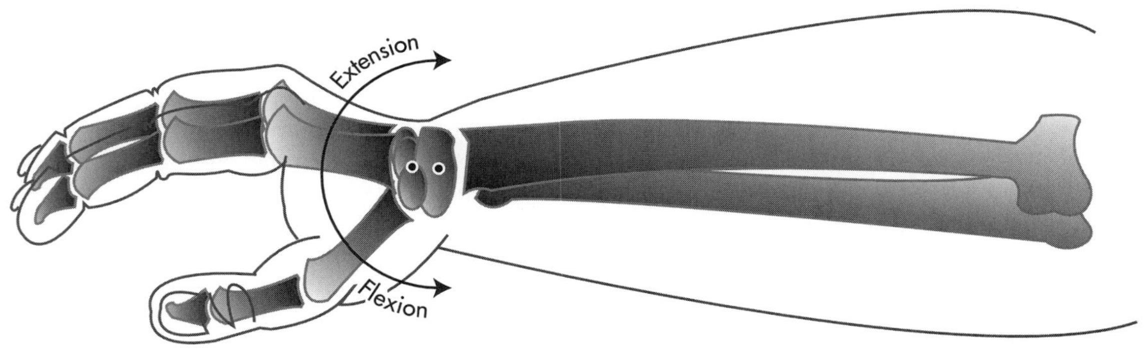

FIGURE **8-1**
Wrist flexion and extension occur at more than one side-to-side axis because wrist articulation is so complex.

Flexors and extensors working in the correct combinations deviate the wrist; therefore no muscle has the word *deviator* in its name. The radial wrist flexors and extensors, lateral to the front-to-back axis, work together to radially deviate. The ulnar flexors and extensors medial to the same axis produce ulnar deviation.

Imagine the hand as a puppet and the muscle forces as strings attached to the four corners of the wrist. The strings balance the hand when the forearm is upright. Without these strings the hand tends to assume flexion, extension, or ulnar or radial deviation. Muscle forces balance each of these gravity tendencies but do not lie directly opposite the tendencies.

Paired wrist muscles function like certain back muscles; two work together to cancel one effect and produce another. Activation of the radial and ulnar wrist extensors balances the wrist in extension. Use of one, for example, the extensor carpi ulnaris, produces combined extension and ulnar deviation because the ulnaris like other wrist muscles functions across two axes. This extensor functions with the extensor carpi radialis longus and cancels the deviation effects, producing balanced extension.

Balanced wrist flexion and radial and ulnar deviation follow the same logical progression. The radial and ulnar wrist flexors—the flexor carpi radialis and flexor carpi ulnaris—contract to flex the wrist. Together they cancel deviation, producing wrist flexion. Radial deviation requires that the two radial wrist muscles—the flexor carpi radialis and extensor carpi radialis longus—cancel each others' flexion and extension tendencies. Likewise, the flexor carpi ulnaris and extensor carpi ulnaris cancel each others' flexion and extension, producing ulnar deviation.

The clinical significance of these normal synergistic relationships is clear. Loss of any one wrist muscle results in severe but predictable wrist imbalance. When ***Eduardo Ybarra*** damaged his radial nerve near the elbow, his extensor carpi ulnaris ceased to function. The OT practitioner expects to see weakness in wrist extension because he has one fewer muscle available. When Eduardo extends his wrist, only his radial wrist extensors function, resulting in weakened wrist extension. In addition, unwanted radial deviation accompanies extension because the extensor carpi ulnaris is unavailable to cancel the deviation effect.

The biggest problem created by loss of the extensor carpi ulnaris is unbalanced, severely weakened ulnar deviation. Without this muscle, Eduardo's attempts at ulnar deviation result in flexion and ulnar deviation by the flexor carpi ulnaris. (The muscle's name—*flexor carpi ulnaris,* or *flexor of carpus (wrist) on the ulnar side*—describes its combined function in the absence of its partner.) Furthermore, Eduardo's ulnar deviation is minimal because the extensor carpi ulnaris is the stronger muscle in ulnar deviation. How can Eduardo lose one ulnar extensor and experience his greatest deficit in ulnar deviation?

Paul Brand, a renowned hand surgeon and author, and Anne Hollister demonstrated the true functions of the wrist muscles.[2] The work shows that many wrist muscles are named for functions quite different than those they actually perform.

Figure 8-2 provides Brand and Hollister's summary[2] of muscle function at the wrist based on moment arms for the various movements. The graph indicates the length of each wrist muscle's moment arm for flexion, extension, and ulnar and radial deviation. Muscles with the longest moment arms for ulnar or radial deviation are at the extreme positions of the x axis. The longest moment arms for flexion or extension are at the extreme positions of the y axis. The farther each muscle is from the intersection, the greater its tendency to perform that function.

The graph clarifies that each named wrist muscle produces two movements. Originally, each muscle was named for the strongest action anatomists believed it produced. The flexors carpi radialis and ulnaris function primarily as their names suggest, which is indicated by their longer moment arms for flexion than for deviation. The same is true for the extensor carpi radialis brevis.

The extensors carpi radialis longus and ulnaris do not adhere to this naming scheme; each has a longer moment arm for deviation than for extension. In fact, the ulnaris has a moment arm for ulnar deviation more than four times that for extension. (Brand[3] suggests that a more appropriate name, such as *adductor carpi dorsalis,* would emphasize deviation instead of extension.) This graphic summary of each muscle's effect on the wrist explains why loss of the extensor carpi ulnaris creates a greater deficit in ulnar deviation than in extension.

BALANCE AFTER TENDON TRANSFER

Surgeons use Brand and Hollister's findings[2] to make decisions about the transfer of function from innervated to noninnervated muscles. In Eduardo's case, a second injury resulted in the loss of all wrist extensor function. His surgeon suggested that Eduardo's pronator teres may replace lost wrist extension. Eduardo's surgeon detached the pronator at its insertion, split it, and reinserted one side onto the distal extensor carpi radialis brevis tendon and the other onto the ulnar side of the fourth metacarpal.

However, a surgical procedure like this involves extensive planning. The pronator teres often is reinserted only onto the extensor carpi radialis brevis tendon distally because this tendon has a lesser moment arm for radial deviation than the extensor carpi radialis longus. Brand and Hollister[2] note that the brevis, although it is less of a radial deviator than the longus, still has a substantial moment arm for deviation (see Figure 8-2). If the pronator is attached only to the brevis, wrist exten-

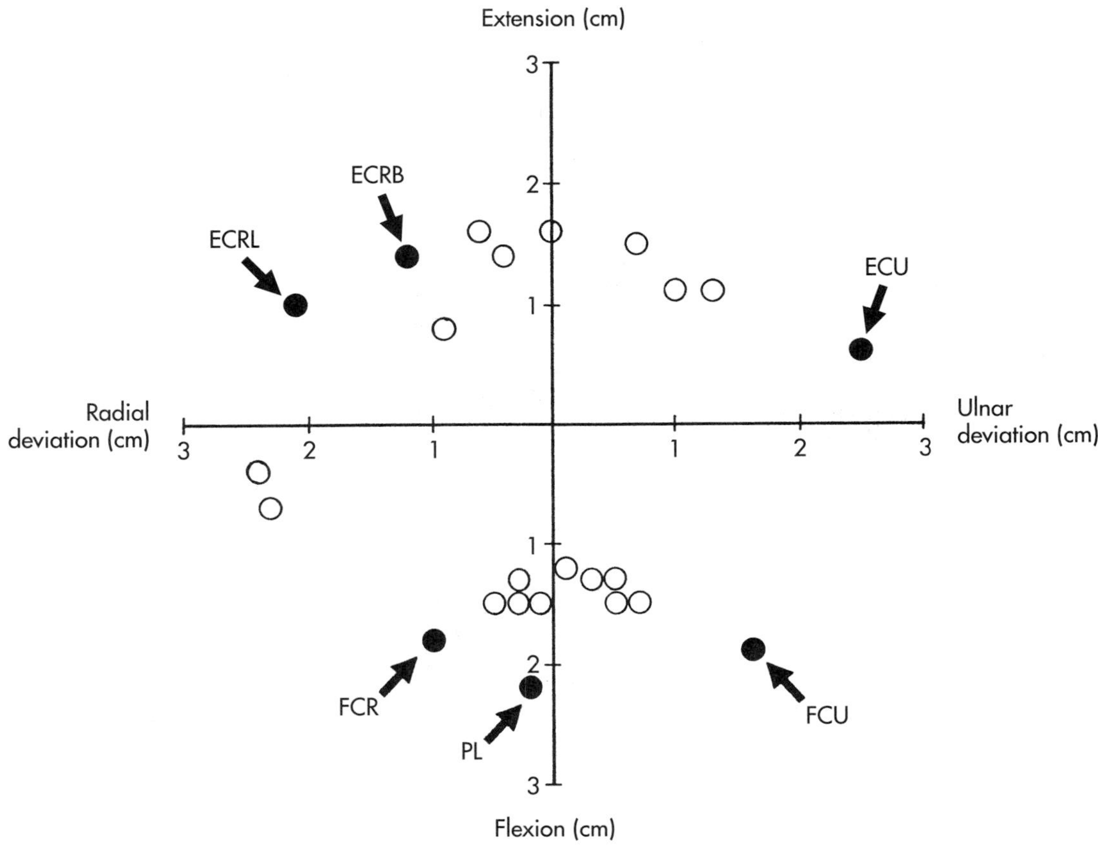

FIGURE **8-2**
Moment arms for the various wrist muscles (extensors and flexors) producing wrist flexion, extension, and deviation. *ECRB,* Extensor carpi radialis brevis; *ECRL,* extensor carpi radialis longus; *ECU,* extensor carpi ulnaris; *FCR,* flexor carpi radialis; *FCU,* flexor carpi ulnaris; *PL,* pollicis longus. (Modified from Brand PW, Hollister A: *Clinical mechanics of the hand,* ed 2, St Louis, 1993, Mosby.)

sion produces unwanted radial deviation, creating wrist imbalance. Eduardo's surgeon followed one of Brand and Hollister's two suggestions[2] for balanced wrist extension. The ulnar insertion on the fourth metacarpal matches the extension moment arm of the brevis. It also provides an ulnar deviation moment arm nearly equal to the radial deviation moment arm of the brevis. The two attachments cancel each others' deviation effects; contraction of the pronator teres then produces balanced wrist extension. Thus Eduardo regains balanced wrist extension through transfer of the pronator teres.

The Hand

The hand is composed of 19 bones (27, including the carpal bones); 18 intrinsic muscles also begin and end in the hand. In addition, 18 more tendons from the extrinsic muscles terminate in the hand. They transmit forces from the long flexors and extensors and the thumb abductor, the bellies of which are located in the forearm. We have considered muscles acting across one or two joints, but the majority of hand muscles cross two or more joints. In fact most extrinsic muscle tendons function across four joints, including the wrist.

Achieving muscle balance in the hand makes wrist balance appear easy. Fingers flex in a variety of grasps, and the weight of each object in the hand creates resistance. Muscles, especially extrinsic muscles, give and take in function, one yielding in passive distal excursion as its antagonist contracts to produce movement. In both grasp and release, the intrinsic muscles balance the effects of long flexors and extensors.

ARCHES

A relaxed hand yields valuable information about its structure. We tend to imagine the hand in action, grasp-

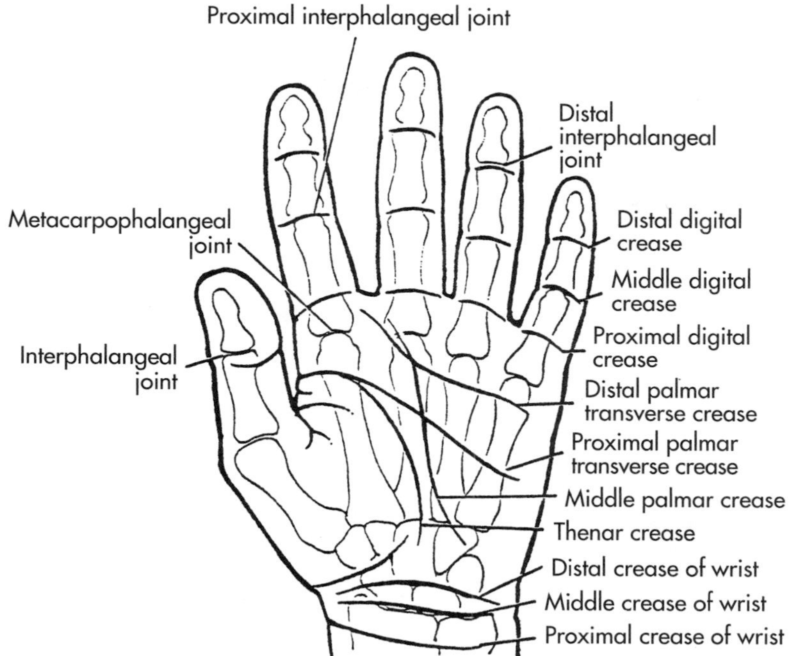

FIGURE **8-3**
Palmar skin creases are related to underlying wrist and digital joints. Metacarpophalangeal joints lie at the level of the distal palmar crease. (From Fess EE, Philips CA: *Hand splinting principles and methods,* ed 2, St Louis, 1987, Mosby.)

ing, opening with a cupped palm, or finely manipulating small objects.

Hands are full of creases, shadows, and curves (Figure 8-3); they have no flat places. Two arches, oriented 90 degrees to each other, furnish the overall curved effect. The **transverse arch** curves from the radial to the ulnar side of the hand. Its apex, or highest point, lies near the head of the third metacarpal (Figure 8-4, *A*). The **longitudinal arch** curves from the wrist to the fingertips (Figure 8-4, *B*). The row of metacarpal heads (2 through 5) is the highest point in the longitudinal arch. This arch is longest at metacarpal number 2 and shortest at number 5 due to the different lengths of the metacarpals and the corresponding metacarpophalangeal (MCP) joints. OT practitioners who fail to appreciate the short length of the longitudinal arch on the ulnar side of the hand create splints that extend too far distally and block flexion of MCP joints 4 and 5.

Both arches change shape as the hand moves to manipulate objects, but its relaxed state is the key to an understanding of hand structure. The radial and ulnar ends of the hand (metacarpals 1, 4, and 5) are more mobile than ligament-bound metacarpal heads 2 and 3. The degree of radial freedom is most obvious in thumb movement. Cup your hand or manually wiggle the fifth metacarpal head in alternating anterior and posterior directions to demonstrate the ulnar side's mobility. Hands must relax into their arches and not be forced into a more flattened position with a splint. Avoid disturbing the basic architecture of these normal arches in any focus on a specific hand problem.

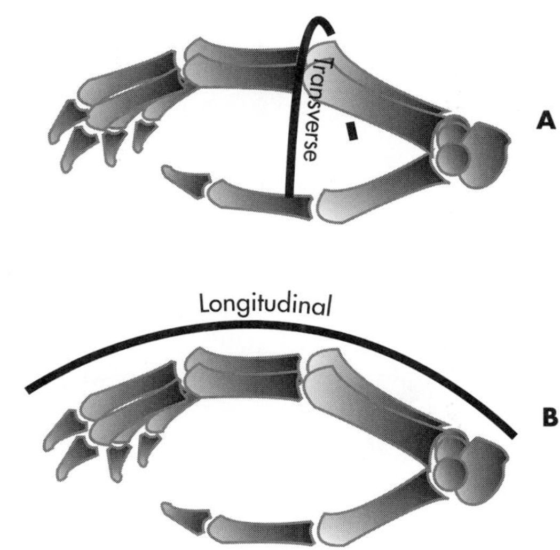

FIGURE **8-4**
The transverse **(A)** and longitudinal **(B)** arches.

ARTICULATIONS

The serial arrangement of finger joints and nearly parallel arrangement of fingers gives the hand its freedom of movement. Fingers 2 through 4 articulate with the metacarpals at the condyloid MCP joints. These joints allow flexion and extension and abduction and adduction. Because of the joint shape and arrangement of ligaments, full flexion of the MCP joints involves maximal stretch of the ligaments and limits abduction and adduction (Figure 8-5 and A Closer Look Box 8-2).

The IP joints of digits 2 through 5 are hinge joints that allow flexion and extension only. These joints move in one fewer plane than the MCP joints, but both proximal and distal IPs are essential for finger-to-palm grasp. The many IP joints alone allow grasp between the digital pads and the distal palm. Working with both types of joints permits a whole-hand grasp that ranges in diameter from smaller than a broomstick straw to larger than a soda can. Normally, flexion and extension of the MCP and IP joints occur together, but muscle function imbalance caused by disease or injury produces isolated and incongruous movement of MCP to IP joints.

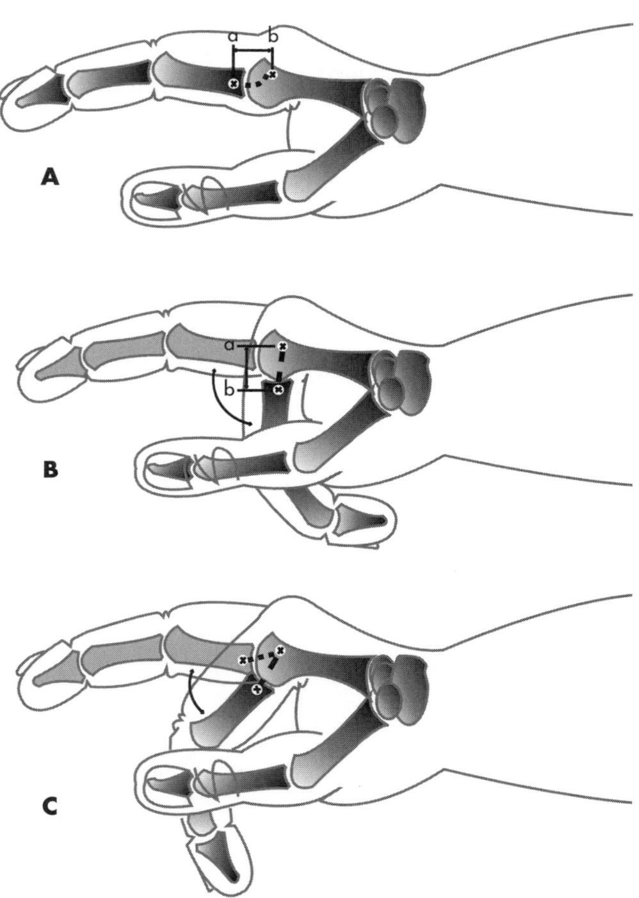

FIGURE **8-5**
A, Points *a* and *b* are close together in the extended position, and the ligament is slack. **B,** The points are farther apart in metacarpophalangeal flexion, and the ligaments are tight. Immobilization in metacarpophalangeal extension allows the ligaments to shorten because the joint cannot move and stretch daily. **C,** After immobilization, the tightening of the shortened ligament restricts metacarpophalangeal flexion as *a* and *b* are separated by the movement of the joint from extension to flexion. The index finger is flexed more in B than in C, in which tight ligaments limit flexion after improper immobilization in metacarpophalangeal extension.

The thumb

Thumb joints differ from their counterparts in the other digits. The lone IP joint of the thumb is a hinge like those in other digits. The MCP joint appears to be a condyloid joint but functions like an IP joint, allowing only flexion and extension. The carpometacarpal (CMC) joint, at the very base of the thumb, functions like a freer version of the MCP joints in the other digits. The CMC's proximal location and freedom of movement make opposition of the thumb possible. (Opposition is the ability to touch the thumb to another finger so that its pad is opposite the digit's pad.)

The thumb acts like an extra index finger, one rotated nearly 90 degrees and attached directly to the wrist at a

BOX 8-2

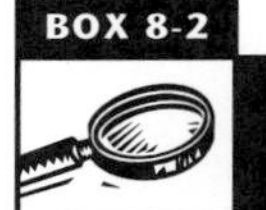

A **CLOSER** LOOK

Tight Joint Positions

The close-packed joint position stretches ligaments tight, preventing further movement and compressing the joint surfaces.[6] If the MCP and interphalangeal (IP) joints must be immobilized (for example, after surgery), each is splinted in its close-packed position—full MCP flexion and full IP extension. This position maximally stretches structures so that scar tissue assumes the length of the tissue in that position. Once the joint is mobile, movement is in the direction of tissue slack, and scar tissue does not limit motion.

If the MCP is immobilized in extension, scar tissue bridging the joint and connecting opposite sides becomes a larger problem (see Figure 8-5). As the MCP flexes, adjacent points on opposite sides of the joint separate because of the shape of the metacarpal head. Flexion stretches scar tissue to its limit early in the movement, and passive insufficiency of the scar tissue prevents good functional range into MCP flexion (extension contracture). In individuals with palmar burns, skin contractures are likely to form if the hand is splinted in MCP flexion. The greater likelihood of skin flexion contracture must be weighed against that of joint extension contracture.

30-degree angle from the palm (instead of in the same plane). The thumb's MCP functions like an IP joint, and the first metacarpal moves freely at the CMC joint, behaving more like a proximal phalanx than a metacarpal. The thumb's CMC joint, not its MCP, can perform both flexion and extension and abduction and adduction. This joint functions more like an MCP than anything else.

The saddle-shaped CMC joint of the thumb deserves special consideration because of its articulation with the distal surface of the trapezium bone. The proximal surface of the first metacarpal conforms to the saddlelike trapezium just as a person riding a horse conforms to its saddle. This articulation allows the thumb to perform flexion and extension and abduction and adduction. This mobility allows the less-mobile MCP and IP joints to perform flexion and extension in many different positions in relation to the palm.

Because of the difference in orientation of the axes of motion, flexion and extension and abduction and adduction of the thumb occur in different planes than those of digits 2 through 5. Instead of a side-to-side axis for flexion and extension, the thumb flexes and extends around an axis oriented front to back in relation to the palmar and dorsal surfaces of the hand (A Closer Look Box 8-3). Thumb abduction/adduction revolves around a side-to-side more than a front-to-back axis. Because of these different orientations, thumb movements differ from movements of the same names in the fingers (A Closer Look Box 8-4).

No discussion of thumb articulations is complete without an examination of opposition. Anatomy describes *opposition* as the ability to touch the little finger with the thumb, but functionally the thumb can touch all the other digits, 2 through 5. Opposition involves movement

BOX 8-3

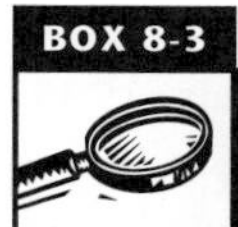

A **CLOSER** LOOK

Directional Terms

As anatomy and kinesiology students, you must learn new directional terms for the body. Synonyms such as ventral for "anterior" and dorsal for "posterior" abound in descriptions of the hand and forearm. You may abandon the original terms because they lack clarity.

As the hand moves around the body, words like anterior and posterior lose their abilities to describe the hand's position in space. For example, the flexor tendons are anterior to the MCP joints only when the palm faces forward. However, these tendons are always on the palmar side of the joints regardless of the hand's position in space. The following are terms used to describe the forearm and hand. Learn all these synonyms because the ideal descriptive term differs with each situation.

ORIGINAL TERM	*SYNONYM*
Anterior	*Palmar, volar*
Posterior	*Dorsal*
Medial	*Ulnar*
Lateral	*Radial*
Adduction (wrist)	*Ulnar deviation*
Abduction (wrist)	*Radial deviation*
Manual digital rotation (digits 2 through 5) at the MCP (turning the palmar surface toward the thumb)	*Supination of digit*
Manual digital rotation at the MCP (turning the palmar surface from the thumb)	*Pronation of digit*

BOX 8-4

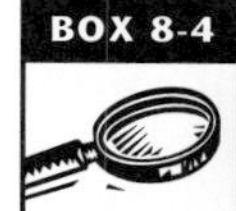

A **CLOSER** LOOK

Thumb Exercises

Thumb movements differ from movements with the same names in digits 2 through 5 because the axis orientation differs. Thus we gain more from kinesthetic learning than from looking at figures.

Supinate your forearm, and lay the hand palm up on a table. Extend the thumb by stretching it out from the palm and touch the table. Think of thumb flexion as sweeping the palm clean. Move the thumb toward the palm and then onto it so that continuation of this flexion movement sweeps across and stays in contact with the palm. Remember that the axis sticks out of the CMC joint with a palmar-dorsal orientation. The plane of the movement is the plane of the palm.

Abduct and adduct the thumb by positioning the forearm in midpronation-supination (neutral) so that you are looking at the hand from the radial side. You should see your thumbnail and the side of the index finger. Adduction, the beginning point of abduction, occurs here with the side of the thumb closest to the fingers in contact with the palm and proximal index finger.

Maintain this thumb orientation without losing sight of the thumbnail and move your thumb from the palm. If you do this with your left hand, the L shape that emerges is full thumb abduction. This motion should form an arc in a plane nearly perpendicular to the palmar plane. The axis sticks out from the base of the first metacarpal (the location of the CMC joint).

of the thumb from the palm, around and then over to another digit so that the pad of the thumb is opposite to the pad of the other digit.

Opposition is a combination of movements rather than a pure movement like flexion. Opposition involves thumb abduction from the palm, thumb flexion in this abducted position, and the appearance of thumb rotation. Kapandji's illustrations[5] describe pure rotation on an axis through the thumb, but Brand and Hollister[2] use the term *circumduction* through a cone-shaped path with an apex at the CMC joint (Figure 8-6). They describe opposition as thumb pronation; supination returns the thumb to the beginning, unopposed position.[2]

Before you begin opposition movement, notice that you can see creases, finger pads, and the side of the thumb but no fingernails. Now touch the thumb to the little finger and watch the thumbnail come plainly into view. Circumduction turns the thumb around and changes your view from the thumb's front and side to its back. This movement occurs at the CMC joint. Pronation of the thumb, slightly different from circumduction at the wrist, gives the saddle joint its third degree of freedom.

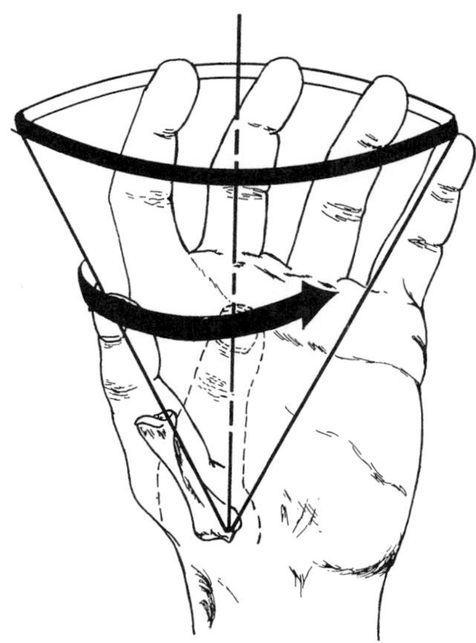

FIGURE **8-6**
Thumb movement occurs around a cone-shaped axis. (From Brand PW: *Clinical mechanics of the hand,* St Louis, 1985, Mosby.)

WRIST AND FINGER COORDINATION

The tendons of the long finger flexors and extensors originate in the forearm and cross the wrist to insert onto the fingers. Brand and Hollister[2] found that the finger muscles, through their long tendons, have overwhelming effects on the wrist (Figure 8-7). Many long finger flexors and extensors have moment arms for wrist flexion and extension as large as those of the wrist muscles themselves. A number of individual "slips" of the extensor digitorum communis are capable of wrist deviation.

The main concern in this discussion is that the finger muscles move both the fingers and the wrist if the wrist is not stabilized. Because the extensor digitorum communis' moment arm affects the wrist, whenever this muscle contracts to extend the fingers, wrist flexors must stabilize the wrist. The same is true of all finger muscles with moments at the wrist.

A look at Eduardo's hand before surgery provides an example. Radial nerve damage paralyzed Eduardo's wrist and finger extensors, and he no longer can extend his wrist and fingers. His grasp also is severely weakened, yet none of the finger flexors used in grasp are paralyzed by radial nerve damage. Why is grasp a problem for Eduardo?

When Eduardo tries to grasp an object, his wrist flexes while his fingers encircle the object. He has so much wrist flexion that he cannot pick up a pencil. Compare Eduardo's grasp pattern with your own to see that wrist extension, not flexion, usually accompanies grasp. The tighter your grip, the more you extend the wrist, sometimes to 40 or 45 degrees (see Figure 8-7).

Active and passive insufficiency

Why can't Eduardo grasp with his wrist flexed? The answer refers to the concept of muscle excursion and its limitations. Every joint movement requires active muscle excursion, and muscles possess only limited amounts of excursion. Because finger flexors are multijoint muscles, without stabilization they flex each of their joints, including the wrist. Wrist flexion requires excursion, so when Eduardo's finger flexors contract to move his fingers, the excursion they use in unintentional wrist flexion is no longer available for finger flexion (Figure 8-8). Eduardo's efforts all result in incomplete finger flexion. The more Eduardo's unstabilized wrist flexes, the less excursion he has for his fingers. Active insufficiency occurs when a multijoint muscle acts at all its joints simultaneously.

Active insufficiency is actually a combination of insufficient excursion and insufficient strength capability. The physiology of muscle contraction is complex, but strength capability encompasses the idea that tension (force) production relates to length. In passive stretch, tension is created in an elastic fiber as its length is increased. Active tissues like skeletal muscles produce tension through shortening in concentric contraction. A muscle's length at the time of contraction affects its ability to produce force (Figure 8-9).

A muscle that has contracted across all its joints simultaneously, like the finger flexors that have flexed the fingers and the wrist, is a muscle trying to produce force

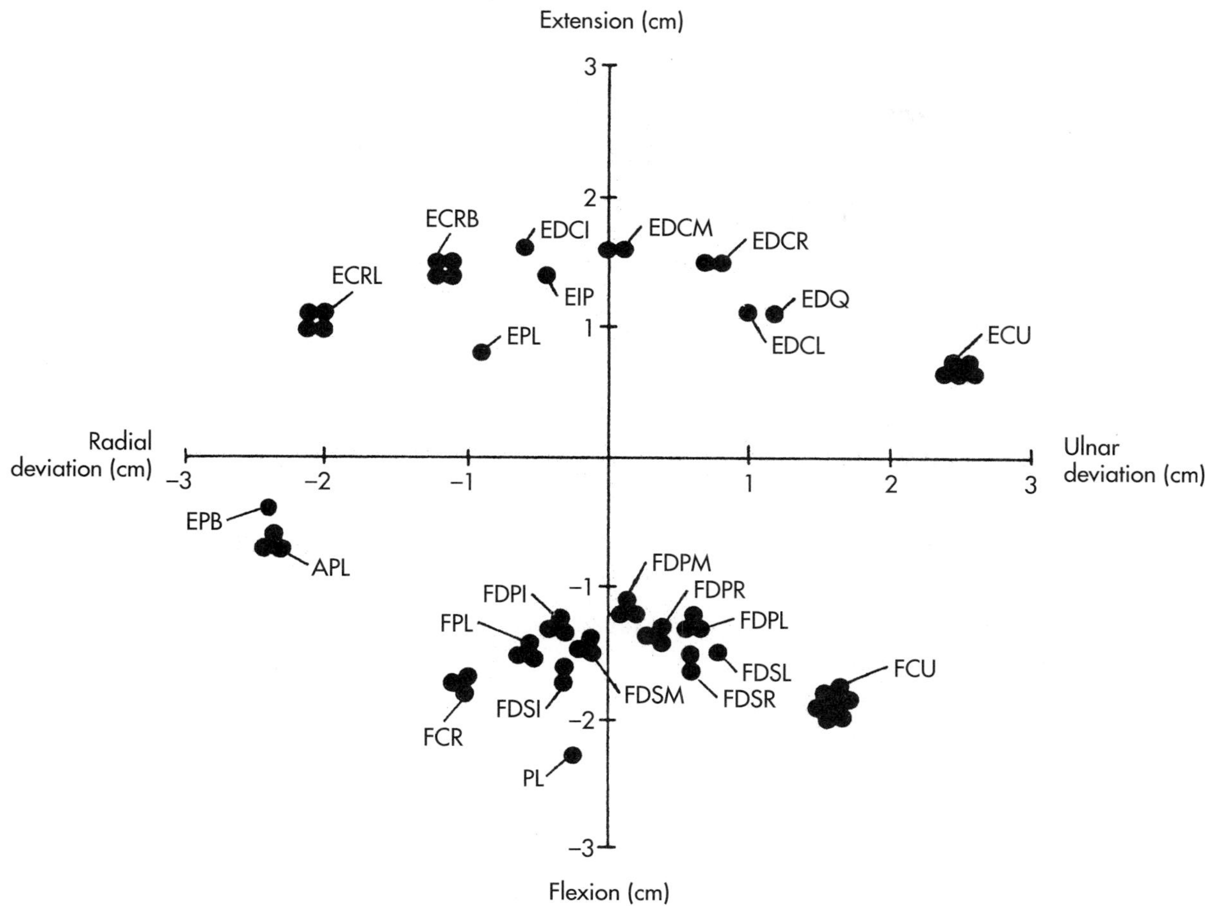

FIGURE **8-7**
This is not an anatomical diagram; it is a simplified mechanical statement of the capability of each muscle to affect the wrist joint. The positions of the tendons to the axes of flexion and extension and ulnar and radial deviation represent their moment arms at the wrist. The number of circles in a cluster indicates the tension capability of that muscle-tendon unit rounded to a whole number. *APL,* Abductor pollicis longus; *ECRB,* extensor carpi radialis brevis; *ECRL,* extensor carpi radialis longus; *ECU,* extensor carpi ulnaris; *EDCI,* extensor digitorum communis (index); *EDCL,* extensor digitorum communis (little); *EDCM,* extensor digitorum communis (middle); *EDCR,* extensor digitorum communis (ring); *EDQ,* extensor digiti quinti; *EIP,* extensor indicis proprius; *EPB,* extensor pollicis brevis; *EPL,* extensor pollicis longus; *FCR,* flexor carpi radialis; *FCU,* flexor carpi ulnaris; *FDPI,* flexor digitorum profundus (index); *FDPL,* flexor digitorum profundus (little); *FDPM,* flexor digitorum profundus (middle); *FDPR,* flexor digitorum profundus (ring); *FDSL,* flexor digitorum superficialis (little); *FDSI,* flexor digitorum superficialis (index); *FDSM,* flexor digitorum superficialis (middle); *FDSR,* flexor digitorum superficialis (ring); *FPL,* flexor pollicis longus; *PL,* palmaris longus. (From Brand PW, Hollister A: *Clinical mechanics of the hand,* ed 2, St Louis, 1993, Mosby.)

in its shortest length. The graph in Figure 8-9, *B* shows that when the muscle is too short, it produces less force. Therefore active insufficiency is a combination of insufficient excursion and insufficient force.

Something else happens simultaneously on the other side of Eduardo's joints when his finger flexors are in active insufficiency. On the extensor side, his extensor digitorum communis experiences maximal stretch. Recall that movement resulting from concentric contraction of the agonists (finger flexors in this case), requires passive excursion of the antagonist (the extensor digitorum communis) stretched distally across the same joints. Eduardo's extensor is in passive insufficiency and cannot stretch across all its joints simultaneously.

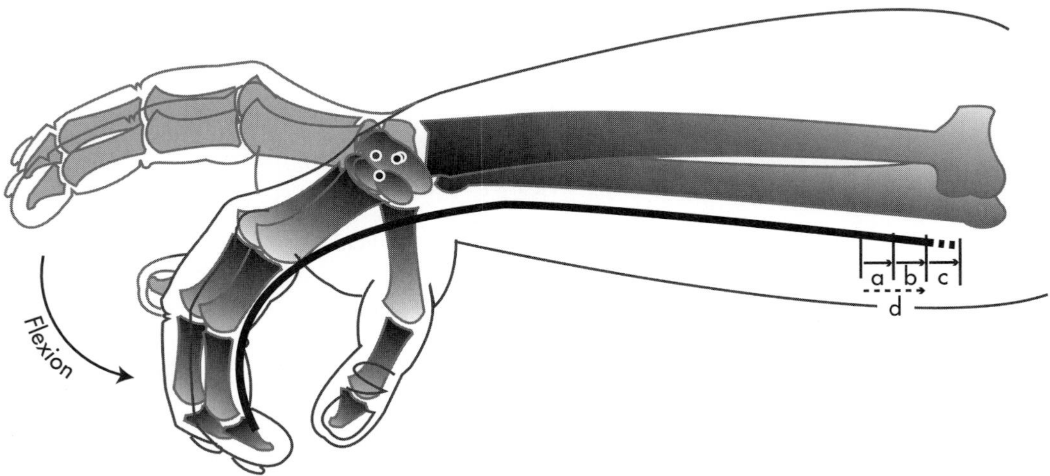

FIGURE **8-8**
Finger flexor excursion is wasted at the wrist. Excursion required for wrist flexion is represented as *a,* and excursion for finger flexion is *b.* With the wrist flexed, an additional amount (*c*) of excursion is necessary to fully flex the fingers. Because the sum of *a* and *b* is the actual excursion necessary for full finger flexion (*d*) and excursion *a* is wasted at the wrist, the fingers cannot fully flex.

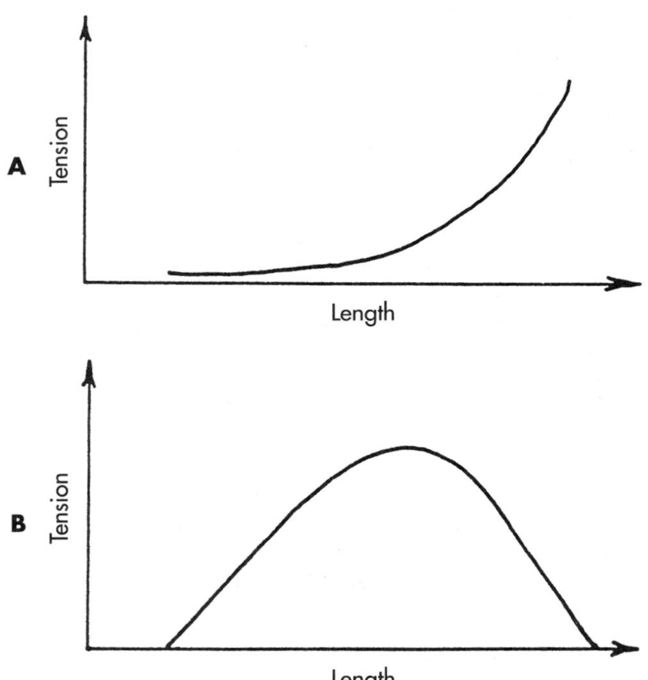

FIGURE **8-9**
A, The general shape of the length-tension curve of a muscle when the muscle is passively stretched. The muscle may require only a little tension to be stretched near its resting length. The muscle requires more tension to stretch less as it nears its elastic limit. **B,** The general shape of active contraction of a muscle fiber. The muscle can produce its highest tension at its resting length. It is able to produce less active tension as it shortens or lengthens. (From Brand PW, Hollister A: *Clinical mechanics of the hand,* ed 2, St Louis, 1993, Mosby.)

Undesirable wrist flexion stretches Eduardo's extensor digitorum communis prematurely. It has enough length to be stretched during full finger flexion but not full finger and wrist flexion. The extensor's inability to stretch further distally limits flexion. Thus two mechanisms inhibit full finger flexion around the object—active insufficiency of the finger flexors and passive insufficiency of the finger extensors.

Passive insufficiency can be advantageous in self-defense. An aggressor holds a weapon tightly with strong finger flexion and wrist extension. Grasping the aggressor's hand and forcing the wrist into flexion maximally stretches the extensor digitorum communis. The tension created pulls the fingers into extension enough to reduce the force of the grip. Because the extensor is not long enough to allow full wrist and finger flexion, the aggressor loses the grip on the weapon.

Tenodesis grasp and release

Passive insufficiency also explains tenodesis-type actions. The self-defense move previously mentioned forced wrist flexion to build passive tension in the extensor digitorum communis. This passive tension caused the fingers to extend slightly, although the fingers actively were flexing to grasp a handle. Consider the effect of passive tension on relaxed fingers. Active and passive wrist flexion stretch the finger extensors, producing enough tension to pull the fingers into extension.

This wrist flexion and finger extension combination is called **tenodesis release** when the passive tension yielding finger extension forces the fingers to release an object. The name is derived from tenodesis surgery, which shortens the long tendons of the fingers and attaches their proximal ends securely to bone. After surgery, the tendons reach passive insufficiency sooner in the movement. Tenodesis movements can occur without the surgery, but surgical shortening increases the finger movement because shorter tissues stretch and build tension sooner than longer tissues build tension. In tenodesis release, wrist flexion causes tension in the extensor digitorum communis. After surgery, less wrist flexion produces sufficient tension on the extensor to cause further finger extension.

Tenodesis grasp works on finger flexor tendons in the same way. Wrist extension stretches the flexor digitorum profundus, producing finger flexion. After a surgeon shortens the finger flexors and attaches them to bone, greater finger flexion accompanies the same amount of wrist extension, improving the grasp's efficiency.

Therefore tenodesis grasp and release can occur without active contractions of the finger flexors and extensors. In each case, passive tension in the finger tendons, not active contraction, causes the finger movement.

Bernice Richards calls her tenodesis grasp a "miracle grip." Because of her C5 quadriplegia, Bernice lost innervation to her finger flexors and extensors and wrist flexors and extensors. Shortly after she arrived in the spinal cord unit of the rehabilitation hospital, Bernice's OT practitioner noticed that she had a small amount of active wrist extension on the left side. This condition, known as "sparing," allows individuals with spinal cord injuries to perform isolated movements beyond the level of the lesion. Bernice used sparing to develop sufficient strength to regain full active wrist extension.

Bernice's doctors originally thought she might need surgery to shorten her finger flexors enough to grasp effectively. OT staff members at the acute hospital where she spent the days immediately after her accident understood how tenodesis grasp worked and were careful to move Bernice through the proper kind of passive range of motion.

These acute-care practitioners understood they must allow the finger tendons to shorten over time after a cervical spinal cord injury. They took care not to stretch Bernice's long finger flexors while maintaining passive range of motion in her wrists. They passively extended Bernice's wrists and at the same time passively flexed her fingers. OT staff members only brought Bernice's fingers into full extension when her wrist was simultaneously flexed. In this way, Bernice maintained extremes of joint range without experiencing tension in her tendons.

The OT staff members in the rehabilitation hospital took this technique one step further, allowing Bernice's flexor digitorum profundus to shorten so that even in full wrist flexion, her fingers maintained some flexion. The added shortening gives Bernice enough tension to hold a microphone in her left hand when she sings.

MUSCLES PRODUCING FINGER MOVEMENTS

Long finger flexors and extensors provide major forces for finger function, but the smaller intrinsic muscles balance undesirable movements in the hand just as the wrist muscles balance movements at the wrist. Despite their strength, the flexors digitorum profundus and superficialis and the extensor digitorum communis produce severely abnormal movements without the balancing effect the intrinsics provide.

Interossei and lumbricals

The lumbricals are often the first intrinsic muscles students of anatomy encounter. The lumbricals are associated with flexion through their origins on the flexor digitorum profundus tendon and extension via their insertions onto an expansion of the extensor digitorum tendon. The lumbricals must be observed in relation to the axes they cross to understand their complex functions. They run anterior to the side-to-side axis for MCP flexion, where their role is flexion. Each lumbrical travels to the radial side of the digit and inserts onto the extensor digitorum communis tendon through an expansive arrangement of connective tissue called the *extensor expansion* (also called the *extensor* or *dorsal aponeurosis* or the *extensor* or *dorsal hood*). This connection allows the lumbricals to extend the IP joints.

The extensor expansion elongates the lumbrical tendon, carrying it posterior to the side-to-side IP axes, where it inserts onto the distal phalanx of each digit. The lumbricals can extend the IP joints via this posterior relationship to the IP axes. In their serpentine travel through the digits the lumbricals pass anterior to and flex the MCP joints and pass posterior to and extend the IP joints.

We think of the palmar and dorsal interossei primarily as finger abductors and adductors. Although these movements are necessary in the manipulation of objects, the interossei are as important as the lumbricals in combining MCP flexion and IP extension.

The interossei originate on sides of the metacarpal shafts and partially insert onto the sides of the proximal phalanx of each finger. This course establishes a radial, or ulnar, relationship to the front-to-back axis at the MCP joint, where the interossei abduct and adduct. Each interosseus also inserts onto the extensor expansion, slightly more proximally than the lumbricals. These insertions lend the interossei the same relationships to axes as the lumbricals, allowing them the same functions, MCP flexion and IP extension.

The lumbricals and interossei share a function, although the pennate fiber arrangement of the interossei makes them stronger muscles than the lumbricals. The cross section of each interosseus is greater than any one lumbrical (Table 8-1). MCP flexion and IP extension in

TABLE 8-1
Comparison of Interosseus and Lumbrical Cross Sections

DIGIT	INTEROSSEUS CROSS SECTION %*	LUMBRICAL CROSS SECTION %
Index finger	First dorsal = 3.2 First palmar = 1.3	First lumbrical = 0.2
Middle finger	Second dorsal = 2.5 Third dorsal = 2.0	Second lumbrical = 0.2
Ring finger	Second palmar = 1.2 Fourth dorsal = 1.7	Third lumbrical = 0.1
Little finger	Third palmar = 1.0 Abductor digiti minimi = 1.4	Fourth lumbrical = 0.1

(Modified from Brand PW and others: Relative tension and potential excursion of muscles in the forearm and hand, *J Hand Surg* 6(3):209-219, 1981.)
*Values represent the percentage of total cross section (force capability) of all the muscles in the forearm and hand. Use them to compare one muscle with another. Notice that each interosseus has a higher percentage of force than each lumbrical and that each digit has two interossei and one lumbrical. The table includes the abductor digiti minimi because it serves as the "interosseus" for the fifth digit.

each digit (2 through 5) have contributions from two interossei and only one lumbrical[4]:

> The combined tension of the two interossei [per finger] is of the same order of a [long] finger flexor. The position of the interossei close to the axis of flexion-extension of the metacarpophalangeal joint limits their moment for flexion-extension, but their significance in the total balance of the hand must be considerable.

A look at two hand clinic clients demonstrates how the lumbricals and interossei work together. ***Yasmeen Harris*** is a 10-year-old girl who sustained serious injury to her right forearm after she crashed through a storm door while playing tag. Surgeons reattached her tendons, but the median nerve did not fully regenerate. ***Zachary Larson*** is a 12-year-old boy who fractured his right elbow when he fell off a skateboard. Zachary's ulnar nerve was crushed and stretched beyond repair.

Yasmeen's median nerve damage paralyzed her first two lumbricals, causing MCP hyperextension and partial IP flexion of her index and middle fingers. Unfortunately, children at her school make fun of her "claw hand." Zachary's ulnar nerve damage paralyzed his interossei, causing a similar appearance in his fingers, especially his ring and little fingers. Because all four fingers are involved, Zachary's nerve damage appears extreme. In contrast, Yasmeen's ring and little fingers are normal. Furthermore, she can move her index and middle fingers better than Zachary can his ring and little fingers. Yasmeen's injury seems less serious than Zachary's, although each injured a major nerve.

Review the motor innervations of the interossei and lumbricals and appreciate the shared functions of the intrinsic muscles. The ulnar nerve supplies all the interossei and the lumbricals to the ring and little fingers. Ulnar nerve damage leaves the ring and little fingers without intrinsic support and removes the interossei from the index and middle fingers, leaving only the lumbricals. Zachary's ring and little fingers are totally unbalanced, and his index and middle fingers are partially impaired. However, median nerve damage removes only the lumbricals to the index and middle fingers. Therefore Yasmeen's two fingers are impaired only mildly because the interossei still support them. Her ring and little fingers are balanced because they retain both interossei and lumbricals.

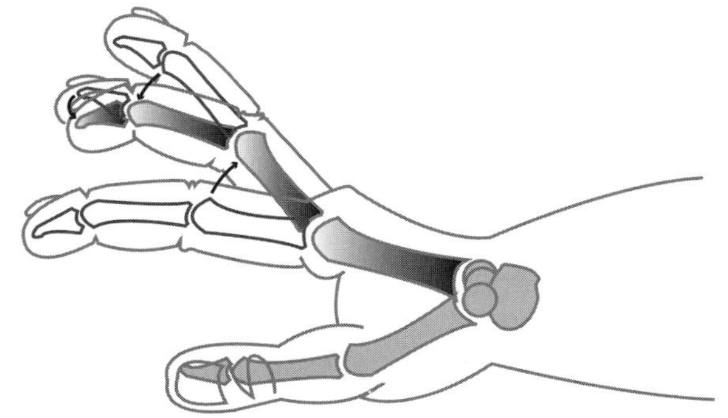

FIGURE **8-10**
Intrinsic minus hand.

Let us use information from the fresh dissection of a nonembalmed cadaver arm to help us understand the imbalances caused by loss of intrinsics, which causes **intrinsic minus hand** (Figure 8-10). By pulling isolated tendons, we see the pure function of one muscle at a time and understand how the lumbricals and interossei balance the pull of the long finger flexors and extensors. An initial pull on the extensor digitorum communis of the index finger results in extension of the IP joints and hyperextension of the MCP joint (Figure 8-11, *A*). Simultaneous pull on the flexor digitorum profundus in an attempt to flex the MCP and correct the hyperexten-

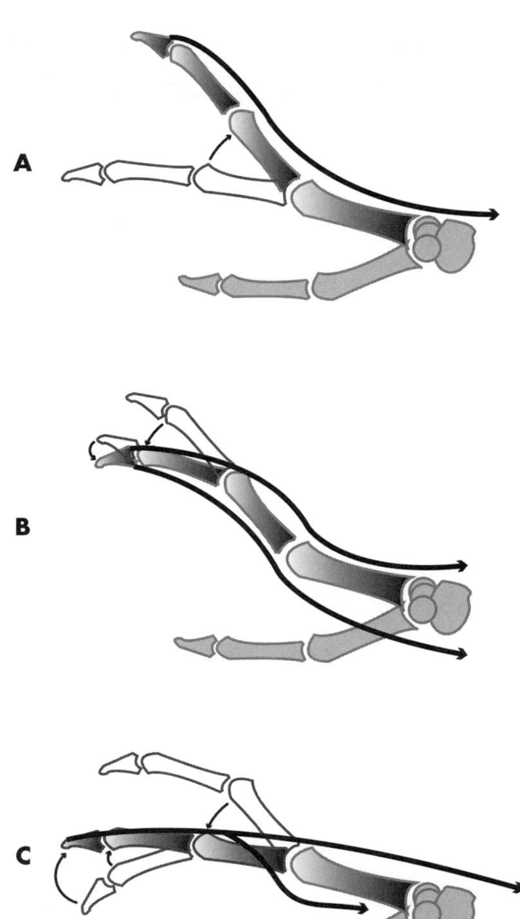

FIGURE **8-11**
Pull of the extensor digitorum alone **(A)** with simultaneous pull on the flexor digitorum profundus **(B).** Simultaneous pull on the first dorsal interosseus and first lumbrical at their insertions onto the extensor expansion **(C).**

sion results in the characteristic claw created by MCP hyperextension and partial IP flexion (see Figure 8-11, *B*). A pull on the first dorsal interosseus and first lumbrical at their insertions onto the extensor expansion immediately corrects MCP hyperextension without causing IP joint flexion (see Figure 8-11, *C*).

This correcting influence of the lumbricals and interossei follows their definition as combined MCP flexors and IP extensors. A finger positioned in MCP hyperextension and partial IP flexion straightens as soon as its lumbrical and interossei activate. Straightening requires MCP flexion (from hyperextension) and IP extension (from partial flexion). In other words, a straight finger is straight because the intrinsics' MCP flexion prevents MCP hyperextension by the extensor digitorum communis. This corrects the claw before it occurs.

Extrinsic and intrinsic function

The fingers flex and extend to close and open the hand via alternate contractions of the flexor digitorum profundus and extensor digitorum communis. Activation of the long flexors and extensors requires synergistic activation of the wrist extensors for hand closure and wrist flexors for hand opening. Synergistic wrist movements prevent undesirable action of the long finger flexors and extensors at the wrist.

The role of the intrinsics is less clear. Basmajian and DeLuca[1] believed the interossei are active any time IP extension accompanies MCP flexion. The lumbricals appear active with IP extension regardless of MCP position and are most active in full IP and MCP extension at the end of hand opening. Basmajian and DeLuca[1] did not notice either intrinsic functioning in hand closure. Brand and Hollister,[2] viewing the intrinsics from a surgical and functional perspective, emphasized the interossei as contributors to grip strength in a closed hand.

Clinical evidence provides a different interpretation of intrinsic function in hand closure. ***Vincent Pearson*** contracted an influenza virus several months ago. Subsequently, he developed Guillain-Barré syndrome, a neurological deficiency, which paralyzed his intrinsic muscles. Vincent's intrinsic minus hands form characteristic MCP hyperextension and partial IP flexion when they are open. The posture of his open hands is consistent with the summary by Basmajian and DeLuca[1] of intrinsic muscle function, but Vincent's lack of intrinsic function has a noticeable effect on hand closure. When he reaches to pick up the newspaper, he begins with MCP hyperextension and IP flexion. His fingers make a shallow sweeping motion as they roll the paper into his palm. Watching Vincent illustrates how poor intrinsic function drastically changes the ability to flex the fingers in a typical grasp.[7]

MUSCLES PRODUCING THUMB MOVEMENTS

The long flexors and extensor of the thumb cross many joints, as do the extrinsic muscles of the other fingers. Various wrist muscles balance the wrist as the thumb moves. The abductor pollicis longus has a long moment arm for wrist radial deviation (see Figure 8-7). Abduct your thumb and palpate the extensor carpi ulnaris tendon distal to the ulnar head. The activity you feel in the tendon indicates how much work it takes to provide ulnar balance, preventing radial wrist deviation from activation of the long thumb abductor.

Muscle combinations, or in some cases isolated muscles, move the thumb joints in specific ways. The IP joint of the thumb is flexed only by the flexor pollicis longus. This flexor's primary function is to pinch at the IP joint.

The flexor pollicis longus can flex the MCP and CMC joints, but the short flexor, short abductor, and thumb adductor play larger roles at these two joints.[2]

Two extrinsic extensors—the extensor pollicis longus and brevis—extend the thumb. The former extends the thumb at all joints and adducts the CMC joint. Because of median nerve damage, Yasmeen cannot oppose her thumb for grasp. She uses an adduction scissors grasp between her thumb and second metacarpal. The flexor pollicis longus, which also has an adduction moment, works with the extensor pollicis longus to generate enough adduction force to allow Yasmeen the ability to grasp most objects.

The third thumb extrinsic, the abductor pollicis longus, helps abduct the thumb but is more of a CMC extensor. Yasmeen's OT intern originally thought the radially innervated abductor pollicis longus would supply some abduction to her thumb and was disappointed to discover this muscle could not bring the thumb from her palm. More experienced OT practitioners noted that although the abductor pollicis longus cannot abduct, it balances the strong thumb adductor, preventing thumb collapse during pinch.[2]

The thenar muscles—the abductor pollicis brevis, opponens pollicis, and flexor pollicis brevis—generally are regarded as thumb-positioning muscles. Thenar muscle loss is associated most obviously with opposition loss. The abductor pollicis brevis abducts the thumb, and the opponens pollicis pronates the first metacarpal in circumduction. The flexor pollicis brevis assists in pronation (flexor and pronator) and is very effective in MCP and CMC flexion.[2] This flexor also is involved in pinch.

The adductor pollicis is stronger than the flexor pollicis longus and has a larger moment arm for CMC adduction than any muscle in the hand at any other joint.[2] This adductor is a flexor and supinator, sharing one and opposing another function of the flexor pollicis brevis (flexor and pronator).

Pinch

Brand and Hollister[2] termed the adductor pollicis the "pinching muscle." It works with the flexor pollicis brevis to stabilize the first metacarpal, and together they provide a foundation for pinching power. This dual component of pinch involves MCP joint flexion and first metacarpal adduction at the CMC joint. The adductor pollicis and flexor pollicis brevis move and hold the base of the thumb so that the long flexor can flex the pad and tip of the thumb against other digital pads and surfaces. Tip and palmar (pad-to-pad) prehension result from this muscle combination.

Key pinch (lateral pinch) places the thumb pad against the lateral side of the index finger near the index proximal IP (PIP) joint. The flexor pollicis brevis and adductor pollicis work together on the thumb MCP and CMC, and the long flexor primarily operates the IP joint. The first dorsal interosseus is equally important in flexion and abduction of the index MCP joint. The first dorsal interosseus stabilizes the index finger so that the thumb has something to pinch against. Brand and Hollister[2] suggest that digits 3 through 5 must flex together under the index finger as a brace in case the first dorsal interosseus fails.

TABLE 8-2
Thumb Use in Grasp

GRASP	THUMB USE
Spherical	Opposition
Cylindrical	Opposition
Power	Adduction against handle or opposition against flexed fingers (fingers flexed around handle)
Precision	Opposition
Hook	None
Scissors	Adduction

Grasp

Grasp (prehension) patterns are identified by appearance. Cylindrical and spherical grasps hold objects of similar descriptions. Power grasps involve forceful grips of objects like hammers. Precision grasps, or pinches, require opposition of the thumb to the other digits, either tip-to-tip (tip prehension) or pad-to-pad (palmar prehension).

OT practitioners must identify which patterns require the thumb and, of those, which require opposition. For example, a scissors grasp (adduction of the thumb to the second metacarpal in a scissors motion) requires thumb adduction only, ignoring the thenar muscles. A hook grasp like that used to hold the handle of a suitcase does not require thumb use. Yasmeen has used the scissors grasp since her median nerve injury (Table 8-2).

Zachary's grasp after ulnar nerve loss is much more impaired (Figure 8-12). This surprised his OT interns because they equated grasp with thumb opposition, mainly a median nerve function. OT practitioners reminded them of the role the ulnar-innervated thumb adductor plays in grasp. Figure 8-12, *B* shows the thumb position without the adductor pollicis' contribution to stabilize the first metacarpal.

Loss of the interossei and the third and fourth lumbricals results in imbalance at the MCP joints of digits 2 through 5. The digits are incapable of the deep sweep necessary to move around objects placed in the palm. The fingertips and volar metacarpal heads hold objects with point pressure (see Figure 8-12, *B*).

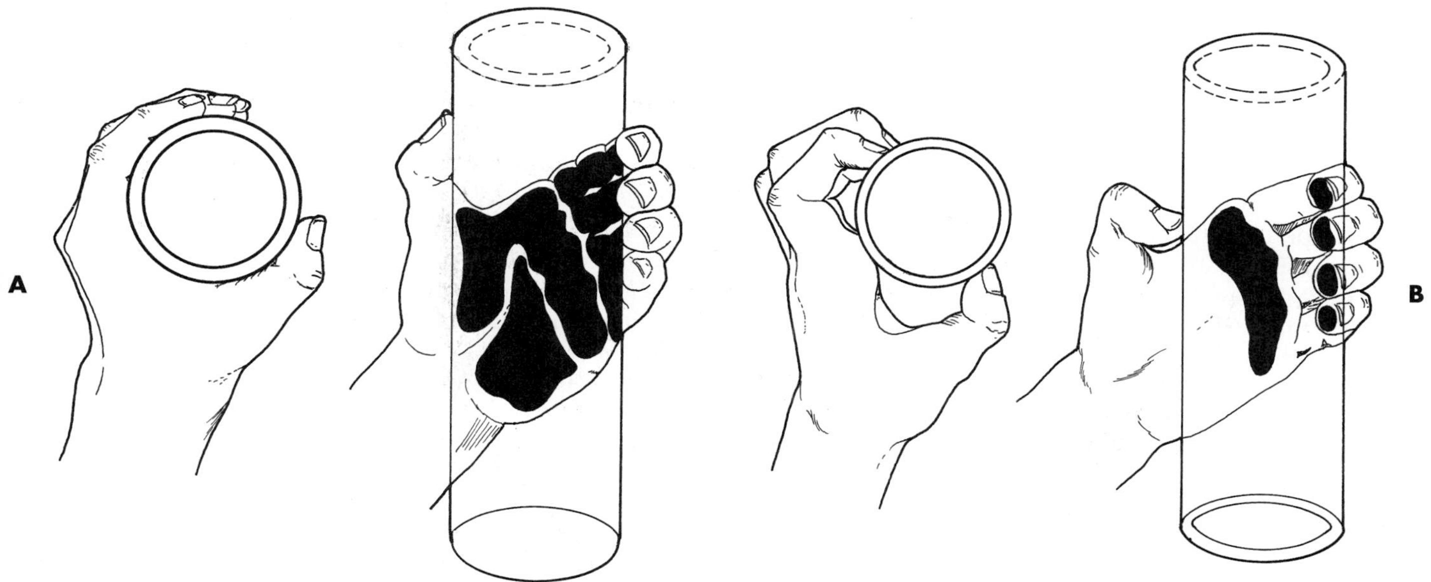

FIGURE **8-12**
A, A normal hand grasps a cylinder. The area of skin contact is marked in black. **B,** A hand without ulnar-innervated intrinsic function limits the area the fingertips and metacarpal heads can touch in grasp. (From Brand PW, Hollister A: *Clinical mechanics of the hand,* ed 2, St Louis, 1993, Mosby.)

Pathological Conditions

Acute orthopedic trauma, nerve damage, and progressive connective tissue disease all disrupt hand function. We saw Vincent's intrinsic minus hand; now we see how changes in the relationships of forces to axes and muscle excursion requirements affect others' hand function.

BOUTONNIERE

Rheumatoid arthritis has disrupted ***Linda Valdez***'s extensor expansion. Blunt trauma to the dorsal aspect of the PIP joint can cause similar connective tissue degradation. Regardless of cause, the mechanics of the problem are the same.

When Linda flexes her finger, it stretches the extensor expansion over the dorsal aspects of her MCP and IP joints. A tear in the extensor tendon dorsal to the PIP causes her PIP joint to protrude through the expansion when passive tension develops in finger flexion. Just as a tear in the knee of a pant leg allows the pants to slip posteriorly on the knee in a deep-knee bend, the extensor expansion slips to the palmar side of Linda's PIP joint. The force of the digit extensor loses its moment arm for PIP extension. As the tendon slips palmarly with more finger flexion, it actually develops a moment arm for PIP flexion (Figure 8-13).

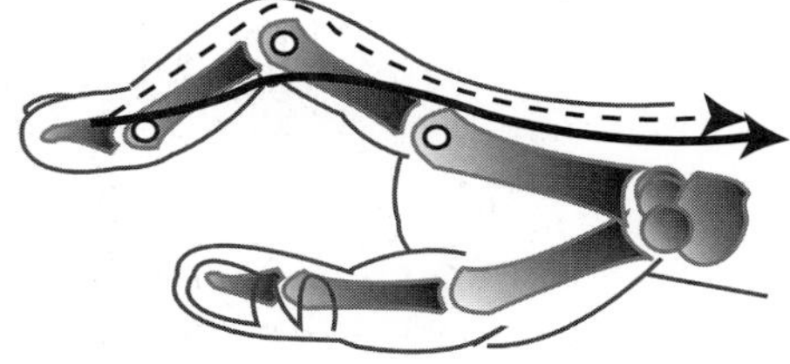

FIGURE **8-13**
The extensor digitorum tendon's route in boutonniere. The normal path *(dotted line)* maintains a dorsal relationship to both interphalangeal joints and the metacarpophalangeal joint. The altered path *(solid line)* after palmar displacement is anterior to the PIP axis, resulting in a proximal interphalangeal flexion moment.

Linda can bend her finger but cannot straighten it (extend the PIP). The more she tries to straighten, the more the extensor digitorum communis flexes the PIP. Eventually, Linda hyperextends her distal IP (DIP) with excessive effort. She is able to passively extend her PIP and hold it straight, using the extensor. Passive extension reestablishes the dorsal relationship of the extensor to the PIP axis, and the muscle once again extends the PIP. Linda can hold her finger straight until the next time she tries to flex her finger in a grasp, when the extensor expansion slips again and the problem reestablishes itself. If Linda decided not to passively extend her finger and left it in flexion, secondary joint contracture would result.

ULNAR DRIFT

Linda's connective tissue disorder also creates ulnar drift. Ulnar drift occurs when the extensor digitorum communis tendon slips off the high, dorsal point of the MCP joint and moves toward the ulnar side (Figure 8-14). The digit or digits follow the drifting tendon, abducting or adducting at the MCP depending on the digit involved. When digits 2 through 5 are involved, the hand takes on a wind-swept appearance and is referred to as "wind-swept hand."

In ulnar drift the force relationship of the extensor digitorum communis tendon to the front-to-back axis for MCP abduction and adduction must be examined. In its normal anatomical position the extensor digitorum communis has no moment for abduction and adduction because it pulls directly through this axis. After slipping ulnarly, the tendon develops a moment at this axis (see Figure 8-14). If the index finger is involved, the tendency is toward adduction; if the long finger is involved, MCP abduction results. OT practitioners use the terms *ulnar deviation* and *ulnar drift* of the MCP to prevent confusion over abduction and adduction. The extensor still can extend the finger, even though its moment arm decreases as it slips palmarly, falling down the MCP joint.

In some cases of long-standing ulnar drift the proximal phalanx slips palmarly off the metacarpal head. This happens for a number of mechanical reasons, including support failure in the dorsal structures. The joint's articulation is altered, but if no contracture has formed, the MCP joint can extend passively after manipulation of the proximal phalanx in line with the metacarpal head. Failure to reduce subluxation before passive MCP extension can damage the joint further, especially when the MCP is splinted with an extension force. Passive extension of the MCP without reduction causes "tilting" (Figure 8-15) and can damage joint surfaces.

BOWSTRINGING

Iris Clark cut the A1 and A2 pulleys of her right index finger when a glass she was washing broke. After the

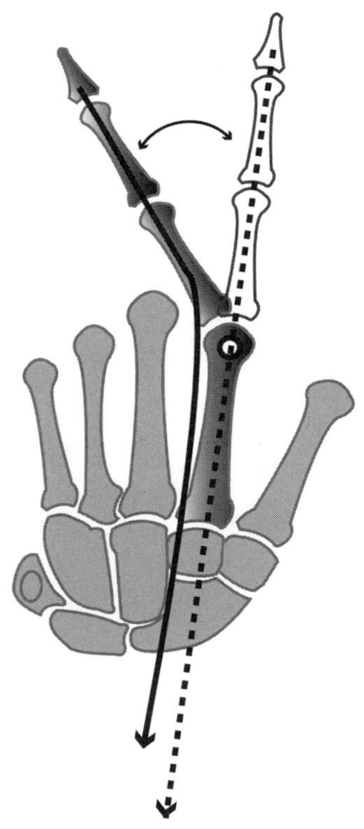

FIGURE **8-14**
Ulnar drift of the extensor digitorum communis tendon and the index digit at the metacarpophalangeal joint.

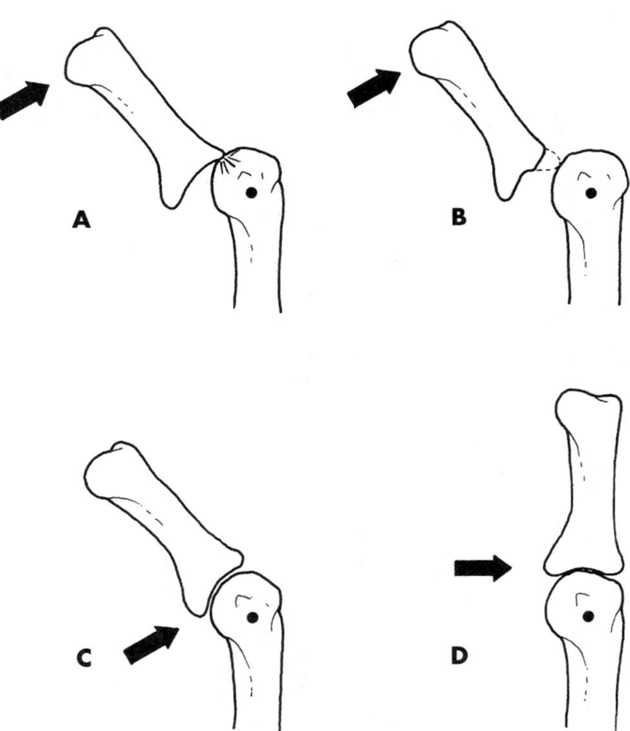

FIGURE **8-15**
The heavy arrows demonstrate force applied to a joint that has a partial subluxation, a block to free gliding, or both. **A** and **B,** Force is applied with a long moment arm, resulting in tilting without gliding and in eventual absorption of the lip of the phalanx. **C** and **D,** Force is applied with a short moment arm (close to the joint), resulting in restored gliding. (Modified from Brand PW, Hollister A: *Clinical mechanics of the hand,* ed 2, St Louis, 1993, Mosby.)

wound healed, she complained that she could not bend her index finger as far as her other fingers. The digital connective tissue pulleys (located proximal and distal to the MCP joint) keep the long flexor tendons in close proximity to the metacarpal and phalangeal bones. When Iris flexes her index finger, the palmar skin at the proximal digital crease elevates and webs out from the bowstringing of the long flexor tendons (Figure 8-16). Pressing on the skin over the tendons pushes the tendon back into its bed, increasing digital flexion.

Early mechanical inspection indicates that bowstringing increases the moment arm of the tendon at the joint. However, this longer moment arm is useless because bowstringing uses the muscle's limited excursion. A tendon or muscle that operates with a long moment arm inserts farther away from the joint; the more distal the insertion, the greater the distance a muscle must travel to move the joint (Figure 8-17).

Pulleys act as functional insertions for muscles and tendons. By passing under the pulley close to the joint, the tendon acts on the pulley to move the bony segment, even though the actual insertion may be two segments down the line (Figure 8-18, *A*).

This functional proximal insertion decreases the excursion necessary for joint movement. Rupture of the pulley effectively changes the insertion of the tendon to a more distal location, in Iris' case the A3 pulley near the PIP joint. Pulling on this more distal insertion requires greater excursion for the same amount of joint movement. In rotary motion, points farther from the axis travel greater distances (see Figure 8-18, *B*). Iris' muscle has a finite excursion, just enough for flexion of all the joints. When her tendon passes through the pulley, the excursion is adequate. Without the pulleys, her available excursion is inadequate to move the distal insertion. Consequently, she has less than full range of motion (less DIP flexion in Figure 8-18, *B*).

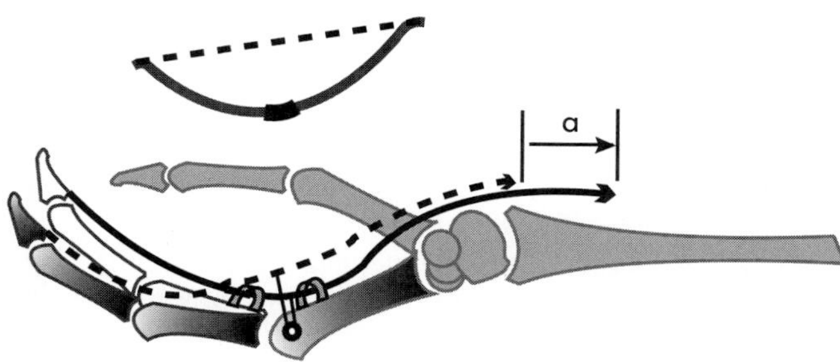

FIGURE **8-16**
The A1 and A2 pulleys normally hold the long flexor tendons close to the volar side of the metacarpophalangeal joint. Bowstringing of a tendon after these digital pulleys rupture changes the joint's mechanics. (The name derives from the appearance of a string on a bow; its natural tendency under tension is to bridge the concavity of the bow, not conform to it.) Note that bowstringing of the long flexor tendon at the metacarpophalangeal joint increases the moment arm but also results in loss of excursion *(a)* and less range of motion into flexion.

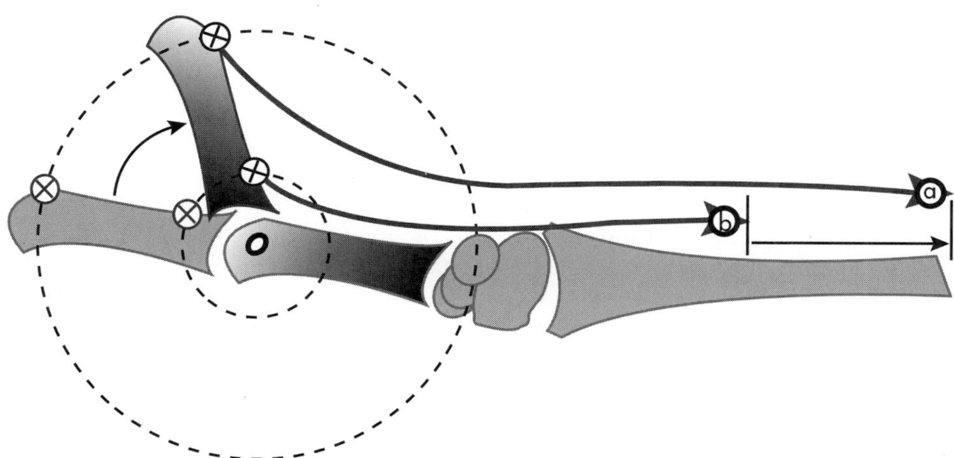

FIGURE **8-17**
Rotary motion dictates that proximal insertions move through less distance than more distal insertions in the same segment movement. The greater the distance the insertion travels, the greater the muscle excursion necessary to move that insertion. Notice that tendon *a* exhibits more excursion than does *b*. Muscles functioning at more distal insertions require more excursion for movement unless the tendon passes through a pulley on the way to its insertion.

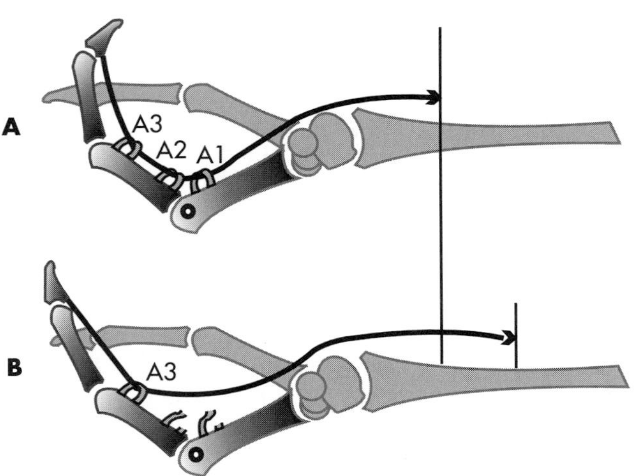

FIGURE **8-18**
The A1, A2, and A3 pulleys act as functional insertions for muscles, even though the actual insertions are more distal. The benefit is joint motion with less excursion **(A).** Rupture of the pulley results in muscle action at the next pulley and greater excursion **(B).**

BOX 8-5

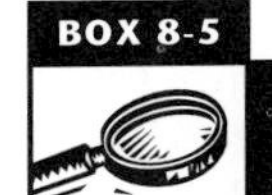

A **CLOSER** LOOK

Increased Range in Tendon Adhesion

Karen Wu *needs a splint for the flexor tendon adhesion at her third metacarpal. The OT practitioner flexed Karen's MCP to create slack to check PIP extension when diagnosing the problem. Now the OT practitioner must splint the tendon under a mild stretch to attain the opposite motion. Because Karen's tendon crosses multiple joints distal to the point of adhesion, the OT practitioner must splint all these joints to produce a stretch. Consider what would happen if the OT practitioner splinted only the PIP in as much extension as possible. After all, Karen can straighten her MCP and DIP joints, but not her PIP.*

As soon as the OT practitioner places the PIP into the splint under tension, the MCP or DIP curls into flexion. (PIP extension pulls the two surrounding joints into tenodesis flexion.) The end result extends the PIP, flexes the MCP and DIP, and leaves the flexor tendon in a relaxed, unstretched state. A successful splint puts all joints distal to the adhesion into extension. This splint places the entire flexor tendon under tension, and no joints are free to relieve it.

JOINT CONTRACTURE AND TENDON ADHESION

Karen Wu, a 15-year-old high school sophomore, comes to the clinic complaining that her right middle finger does not straighten or bend all the way. The OT practitioner evaluating Karen's hand has a number of ideas about what is causing her problem. Karen says that she broke her hand several months earlier. Because Karen lacks external scarring and her skin moves freely over the surface of her dorsum and palm, the OT practitioner concentrates on two very distinct possibilities—joint contracture and tendon adhesion.

The practitioner manipulates Karen's third finger to determine which condition is causing her problem. Joint contractures involve the joint itself. Moving a joint with a contracture does not affect the position or movement of other joints in the sequence. Tendon adhesions, however, involve the tendon and do affect proximal and distal tendon excursion necessary for movement of all the joints the tendon crosses.

Karen's medical record shows she fractured the third metacarpal shaft 3 months ago, and the OT practitioner suspects flexor tendon adhesion at the site of the healed fracture may be Karen's problem. First, however, the practitioner must prove this theory.

Karen complains of limited ability to actively and passively extend the PIP. First, the OT practitioner positions Karen's MCP and DIP joints in flexion to create slack in the flexor tendon. The practitioner then attempts passive extension of the PIP. If Karen's problem is tendon adhesion; her PIP joint can move freely into extension. The slack created distal to the adhesion allows the flexor tendon sufficient excursion for PIP extension (A Closer Look Box 8-5).

The OT practitioner verifies the adhesion by evaluating proximal excursion because an adhesion blocks both distal and proximal excursion. Active PIP flexion requires proximal excursion of the flexor tendon. A tendon adhesion prevents such active flexion. After checking Karen's passive PIP extension, the OT practitioner asks Karen to try flexing (bending) her finger. Karen is unable to actively flex any distal joints, but the OT practitioner can move them passively into full flexion. Passive flexion verifies proper joint function, and the lack of active flexion is due to an adhesion that blocks excursion.

If Karen had limited passive and active PIP extension regardless of MCP position and unlimited active joint flexion, the OT practitioner would diagnose Karen with PIP joint flexion contracture.

Of course, long-standing tendon adhesions can produce joint contractures. It is possible for an individual to have both, one discovered only after the other has been treated successfully.

Torque range of motion

OT practitioners have been measuring passive range of motion (PROM) since Bird T. Baldwin's work at the beginning of the twentieth century. Most practitioners assume measurements with a goniometer are fairly accurate, but PROM assessment in joints stiffened by edema or contracture is especially vulnerable to inaccuracy. Disuse of any joint may result in contractures of skin, fat, or periarticular tissue. In these instances, PROM measurements depend on how much force the OT practitioner is comfortable using.

Torque range of motion tries to control and document the amount of force used in PROM evaluation. Whenever a joint is passively ranged to its maximal point, equilibrium of torques is demonstrated. When an MCP joint is pulled into extension using some amount of force at a specific distance from the joint, a torque of extension is created. The stiff tissue limiting this attempt creates a torque of flexion. At the endpoint of range, torques in each direction are equal.[2]

Sometimes change cannot be measured on the goniometer, yet the joint is easier to move. Torque range of motion simply quantifies that feeling. Because force is used to produce joint motion, it can be measured. Pulling on the segment with a small force gauge (Figure 8-19) can measure range. Hanging a known weight (force) on a segment is an alternative type of PROM measurement (Figure 8-20).

These measurements allow OT practitioners to report both the range and the amount of force necessary to produce movement. These data generate a curve called a *torque-angle curve,* which is used to report the amount of torque needed to bring the joint into different positions or joint angles (Figure 8-21). OT practitioners use these results to decide whether to continue therapy or try an alternative treatment (Figure 8-22).

Even using torque range of motion, different OT practitioners evaluating the same person may end up with different results that do not indicate change in the client. ***Fred Jackson*** is an engineer who visited the hand clinic after MCP joint replacement. He did not receive therapy immediately after the surgery as he should have, so his hand tightened into a dysfunctional flexion pattern. The OT practitioner who sees Fred on the first day determines that it takes 600 g to pull his MCP from 90-degrees flexion to 30-degrees flexion (60-degrees extension). The next week a different OT practitioner finds that it takes only 300 g to move the MCP the same distance. The first therapist placed the force gauge loop on the PIP crease, giving his force a moment arm of 3 cm. The second therapist placed the loop at the DIP crease, applying force at about twice the distance from the MCP axis.

The two OT practitioners could have avoided this miscommunication by either documenting where the force gauge was applied or converting the force to torque. Conversion is simple; multiply the amount of force used by the moment arm. The first measurements convert to

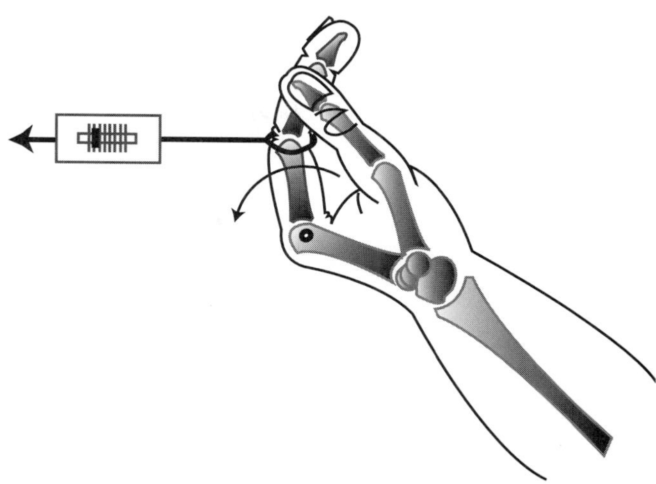

FIGURE **8-19**
A small "fish scale" force gauge quantifies the force involved in joint range.

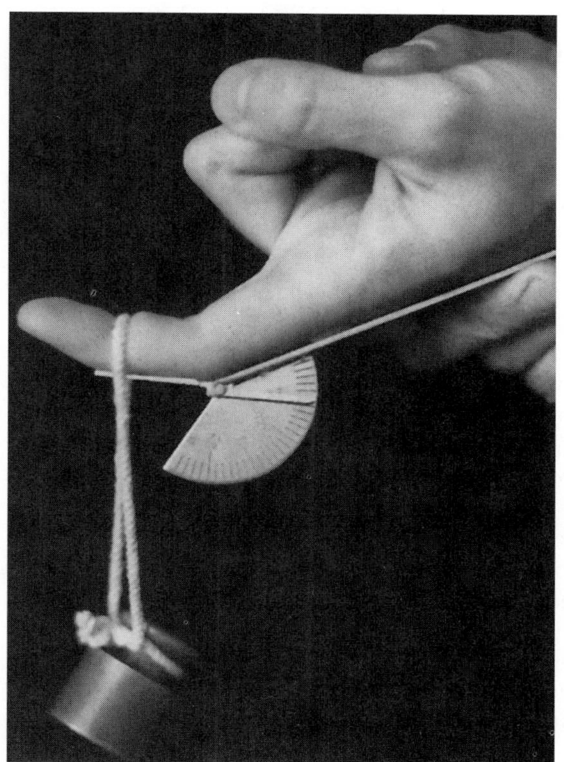

FIGURE **8-20**
One simple way to obtain a torque-angle measurement is to position a hand so that a hanging weight of, for example, 250 g, pulls at a right angle to a segment of a finger and at a finger crease. Alternatively, the weight may be hung over a pulley wheel so that the string is horizontal and the hand is more easily positioned. (From Brand PW, Hollister A: *Clinical mechanics of the hand,* ed 2, St Louis, 1993, Mosby.)

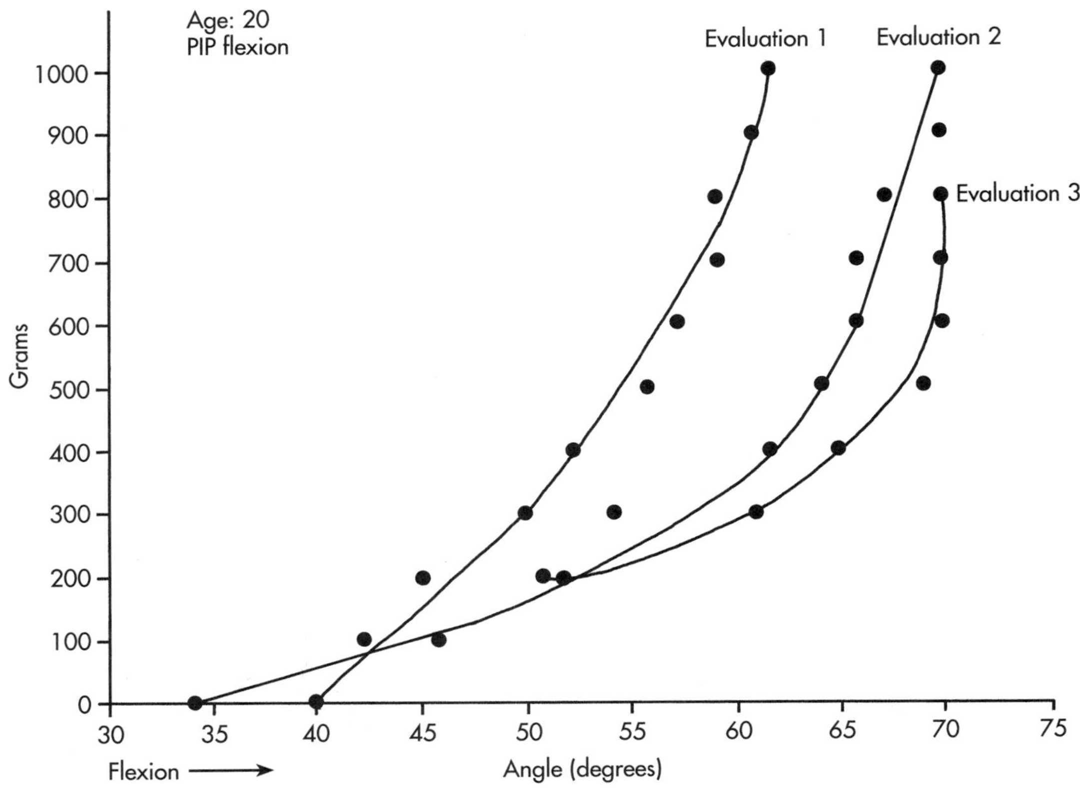

FIGURE **8-21**
This record of a patient's stiff finger shows three torque-angle curves, each one separated by 2 weeks of treatment. The last curve shows a vertical segment at high torque. This led to a decision to discontinue treatment. *PIP,* Proximal interphalangeal. (Modified from Brand PW, Hollister A: *Clinical mechanics of the hand,* ed 2, St Louis, 1993, Mosby.)

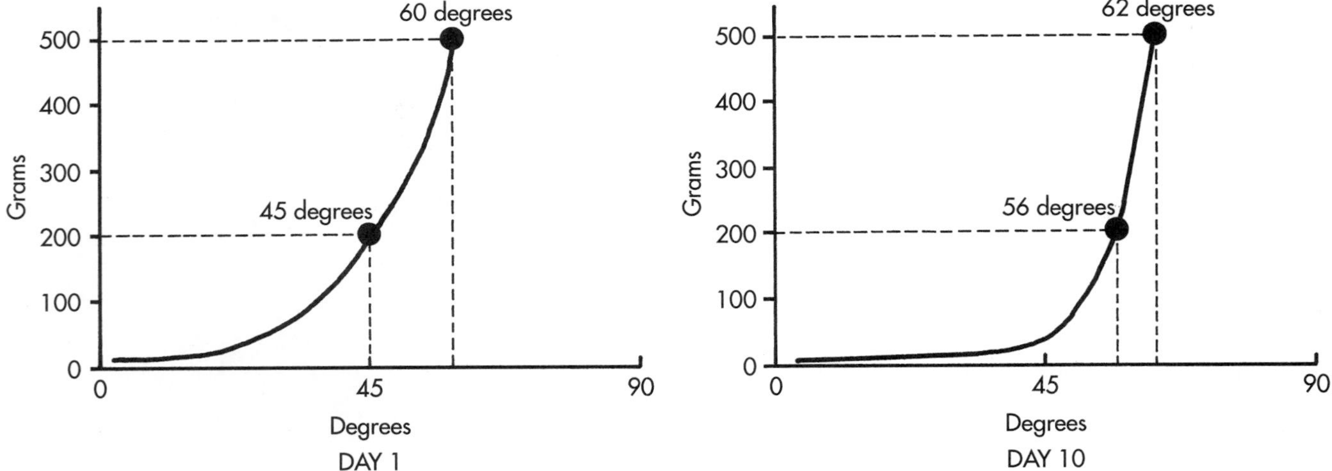

FIGURE **8-22**
The torque-angle curve of this contracted proximal interphalangeal joint shows a gentle, nonspecific curve. After 10 days of therapy, the angle of extension at 500 g has increased only 2 degrees, whereas the angle at 200 g has increased 11 degrees. The shape of the curve has changed to one typical of tough tenodesis, with a steep, straight terminal section. The 10 days of therapy improved the disuse contracture of the skin and fat but made no difference in the underlying tenodesis that was unmasked. (Modified from Brand PW, Hollister A: *Clinical mechanics of the hand,* ed 2, St Louis, 1993, Mosby.)

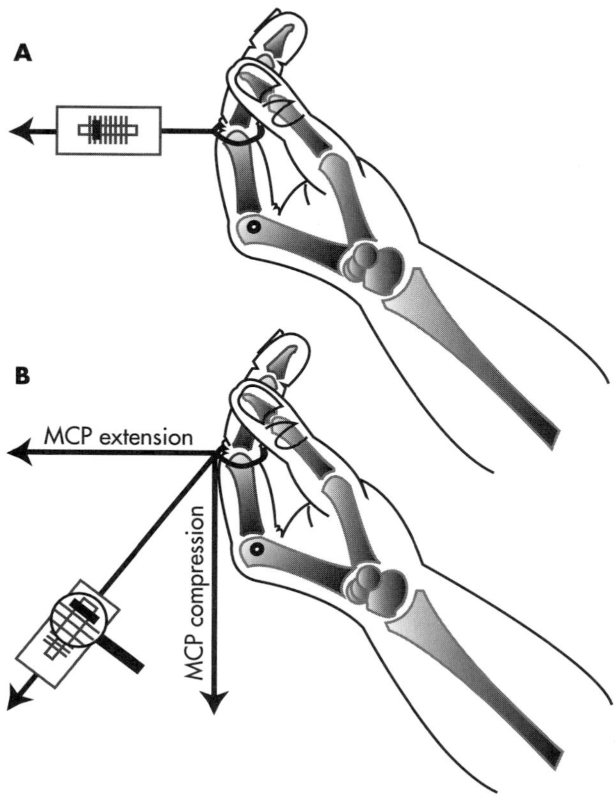

FIGURE **8-23**
Accurate measurement of the force required for passive metacarpophalangeal extension relies on a 90-degree pull on the proximal phalanx **(A).** Pulling with a force oriented at an angle other than 90 degrees wastes the force in a linear effect, in this case, compression. The OT practitioner must increase the amount of force to passively range the joint. (Note that the force reading under the magnifying glass **[B]** is greater than the first force-gauge reading.) This additional force inflates the value, mistakenly representing an increase in joint stiffness. *MCP,* Metacarpophalangeal.

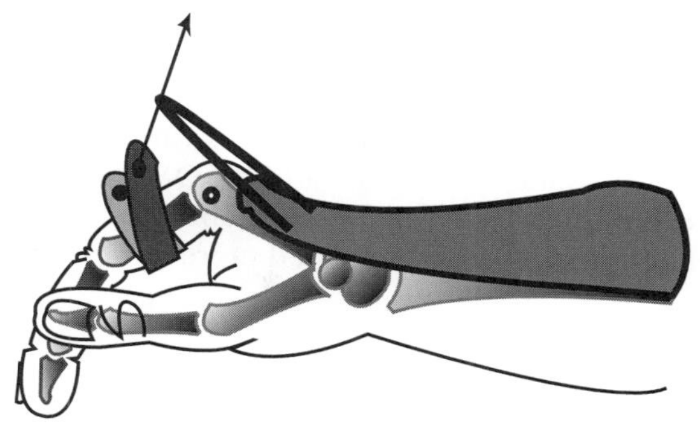

FIGURE **8-24**
Inaccurate outrigger adjustment causes dynamic force to pull at angles other than 90 degrees. In this case the outrigger is too short, and the cuff slips proximally.

BOX 8-6

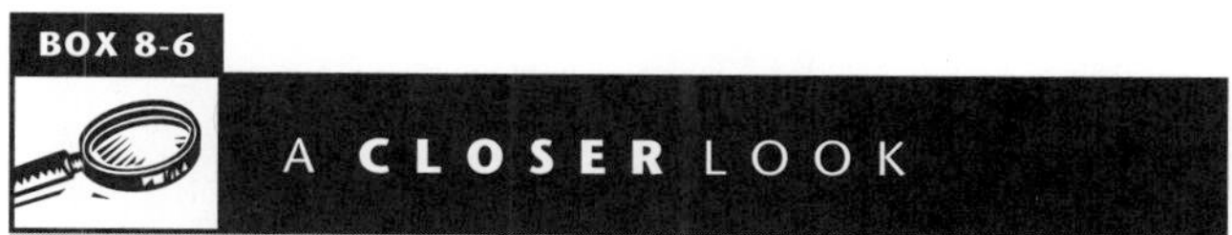

Force Angles in Splinting

Fred Jackson *wears a dynamic extension outrigger splint after MCP joint replacement surgery. He complains that one of the finger cuffs on his splint keeps slipping. The OT practitioner knows immediately that the rubber band attached to the cuff is not at a 90-degree angle to Fred's proximal phalanx. A force applied at 90 degrees to a segment pulls in the intended direction without causing the cuff to shift. If the cuff slips proximally, the force angles toward the hand because the outrigger is too short (see Figure 8-24). Slipping distally implies the outrigger is too long. The OT practitioner adjusts Fred's splint to ensure a true 90-degree pull.*

Because a dynamic force applied at an angle other than 90 degrees means part of the force pulls the segment into an undesirable movement, the OT practitioner does not know how much force the splint actually administers in the intended direction. The undesirable movement (force component) pulls parallel to the segment, sliding the cuff from position. If the rubber band pulls with 200 g, anything less extends the MCP. Instead of applying another rubber band to make up for the wasted component, the OT practitioner adjusts Fred's outrigger to pull at 90 degrees. Now all 200 g pull in the intended direction.

1800 g-cm (600 g × 3 cm). The second also convert to 1800 g-cm (300 g × 6 cm). Many torque-angle curves are reported in terms of force not torque because OT practitioners prefer to record the force as it appears on the gauge. They either document the moment arm or follow a protocol that standardizes the moment arm by stipulating where to place the loop on the finger.

Because he is an engineer, Fred is aware that force gauges must be used at 90-degree angles to prevent errors in measurement. He notes that the first therapist pulled the force gauge at a 90-degree angle to the proximal phalanx, the segment being moved. The third time Fred visited the clinic, a third, less-experienced practitioner was more careful to place the loop at 90 degrees but was less careful to maintain that angle. That practitioner recorded more force than necessary. A force oriented at 90 degrees is a pure rotary force (Figures 8-23 and 8-24 and A Closer Look Box 8-6). Orienting that same force at an angle other than 90 degrees causes part of the force to have a linear effect into or from the joint. (Remember that most of the effect of the back extensors is linear.)

When the less-experienced OT practitioner pulled at an angle other than 90 degrees, part of the force was wasted in the linear effect, which did not help the attempted MCP extension, a rotary motion. Because of this waste, more force was needed for joint PROM and the joint appeared to have stiffened. The problem was that the less-experienced practitioner used more force than necessary.

The Ergonomics of Grasp

Wendy Dabdoub, who has carpal tunnel syndrome, works in a warehouse and must constantly handle produce averaging 12 cm in diameter. A job-site analysis determined that Wendy must apply 4.4 kg of force to maintain her grasp on the produce. Wendy demonstrates a full-hand grasp in the clinic (Figure 8-25). However, observation at the work site reveals that most times she holds the produce

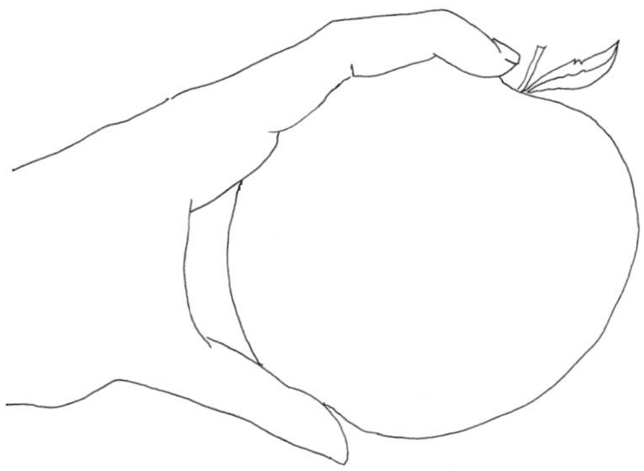

FIGURE **8-25**
Wendy uses the whole hand to grasp the apple.

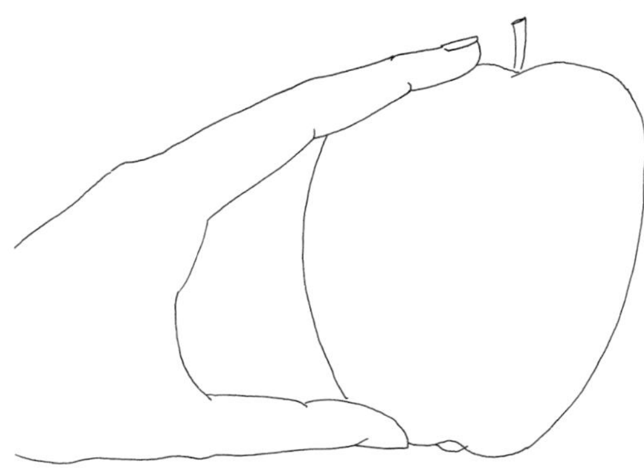

FIGURE **8-26**
Wendy uses a partial-hand grasp to hold the apple.

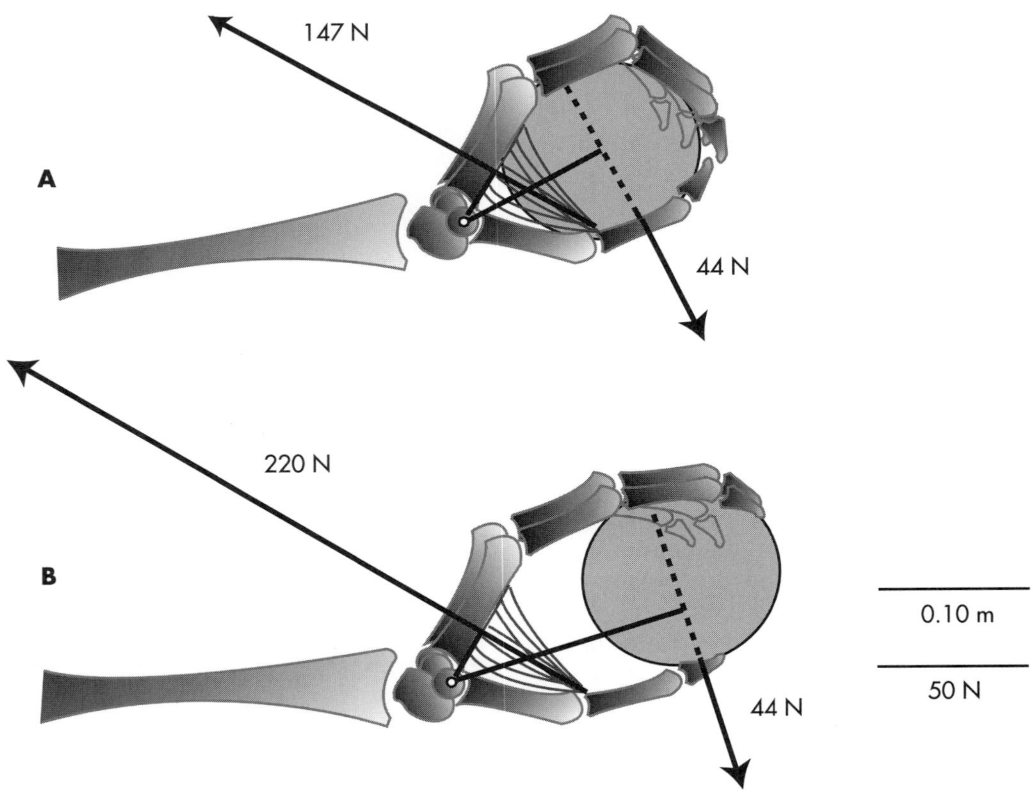

FIGURE **8-27**
Vector diagrams show force needed to maintain the different grips. **A,** Whole-hand grasp. **B,** Partial-hand grasp.

with a partial-hand grasp, making contact primarily with the distal phalanges of her fingers (Figure 8-26).

Measurements reveal that both grasps involve 70 degrees of thumb abduction. Using a whole-hand grasp, Wendy distributes resistance force equally along the palmar surface of her thumb, centered at the level of the proximal phalanx. The resistance is oriented approximately 90 degrees to the proximal phalanx, 10 cm from the CMC joint. With the partial-hand grasp, Wendy applies resistance force more distally, centered at the distal phalanx of the finger, 90 degrees to the finger pad and 15 cm from the CMC joint.

The thumb and thumb adduction maintain gripping force. The tendon of the adductor pollicis inserts on the base of the proximal phalanx. With the CMC in this abducted position, the combined fibers of the adductor tendon pull at a moment arm 3 cm from the axis for adduction (Figure 8-27).

Solve this equilibrium-of-torques problem using resistance (R), moment arm (MA), and the adductor pollicis (AP). Converting kilograms to newtons, equate the torque created by the resistance (R × RMA) with the torque created by the force of the adductor pollicis (AP force × muscle MA).

Whole-hand grasp:

$$44\text{ N} \times 10\text{ cm} = \text{AP force} \times 3\text{ cm}$$

$$\frac{440\text{ N-cm}}{3\text{ cm}} = \text{AP force}$$

$$\text{AP force} = 147\text{ N}$$

Partial-hand grasp:

$$44\text{ N} \times 15\text{ cm} = \text{AP force} \times 3\text{ cm}$$

$$\text{AP force} = \frac{660\text{ N-cm}}{3\text{ cm}}$$

$$\text{AP force} = 220\text{ N}$$

The partial-hand grasp requires the adductor pollicis exert more than 74 N greater force than the whole-hand grasp because the moment arm of the resistance is longer. For the same reason the finger flexors also must work harder. The added strain of the partial grasp aggravates Wendy's carpal tunnel condition, especially when combined with the wrist flexion movements necessary on the job. The OT practitioner educates Wendy about the damaging nature of a partial-hand grasp and encourages her to use a whole-hand grasp.

Summary

The wrist and hand are amazing structures. Their functions help us clarify and elaborate our anatomical knowledge. We see that muscle balance at the wrist and MCP joints is critical. Grasp and manipulation require even more complex systems of balance. Unless the many muscles work together, hand function falters. Basic concepts of hand kinesiology form the foundation for clinical diagnosis and treatment.

Applications

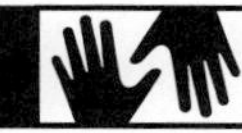

APPLICATION **8-1**
Balanced Wrist Function

Palpate your flexor carpi radialis and flexor carpi ulnaris tendons at the wrist, just proximal to the wrist flexion creases. Perform straight wrist flexion and note tension in both tendons. While holding this position, move the hand slowly toward ulnar deviation and note what happens. Why? Next, from ulnar deviation, slowly move back to flexion, then to radial deviation. What happens to the tension in each tendon? Why?

APPLICATION **8-2**
Shorter Longitudinal Arch

Trace the outline of your hand with the palm up. Make sure your hand is straight on the paper, with its ulnar border parallel to the paper's edge. Before lifting your hand off the paper, mark the location of the proximal palmar crease on the radial side and the distal palmar crease on the ulnar side. Take another piece of paper and cover your drawing. Slowly move the top sheet down, keeping the vertical edges together. Stop when you uncover one of the palmar crease markings. What do you notice?

See Appendix C for solutions to Applications.

REFERENCES

1. Basmajian JV, DeLuca CJ: *Muscles alive: their functions revealed by electromyography,* ed 5, Baltimore, 1985, Williams & Wilkins.
2. Brand PW, Hollister A: *Clinical mechanics of the hand,* ed 2, St Louis, 1993, Mosby.
3. Brand PW: Relative tension of the muscles of the forearm and hand. Presented at *The insensitive hand: biomechanics of deformity,* Careville, La, 1987.
4. Brand PW and others: Relative tension and potential excursion of muscles in the forearm and hand, *J Hand Surg* 6(3):209-219, 1981.
5. Kapandji IA: *Physiology of the joints,* ed 5, New York, 1982, Churchill Livingstone.
6. MacConaill MA, Basmajian JV: *Muscles and movements: a basis for human kinesiology,* Baltimore, 1969, Williams & Wilkins.
7. Smith LK and others: *Brunnstrom's clinical kinesiology,* ed 5, Philadelphia, 1996, EA Davis.
8. Soderberg GL: *Kinesiology: application to pathological motion,* Baltimore, 1986, Williams & Wilkins.

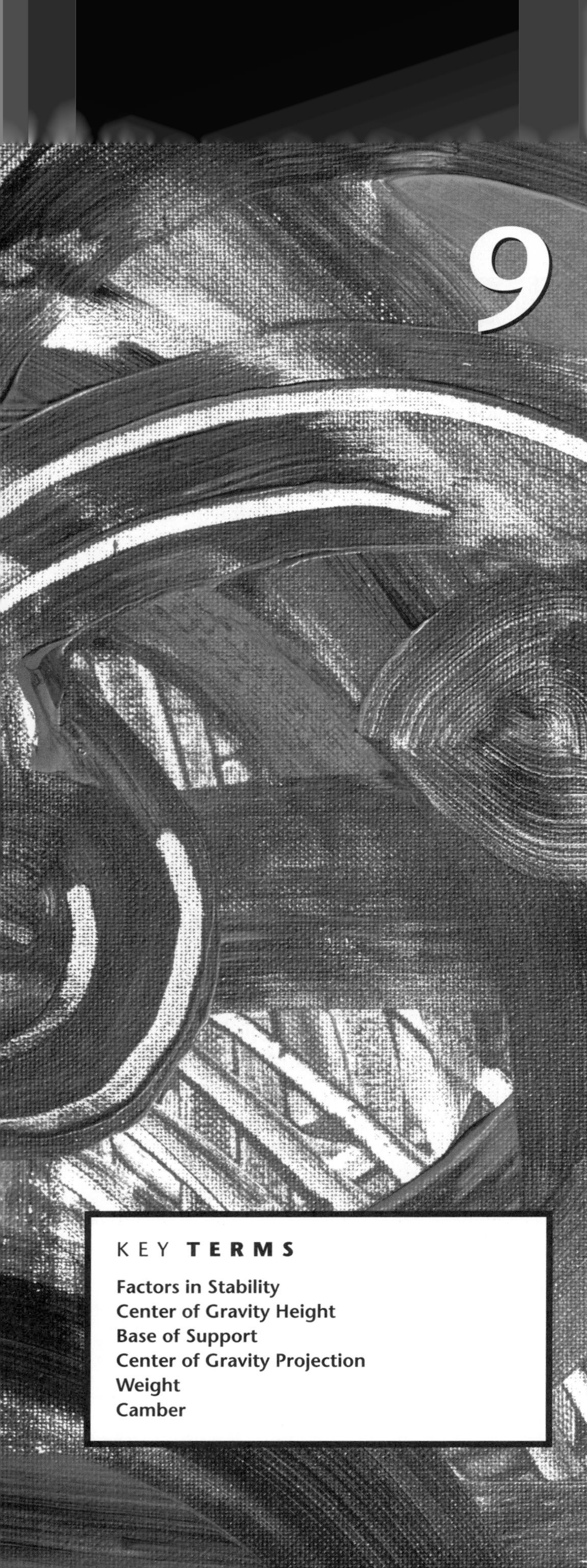

9 The Lower Extremity

KEY **TERMS**

Factors in Stability
Center of Gravity Height
Base of Support
Center of Gravity Projection
Weight
Camber

CHAPTER **OUTLINE**

MUSCLE USE
BALANCE
Weight Bearing
Balance at the hip
Gravity and muscle use
Balance at the knee and ankle
Gravity and muscle use

FACTORS IN STABILITY
Cerebral Vascular Accident
Threats to balance
Transfers
Toilet transfer
Wheelchairs
Semirecliners
Wheels
Instability after amputation
Adjustments affecting stability and pressure

NORMAL GAIT AND VARIATIONS
Running
Jumping and Hopping
Crawling and Climbing

BIOMECHANICAL ANALYSIS

SUMMARY

I *ndividuals walk in upright positions,* leaving their hands free to explore and manipulate the environment. The lower extremities must carry the weight of the body, moving it from place to place. Lower extremities also help maintain balance and equilibrium.

The legs connect to the rest of the body through the articulation of the femur and pelvis at the hip joint. The lower extremities affect vertebral alignment via the pelvis, so muscle length across the knee and hip can influence both standing and sitting posture. The hip itself provides stability and mobility. The knees bring the body closer to or farther from the ground and support the body weight at all positions between the extremes. The ankles and feet form a series of bony articulations that support the body's weight and allow movement. The foot supports the weight of the body in part through arches that act like springs. The longitudinal arch lengthwise and the transverse arch widthwise together form the hollow that exists between the heel and the ball of the foot. These arches absorb the forces created when the body stands still or moves.

Muscle Use

Muscles function at the hip according to their relationships with the axes of motion. Muscles anterior to the hip's side-to-side axis flex when they contract concentrically against resistance. These include the rectus femoris, sartorius, pectineus, tensor fasciae latae, and iliopsoas. Hip extensors lie posterior to the side-to-side axis and include the gluteus maximus and hamstrings (the biceps femoris, semitendinosus, and semimembranosus). In open-chain functions these flexors and extensors move the thigh in relation to the trunk at the hip joint.

Like the upper extremity, closed-chain movements stabilize the distal segment, causing muscles to move their proximal origins. Closed-chain movements play large roles in the lower extremities because weight bearing often stabilizes the foot. Instead of moving the thigh, hip flexors often bring the trunk toward the thigh in closed-chain hip flexion. In an upright position, gravity's downward pull on the trunk causes closed-chain hip flexion; the hip extensors often contract eccentrically to control this movement.

Besides moving the thigh or trunk, hip flexors and extensors maintain the lumbar curve. The iliopsoas, with its attachments to the lumbar vertebrae and pelvis, is a key postural muscle. It pulls anteriorly on its origins at the lumbar vertebrae and ilium to reinforce both the lumbar curve and the anterior pelvic tilt associated with good posture.

On the opposite side of the hip axis the hamstrings affect pelvic tilt via their attachments to the ischial tuberosity. Tight hamstrings limit forward pelvic movement (closed-chain hip flexion) in toe touches, flattening the lumbar curve.

Finally, the hip flexors and extensors interact with gravity in upright sitting, controlling the trunk through their attachments to the pelvis. Hip flexors maintain anterior and posterior trunk balance by counteracting the extension effect of gravity at the hip's side-to-side axis. Hip extensors activate when gravity pulls the upper body into flexion, preventing forward movement of the trunk (closed-chain hip flexion).

Hip abduction and adduction serve as open- and closed-chain motions, primarily interacting with gravity's pull on the upper body at the hip. The gluteus medius and gluteus minimus, together with the adductor group—the pectineus, gracilis, and adductors magnus, longus, and brevis—maintain lateral stability and trunk balance over one leg as individuals walk, run, and perform other movements. They also maintain active sitting balance in side-to-side and diagonal weight shifts. The two gluteal muscles pull the trunk from the body's midline, and the adductor group pulls it toward the midline.

Six small rotator muscles hold the femur firmly in the hip joint just as the rotator cuff muscles of the glenohumeral joint hold the humerus in place. The obturators internus and externus, gemellus superior and inferior, quadratus femoris, and piriformis all originate on the lower pelvis and insert onto or near the greater trochanter of the femur. The neck of the femur serves as a long lever arm, allowing the muscles to generate large amounts of torque. These six muscles either laterally rotate the femur or balance the pelvis and trunk over the lower extremity.

The hip adductors also medially rotate the hip. They vary in length and attach along the shaft of the femur in front of that muscle's mechanical axis for rotation. Depending on the femur's position, hip abductors also have effective moment arms for medial rotation. Together, the medial rotators turn the thigh inward and assist in diagonal balance and weight shifts.

The quadriceps femoris is the primary muscle used in kicking movements (open-chain extension), but it mostly performs closed-chain knee extension, supporting the body weight against gravity. A large muscle, the quadriceps femoris is composed of four parts—the vastus medialis, lateralis, intermedius, and rectus femoris. Of the four, only the rectus femoris originates on the pelvis, crossing the hip joint anteriorly. The others originate on the medial, lateral, and intermediate surfaces of the femur as their names imply. All four converge and insert into the central patellar tendon, which encloses the patella and attaches to the tibia. A multijoint muscle, the rectus cannot simultaneously extend the knee and flex the hip (active insufficiency). It functions best as a knee extensor with simultaneous hip extension, as in the downward stroke of bicycle pedaling.

Posteriorly, the hamstrings are knee flexors. Like the rectus femoris in front, the hamstrings cross two joints, and simultaneous knee flexion and hip extension create active insufficiency. Therefore the hamstrings function best as knee flexors when the hip is flexed simultaneously.

At the ankle the large triceps surae—the soleus and two heads of the gastrocnemius—plantar flexes the ankle. The gastrocnemius originates on the distal femur and can flex the knees. The gastrocnemius and soleus together insert onto the calcaneus through the tendo calcaneus, or "Achilles' tendon." These muscles support the weight of the body and provide sufficient force so that an individual can stand on the balls of the feet when reaching high above the head. Originating on the lateral tibia, the peroneus tertius and extensors hallucis longus and digitorum longus assist the major dorsiflexor, the tibialis anterior.

Inversion and eversion movements help stabilize the foot on uneven ground and allow body weight to shift from side to side when an individual stands or moves. The tibialis anterior and tibialis posterior run medially across the ankle and pull the sole of the foot inward into inversion, or supination. Their insertions onto the medial tarsal bones help maintain the arches and distribute body weight to the lateral sides of the feet.

The peroneus longus and peroneus brevis pull the sole of the foot outward into eversion. These muscles originate on the fibula and insert onto the lateral tarsal bones. They distribute body weight onto the medial side of the foot by everting, or pronating, the foot during weight bearing.

The foot, like the hand, has a number of intrinsic and extrinsic muscles that insert distally onto its multiple phalanges. The lumbricals and interossei help maintain balance by flexing the metatarsophalangeal joints and extending the interphalangeal joints. They keep the toes in contact with the ground as an individual stands and moves. The flexor hallucis brevis and extensor hallucis longus similarly balance the big, or great, toe.

Intrinsic and extrinsic toe flexors, extensors, abductors, and adductors also help maintain balance by allowing the toes to grip the ground. With enough practice, toe muscles can produce movements similar to those of the fingers. For some individuals without upper extremities the functional ability of the intrinsic and extrinsic toe muscles approaches that of the hand.

Balance

Unexpected encounters demonstrate the ability of our muscles to anticipate movement. After a surprising jolt or shove, the muscles almost instantaneously correct themselves. Anticipation is more evident when one step in a staircase is higher than the others, causing individuals to stumble. Ancient Romans used this trick to protect their temples and palaces with long flights of such stairs. Invading armies, running too fast for their normal anticipatory mechanisms to function, would trip, giving the inhabitants a chance to defend themselves.

As the body moves in and out of various positions, muscle groups in the lower extremity continually respond to the body's changing center of gravity. The downward pull of gravity stimulates receptors in equilibrium reactions, which generate weight-bearing adjustments as an individual moves from standing to stooping to balancing the body on one foot. Drawing the force of gravity in any lower-extremity position can establish its effect on each weight-bearing joint. Determining the muscle responsible for balancing gravity's effect is based on equilibrium of torques.

WEIGHT BEARING

The hip joint is a classic ball-and-socket joint in which the ball-like head of the femur sits firmly in the cuplike acetabulum of the pelvis. A series of ligaments form a tough, fibrous capsule that reinforces the joint. The iliofemoral ligament comprises the front of this capsule between the greater and lesser trochanters of the femur. The configuration of the hip permits motion around three separate axes—flexion and extension at the side-to-side axis, abduction and adduction at the front-to-back axis, and rotation at the up-to-down axis running from the femoral head to the condyles.

The hip joint, together with the bones and other joints of the lower extremity, must support the weight of the rest of the body and any added weight an individual holds or carries on the back. The lower extremities also must absorb and adapt to the added forces movement produces. The bones involved are very sturdy; many have curves and arches that allow them to handle large amounts of force and stress. Muscles and ligaments of the lower extremities must sustain large forces efficiently over extended periods.

Balance at the hip

The combined weight of the upper body—the head, torso, and upper extremities—balances against gravity at the hip. Typically, gravity induces hip flexion, extension, abduction, or adduction because of the joint's three degrees of freedom. Direction depends on the upper body's alignment in relation to the hip joint. If the upper body's center of gravity falls anterior to the side-to-side axis, gravity's effect is flexion and the hip extensors (the hamstrings and gluteus maximus) equalize gravity's flexion torque.

If the center of gravity falls posterior to the side-to-side axis, gravity's effect is extension, balanced by the flexion torque the hip flexors—the pectineus, iliopsoas, and rectus femoris—create. In each case, gravity causes closed-chain hip movement, and the trunk flexes or extends toward the femur as opposed to the femur flexing or extending toward the trunk. (Open-chain motions produce kicking and swinging movements.) These balancing acts involve isometric muscle contractions that counteract gravity, so no movement occurs.

Weak muscles make upper-body balance at the hip difficult to achieve. ***Crystal Turner,*** a 4-year-old girl, has low muscle tone. Because her abdominal muscles and hip flexors are weak, Crystal locks her knees in extension and leans backward when she stands upright. This position places her upper body's center of gravity slightly behind the hip joint. Crystal's iliofemoral ligament balances the extension effect of gravity and prevents extension beyond the upright position (Figure 9-1).

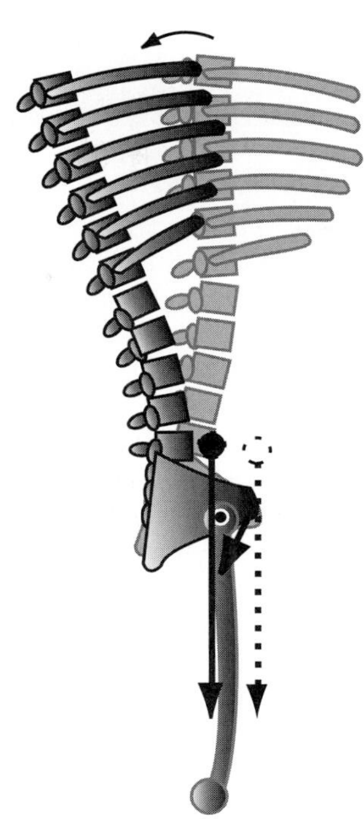

FIGURE **9-1**
The anterior hip ligament (iliofemoral ligament) helps maintain upright posture when hip flexors are weak or absent.

Although her hip muscles are weak, Crystal can control forward bending. She shifts her weight slightly forward, and the hip extensors eccentrically contract to control her upper body as it bends forward in closed-chain hip flexion. Via concentric contraction, these extensors also return her upper body to an upright position with closed-chain hip extension. She can stop at any point and hold the position with an isometric contraction of the hip extensors. Crystal's hip extensors maintain her upright posture in much the same way they do in an individual with normal muscle strength and tone. Only the last step, slight overextension of the hip, differs from normal muscle use. Even with normal hip-flexor strength, the hip extensors interact with gravity to lower and bring the upper body erect.

Because of her weak hip flexors, backward inclination of the trunk is a safe position for Crystal and forward leaning is a controlled movement. However, for ***Alex Fecteau,*** a 6-year-old with newly diagnosed muscular dystrophy, weak hip extensors cause different problems. He cannot incline the trunk forward because ligaments on the posterior side of the hip joint do not tighten and stabilize the hip until the very end of the hip-flexion range. If Alex's center of gravity moves anterior to the hip joint, gravity-induced, closed-chain hip flexion accelerates downward until passive stretch of the hamstrings finally halts gravity's flexion torque. Alex must use his available upper-extremity strength to "climb up" the thighs into erect posture. Using the arms to push the body erect (Gower's sign) is a classic early symptom of muscular dystrophy.[1]

To understand gravity's effect on the hip's front-to-back axis for abduction-adduction, stand on one foot. Lean on the weight-bearing leg, which shifts gravity lateral to the abduction and adduction axis, and you can feel isometric contractions of the pectineus, gracilis, and three hip adductors in the medial thigh (Figure 9-2). As weight shifts toward the non–weight-bearing leg, gravity pulls the body into closed-chain hip adduction and you can feel the hip abductors, gluteus medius, and tensor fasciae latae activate to balance gravity's adduction torque. Closed-chain hip adduction has a ligamentous checkpoint in the iliotibial tract. The ligament itself balances against gravity and tolerates about 20 degrees of hip adduction before the tensor fasciae latae must contract (Figure 9-3 and A Closer Look Box 9-1).

Gravity and muscle use

In Figure 9-4, ***Iris Clark,*** who weighs 60 kg, must balance on her right foot to reach into an overhead cabinet. Gravity adducts the hip in this closed-chain position, and the hip abductors contract isometrically to balance this effect.

In this position, her body weight is in equilibrium with the force of her abductors. Specific moment arms help

BOX 9-1

A **CLOSER** LOOK

Orthopedic Hip Problems

The head and neck of the femur form an angle about 125 degrees to the shaft called the neck-shaft angle. *If the bone forms with a neck-shaft angle greater or less than 125 degrees, it affects the alignment of the entire lower extremity distal to the hip. An angle of more than 125 degrees is called* coxa valga *and results in a bowlegged appearance. The original problem begins where the proximal femur connects to the pelvis at the hips (os coxae), but evidence of the problem is distal outward projection of the femurs (valga). An angle less than 125 degrees is called* coxa vara *and produces a "knock-kneed" appearance because the distal femurs project inward.*

The same terms appear to describe opposite actions at the knee (genu). Genu vara describes inward projection of the distal tibia associated with a bowlegged appearance. Coxa valga and genu vara both describe a bowlegged appearance; they represent opposite problems at two different joints. The same is true of coxa vara and genu valga; both are associated with knock-kneed appearances.

determine how much force the hip abductors must use. Iris' center of gravity lies to the left of the spine at about lumbar vertebra 3 (L3), approximately 8 cm from the axis of motion at the hip. The hip abductor force has a 5-cm moment arm from the axis of motion. The right upper extremity's centers of gravity lie at various distances from the hip joint—45 cm in the hand, 40 cm in the forearm, and 25 cm in the upper arm.

The weight of the head, trunk, and left extremities generates an adduction tendency equal to hip abduction combined with the right upper extremity's tendency to lean the trunk to the right in closed-chain hip abduction (see Figure 9-4, *B*). Converting centimeters to meters and kilograms to newtons, calculate the force the hip adductors must exert:

$$600 \text{ N} \times 0.08 \text{ m} = (4 \text{ N} \times 0.45 \text{ m}) + (9 \text{ N} \times 0.40 \text{ m}) + (16 \text{ N} \times 0.25 \text{ m}) + 0.05 \text{ m} \times \underline{\qquad} \text{ N}$$

$$48 \text{ Nm} = (1.8 \text{ Nm} + 3.6 \text{ Nm} + 4 \text{ Nm}) + 0.05 \text{ m} \times \underline{\qquad} \text{ N}$$

$$48 \text{ Nm} - 9.4 \text{ Nm} = 0.05 \text{ m} \times \underline{\qquad} \text{ N}$$

$$\frac{38.6 \text{ Nm}}{0.05 \text{ m}} = 772 \text{ N}$$

Iris' outstretched right arm decreases the amount of force her hip abductors need because its weight combines with the force of the hip abductors to abduct the right hip. If Iris' left hand were stretched out, it would

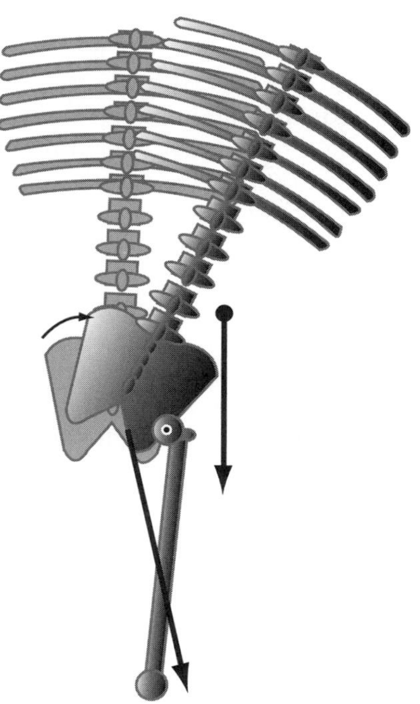

FIGURE **9-2**
Gravity's abduction torque (abduction moment) at the front-to-back hip axis is balanced by the isometric contraction of the hip adductors.

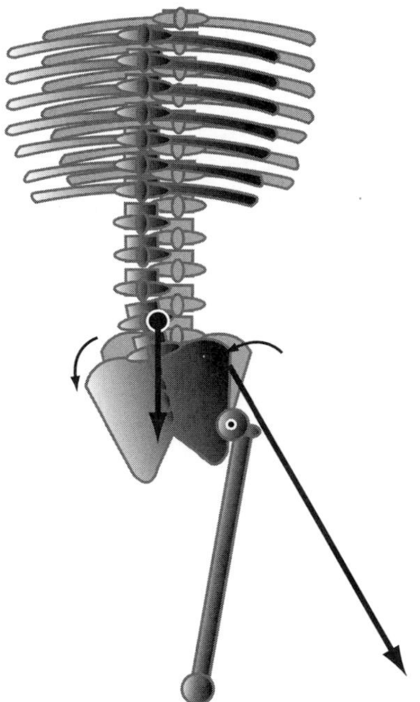

FIGURE **9-3**
Closed-chain hip adduction (pelvic obliquity) occurs when gravity's adduction effect is unbalanced by contraction of the hip abductors. The lateral hip ligament prevents further hip adduction.

shift her body's center of gravity farther from the spine and create a longer moment arm for hip adduction. Then Iris' hip abductors would have to increase their force to match the added adduction tendency. If Iris put her left hand on the countertop, weight bearing would create an upward reaction force that would decrease her body's adduction torque on the hip joint. Iris' hip abductors would contract less forcefully to balance her body at the hip joint, making their job easier. Thus upper extremities help maintain balance and decrease the amount of lower-extremity effort.

Balance at the knee and ankle

The same closed-chain analysis can be applied to ligament stretch, recoil, and isometric muscle contraction acting on the knee and ankle. The knee, a condyloid joint, allows flexion and extension at the side-to-side axis and rotation around the up-to-down axis. Gravity primarily affects the side-to-side axis.

Crystal's weak muscle tone causes her to project her upper body's center of gravity anterior to the knee's side-to-side axis by assuming lordosis and slightly hyperextending her knees. In this position, Crystal's center of gravity has an extension moment, and the extension torque is balanced by the posteriorly placed knee ligaments and knee flexors, the hamstrings and gastrocnemius. Because her knee's ligaments prevent extension beyond the upright, knee-extended position and her iliofemoral ligament prevents hip extension, Crystal can "hang on" her ligaments to stand. As long as the liga-

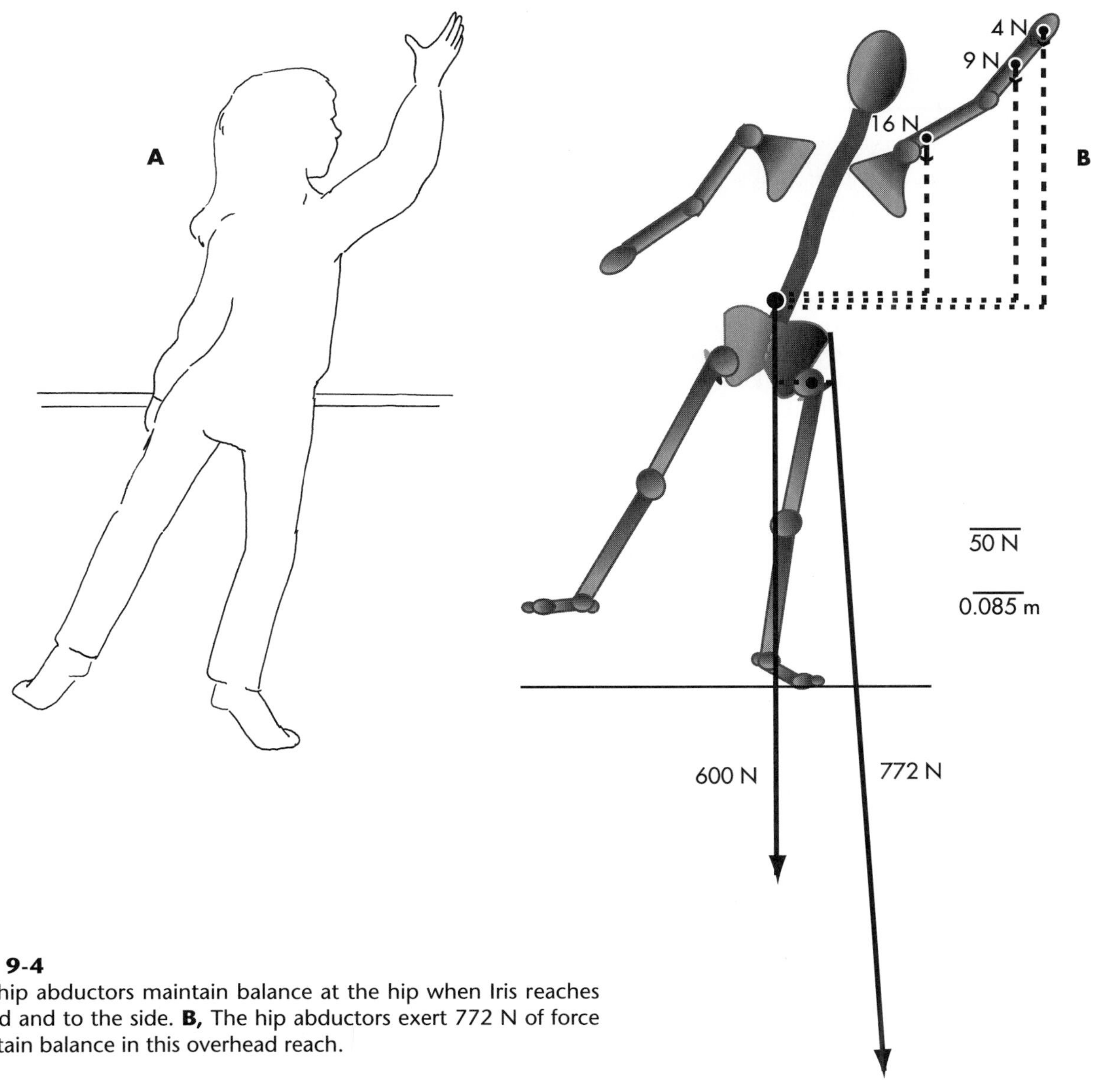

FIGURE **9-4**
A, The hip abductors maintain balance at the hip when Iris reaches overhead and to the side. **B,** The hip abductors exert 772 N of force to maintain balance in this overhead reach.

BOX 9-2

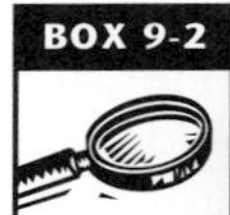

A CLOSER LOOK

Toe Extension in Balance

Stand straight up, feet together, and sway backward just enough that you begin to lose your balance. Notice that your toes curl up as you try to stop yourself from swaying too far backward. What purpose does this serve?

Toe extension is a sign that your body's center of gravity has fallen behind the ankle's axis for dorsiflexion and plantar flexion. The dorsiflexors pull the body forward at the ankle (closed-chain dorsiflexion). Newton's law states that the segment with the least mass moves first. Before the dorsiflexors, including the long toe extensors, can pull the entire lower extremity forward onto the foot, the toes extend. If you lean back too far for the dorsiflexors to be effective, taking a step back helps you maintain balance.

ments remain intact, Crystal's weight is stable on her hyperextended knees. She can stand upright, even on one leg (unilateral weight bearing), with minimal or no muscle contraction.

As in the hip, no ligament balances against gravity-induced knee flexion. When the upper body's center of gravity projects posterior to the side-to-side axis, isometric extensor contractions balance the knee. The quadriceps femoris, attaching onto the tibia distally through the patellar tendon, balances against knee flexion through its proximal attachments on the femur and pelvis.

At the ankle, two muscle groups balance movement at the side-to-side axis for dorsiflexion and plantar flexion. When gravity falls anterior to this axis, posteriorly placed plantar flexors—the gastrocnemius, soleus, and tibialis posterior—activate. When gravity projects posteriorly, ankle dorsiflexors—the tibialis anterior and long toe extensors—equalize gravitational torque on the other side of the axis (A Closer Look Box 9-2). In each case the body's weight stabilizes the feet, so these muscles act on their origins to pull the body forward or backward over the ankle. These closed-chain effects on the ankle are less clear than those on the knee and hip.

Open-chain ankle movements in which the toes rise up (open-chain dorsiflexion) or point down (open-chain plantar flexion) are most familiar. Closed-chain dorsiflexion and plantar flexion occur because body weight stabilizes the distal end of the chain (foot). Closed-chain ankle dorsiflexion and knee flexion occur together in a deep knee bend. The angle decreases between the dorsum of the foot and the lower leg, just as it does in open-chain dorsiflexion (Figure 9-5). Just as eccentric contraction of the knee extensor (quadriceps) controls knee flexion with gravity, eccentric contraction of the plantar flexor controls ankle dorsiflexion in a deep knee bend.

Concentric contractions also produce closed-chain movements at the ankle during fine adjustments for balance in weight bearing. As the dorsiflexors shorten, they pull the tibia forward toward the dorsum of the foot. Slight knee flexion sometimes accompanies this adjustment. Plantar flexors shorten to pull the tibia backward, and the knee extends.

During open-chain plantar flexion, the toes point in the air (when the body does not bear weight), but during closed-chain plantar flexion, the body stands on its toes. Toes, the distal ends of the lower-extremity chain, are planted, and the entire body including the heel moves in relation to them.

Gravity and muscle use

We demonstrate closed-chain plantar flexion when we reach toward an overhead cabinet. We examined the effect of overhead reaching on Iris's hip joint earlier, but now we consider its effect on the ankle. Iris weighs 60 kg (Figure 9-6, *A*), and most of that weight shifts onto the ball of her right foot as she reaches high above her head. We can assume that Iris's center of gravity lies slightly to the left of her spine at about L3. It projects downward posterior to the metatarsophalangeal joints, producing a force vector for closed-chain dorsiflexion. This vector has a moment arm of 8 cm (from Iris's center of gravity projection to the location of the pivot point at her metatarsophalangeal joint [Figure 9-6, *B*]). The gastrocnemius and soleus muscles must produce equal torque toward plantar flexion to support Iris.

Because the force of gravity acting on the body falls closer to the axis of motion than the force of the muscles acting against gravity, plantar flexion is an example of a second-class lever. Iris's muscles have the mechanical advantage because they work almost twice as far from the axis (pivot) as her body weight. Iris's muscles have leverage over gravity; therefore equilibrium of torques helps determine how much muscle force she needs to balance on her toes. Converting centimeters to meters and kilograms to newtons, calculate this force:

$$600 \text{ N} \times 0.08 \text{ m} = \_\_\_\_ \text{ N} \times 0.15 \text{ m}$$

$$48 \text{ Nm} = \_\_\_\_ \text{ N} \times 0.15 \text{ m}$$

$$\frac{48 \text{ Nm}}{0.15 \text{ m}} = 320 \text{ N}$$

Because of their longer moment arms, Iris' muscles exert about half the force of gravity to raise her body's weight.

Gravity's projection determines responsive muscle activity for the maintenance of upright posture at specific

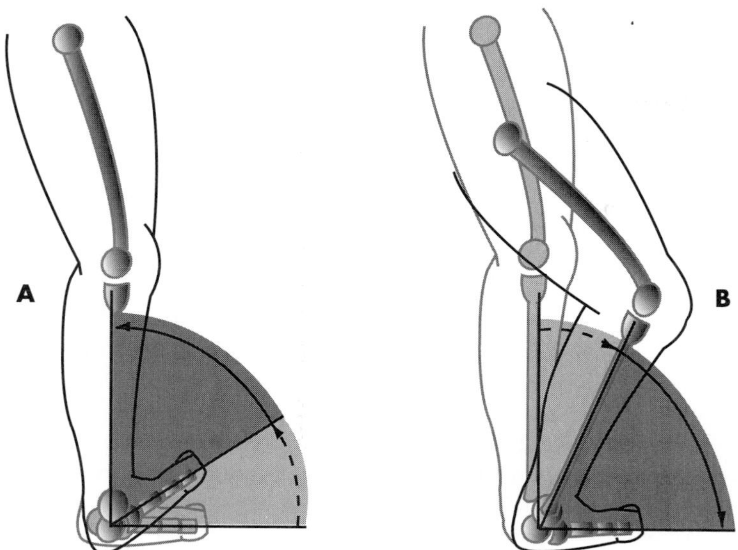

FIGURE **9-5**
The decreasing angle indicates open-chain dorsiflexion **(A)** and closed-chain dorsiflexion **(B).**

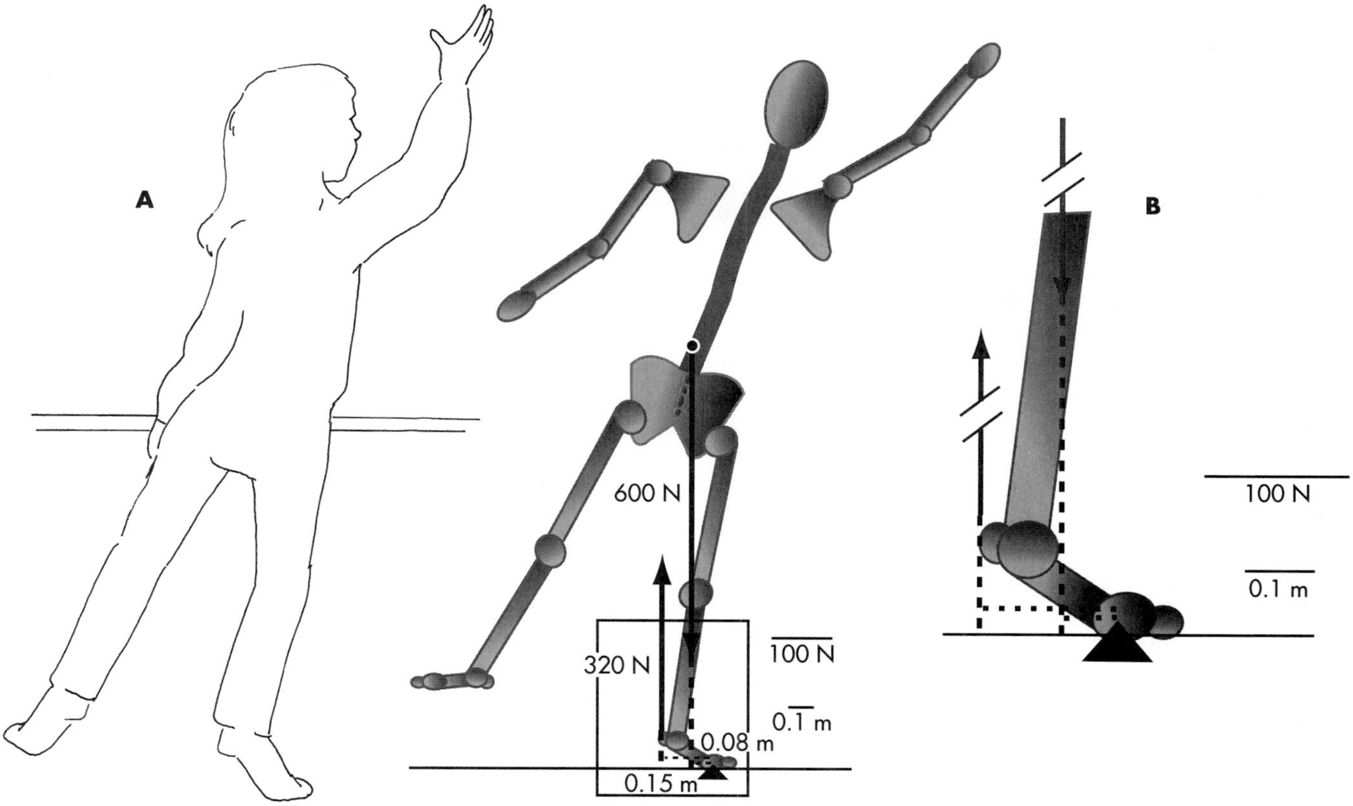

FIGURE **9-6**
A, As Iris reaches into an overhead cabinet, she shifts the weight onto the ball of one foot, which involves plantar flexion of the weight-bearing ankle. **B,** The gastrocnemius and soleus exert 320 N of force to produce closed-chain plantar flexion and raise the total body weight onto the balls of the feet.

joints. It affects the body's ability to maintain overall balance and is one of four **factors in stability.**

Factors in Stability

What determines whether an individual falls or maintains balance? Why does an individual fall during a wheelchair or mat transfer? Why is curb-hopping in a wheelchair so difficult? Exploring the factors that affect stability in a gravity-controlled environment provides answers to these questions.

Imagine yourself standing on a thin ledge of rock, high on the face of a mountain. Would you stand tall or crouch down low? Would you place your feet close together or spread them apart? Would you lean forward, backward, leftward, or rightward or plant yourself directly over your feet? Would you take off your belt pack or keep its weight around your waist? In each case the second selection represents the most stable choice. These answers demonstrate the four factors that affect stability.

Physical bodies are more stable when **center of gravity height** is lower. Notice that toddlers begin to walk by bending at the knees and hips, lowering the center of gravity. Stability depends on a wide stance, or **base of support,** like the one toddlers adopt. The third factor, the **center of gravity projection,** exhibits interplay with the base of support. Standing straight up on the ledge of rock maintains the center of gravity projection through the base of support. Leaning over projects the center of gravity into dangerous zones.

Balance depends on a center of gravity projection. When this projection falls outside the base of support, balance is lost. Efforts to recover are attempts to replace the center of gravity projection within the base of support. For example, if someone pushes you from behind, you may step forward in the direction of the impending fall, increasing your base of support so that the projection once again falls within it. You also may lean backward to place the projection back within the original base of support.

The fourth factor in stability is **weight.** From Newton's law and from our own experiences, we know that the more massive an object, the more difficult it is to move. Traditional Japanese Sumo wrestlers demonstrate mastery of stability and weight, and high-heeled shoes represent disregard for these factors (A Closer Look Box 9-3).

CEREBRAL VASCULAR ACCIDENT

Stability is often a concern in poststroke rehabilitation. As an individual reaches into an overhead cabinet while standing, stability is challenged. After a cerebral vascular accident (CVA), these challenges are accentuated through asymmetrical weight bearing. Challenges to stability occur on an even more basic level as the individual attempts to sit upright and unsupported on a mat table.

Threats to balance

Mary Smith has a left-side hemiplegia, the result of a right-side CVA several months ago. In the course of her therapy, Mary spends time every day on a mat table in Maple Grove Skilled Care Facility. Her base of support is the area at which her buttocks and posterior thighs contact the mat surface (Figure 9-7). Mary's thighs and buttocks form a deep, front-to-back base of support, but the weight of her upper body concentrates at the rear of that base. In other words the projection of Mary's center of gravity lies near the posterior border of her base of support. This projection is inherently unstable. It must be moved to the base's center for greater stability.

The posterior location of Mary's center of gravity projection means she can sway only a little backward before her upper body projection falls outside the posterior border of her base of support. As long as Mary's projection is within her base, the mat's upward push into her body through the base of support balances her upper-body weight's downward pull. An outside projection means that gravity pulls down in a place at which nothing pushes up to hold her trunk erect. No wonder Mary seems fearful of sitting unsupported on the mat.

Normally, projecting the center of gravity backward outside the base of support produces two typical responses: Trunk flexors can overcome the extension effect of gravity and pull the upper body forward so that the center of gravity projects through the original base or both shoulders can extend to place the hands posteriorly, extending the base of support and allowing the center of gravity to project through the new, deeper base.

These typical responses are more difficult for Mary because she sustained motor impairments after her CVA. Mary has left-side hemiplegia, and her trunk muscles activate asymmetrically. As the right trunk flexors contract, part of her trunk rotates to the left and flexes laterally to the right instead of flexing forward symmetrically. She can extend her right shoulder backward but can move her left arm only minimally to her left side, where it lies with wrist flexed, bearing weight on the dorsal surface. Because of motor impairment, her left arm is unable to hold its full share of the upper-body weight. Thus she extends the base of support on one side only. The projection of her trunk's center of gravity falls to the left side of her deeper but narrower base of support.

In addition, Mary's altered sensation and motor function after her CVA have changed her perception of midline. She tends to lean to the right, shifting the side-to-side dimensions of her base of support and bringing her center of gravity projection closer to the right. This in-

BOX 9-3

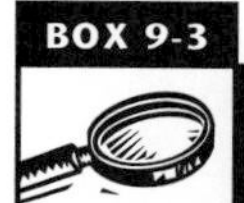

A **CLOSER** LOOK

High-Heeled Shoes and Stability

High-heeled shoes seem designed to make walking difficult because they violate all four stability factors. High heels raise the center of gravity and shift weight forward onto the toes. Pointed toes narrow the base of support in front, and small heels provide an unnaturally narrow base of posterior support. The narrow side-to-side base of support translates into a tendency toward ankle inversion or eversion. The higher the heel, the shorter the front-to-back dimension at the base of support.

The center of gravity projection moves toward the front of an ever-narrowing base of support; therefore the pelvis tilts anteriorly, creating lordosis to move the shoulders behind the pelvis and shift the center of gravity projection posteriorly into the base of support. Body weight does not change, but its application becomes directed into a small area with an extremely high force. Thus high heels are rough on floors and make walking nearly impossible on any outdoor surface but the hardest of packed dirt.

High heels progressively decrease stability and transform weight bearing and walking into hazardous and potentially damaging experiences. Narrowing the base of support in front and back makes it more difficult for each foot to shift weight from the sole to the lateral border of the foot in stance. The arch tends to collapse into inversion after years of use. Shortening the base of support makes lordosis essential to keep the center of gravity projection within the base of support. Prolonged lordosis causes shortening of the hip flexors and can damage the lumbar disks. Raising the heels raises the center of gravity and places the entire unstable mass onto the bones of the forefoot. These small bones were meant to distribute weight over a larger area, buttressed by a shock-absorbing arch. They sustain serious damage when massive forces are concentrated in areas the size of ice-cream cones.

Constant wearing of high heels causes the Achilles tendon to shorten and eventually makes the wearing of flat shoes impossible. Gait is altered, so the swing phase stops short. If not otherwise stretched, the hamstrings shorten. Shortened gastrocnemii, shortened hamstrings, and weakened quadriceps form a triad that leads to lower-back injury in the lifting of even the lightest weights.

creases her risk of falling. As she leans far enough to the right so that her projection falls outside the base, she loses her balance. Her impaired responses diminish her capacity to recover stability and increase her probability of falling.

Mary has similar difficulties standing because she cannot assume a symmetrical stance. Even when both feet are on the ground, Mary's base of support is altered by the unreliability of her left lower extremity. Her functional base of support extends around her right foot only, giving her less than half the normal base other individuals have to stand. Mary's narrow base of support and her impaired ability to shift weight right or left through upper-body movements make it difficult for her to maintain her center of gravity projection through the base of support.

Mary's asymmetrical weight bearing also compromises her ability to reach into overhead cabinets. Raising her right hand over her head and forward moves Mary's center of gravity upward and forward. Therefore her straight-down projection is likely to fall outside the base of her support, causing her to lose her balance. Mary could use a cane, placing it forward to extend her base of support and compensate for her more forward center of gravity projection. However, to accomplish this purpose, she would have to hold the cane in the same upper extremity she uses to reach into the cabinet. The cane then would offer her little support as she reaches.

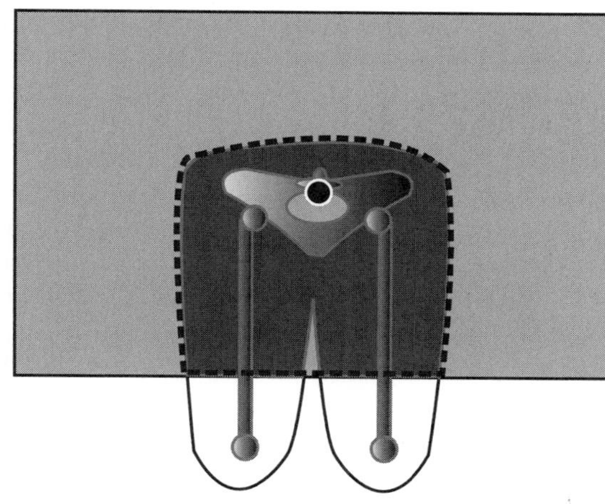

FIGURE **9-7**
Mary's base of support when she sits on a mat table.

TRANSFERS

The factors in stability come into play each time Mary transfers from her wheelchair to her bed or the mat table

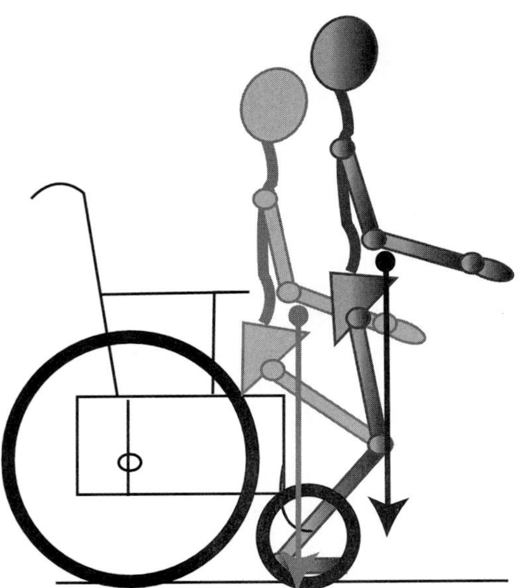

FIGURE **9-8**
Mary's transitional base of support is too close to the wheelchair. Once she stands, she has difficulty preventing her center of gravity from projecting in front of her transitional base of support.

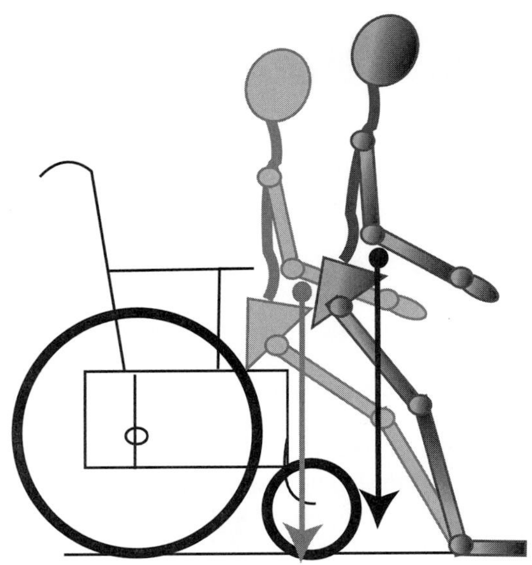

FIGURE **9-9**
Mary's transitional base of support is too far forward. When she moves to stand, she must travel forward more than is possible. Mary finds that with too little momentum, her center of gravity projects behind the transitional base.

to her wheelchair. A transfer moves the center of gravity from one base of support to another, sometimes with a transitional base in the middle. Only as long as her center of gravity projection moves from one base to another without more than a momentary projection between the old and new bases of support can Mary maintain her sense of balance.

As Mary transfers from her wheelchair to the mat table in a stand-pivot movement, the four points at which the wheels contact the wheelchair outline her existing base of support. Her target base is the mat table. A box drawn around the outer edges of Mary's shoes outlines this transitional base of support. Because the OT practitioner supports Mary, the OT practitioner's shoes enlarge the transitional base. Mary and her OT practitioner share this base for a short time.

One day Mary almost fell during a transfer because the OT practitioner placed Mary's feet too close to the wheelchair. While pulling Mary forward in her seat to prepare for the transfer, the OT practitioner placed Mary's feet on the ground between the chair's two front casters, nearly tucked under the chair. As soon as Mary stood up, her center of gravity projected to the very front edge of the transitional base (Figure 9-8). Mary felt like she was falling forward, and the OT practitioner began to fall backward. The OT practitioner then sat Mary back down in the chair.

During the next transfer attempt the OT practitioner overcompensated and placed Mary's feet too far in front of her knees. The transfer required too much forward travel, and Mary felt her gravity projection fall behind the transitional base (Figure 9-9).

Often, OT practitioners in similar situations make a strong, sudden rotation to complete a transfer rather than stop it. This maneuver requires a ballistic-type muscle contraction in the OT practitioner's lower back and generally leads to a low-back injury. Easing a client back into the original position or onto the floor are better options.

The most stable stand-pivot transfer involves consideration of placements at all three bases of support before movement begins. The OT practitioner moves the chair and mat as close together as possible without restricting the practitioner's own base of support. The client scoots forward in the chair, with the feet directly under the knees. As soon as the client's knees and hips extend into standing, the center of gravity projection is automatically through the center of the transitional base. The client easily can move onto the mat if the chair is close enough to the mat. The client is able to pivot and begin flexing the hips and knees. The center of gravity projects behind the feet, but the mat supplies the final base of support.

Meanwhile, the OT practitioner's stability must be ensured. Reaching out too far in front puts the practitioner at a disadvantage and requires forward leaning. The OT practitioner's center of gravity moves anteriorly and projects near the front of the base of support (Figure 9-10, *A*).

As more assistance is provided, the OT practitioner is pulled increasingly toward the client. The OT practitioner should anticipate the forward weight shift and adjust the stance before a transfer by moving as close to the

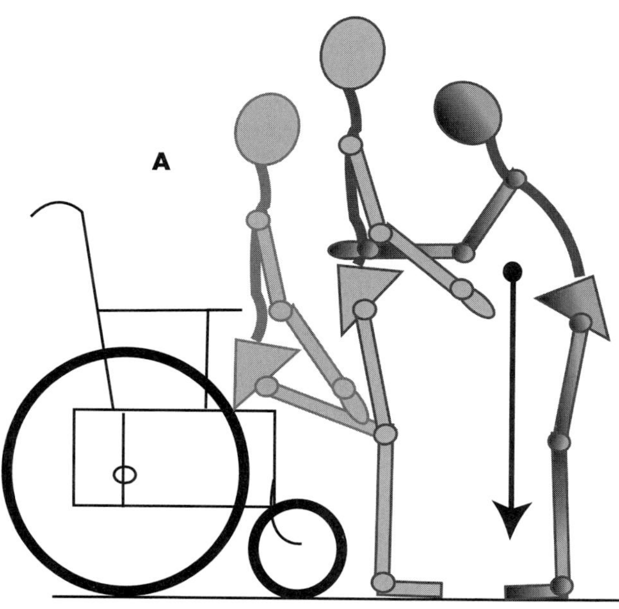

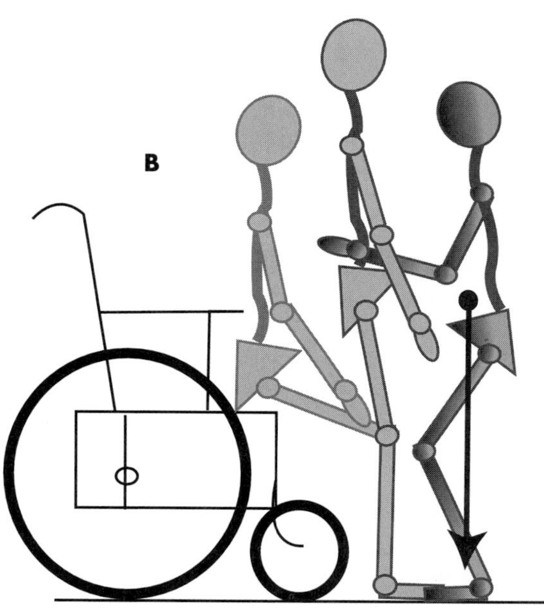

FIGURE **9-10**
A, Leaning and reaching forward to assist the client moves the OT practitioner's center of gravity projection too far forward relative to the base of support. **B,** Standing close and bending at the knees keeps the OT practitioner's projection more centralized in the base of support and decreases the risk of falling.

client as possible. Instead of leaning forward and down to reach for a transfer belt and assist, the OT practitioner bends the knees and maintains the center of gravity projection through the base of support. The OT practitioner reaches forward with the upper extremities only, to prevent forward shift of the practitioner's center of gravity.

BOX 9-4

A **CLOSER** LOOK

Transfers as Therapy

Transfers often are performed hastily. Instead of viewing transfers simply as part of getting the client to the clinic to begin therapy, think of them as opportunities to improve body awareness, strength, balance, impulse control, and sequencing skills. Transfers are one form of therapy and involve more than movement from one place to another.

Engage clients in the transfer for full therapeutic value. Talk to clients about the transfer before, during, and after it occurs. Before the transfer, review the steps and reassure clients about safety. Instruct the clients in the importance of wheelchair positioning and proper use of transfer belts.

Engage the help an aide, who can watch and provide standby assistance. Use clear physical and verbal prompts during the transfer. In stand-pivot and sliding-board transfers, pause for quick assessments when reaching the transitional base of support, and after completing the transfer, assess the full process while the experience is still fresh in your mind.

Above all, do not use transfers as opportunities to prove your strength and experience. Taking time to assist clients in transfers may save time later. Poor judgments present unnecessary risks to clients and threaten the trust between the client and the practitioner.

This keeps the practitioner's projection closer to the center of the base of support (Figure 9-10, *B*).

In moderate- to maximum-assist transfers the weight of the client becomes a forward drag that moves the OT practitioner's center of gravity projection to the front edge of the base. This unstable situation puts both the OT practitioner and the client at risk of falling. The OT practitioner anticipates and balances this added weight; the practitioner's posterior weight shift is synchronized with the amount of assistance the practitioner provides. A posterior weight shift provides a supportive lifting force far superior to that of upper-body strength. The net effect maintains the OT practitioner's center of gravity projection through the center of the base and provides assistance using body weight rather than upper-body strength (A Closer Look Box 9-4).

Toilet transfer

The hamstrings originate on the ischial tuberosity of the pelvis and continue down the back of the leg to attach onto the tibia. Together with the gluteus maximus, they extend the hip as the quadriceps femoris extends the

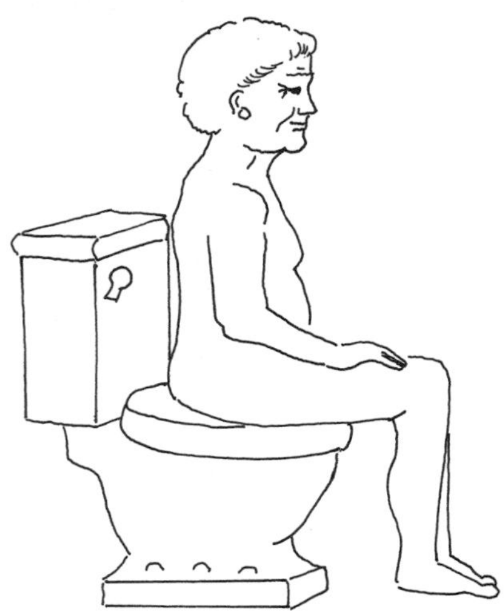

FIGURE **9-11**
Mary tries to stand from an erect sitting posture.

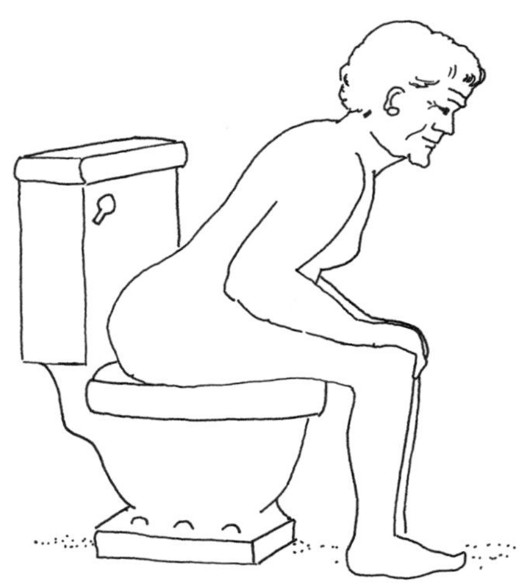

FIGURE **9-12**
Mary tries to stand by leaning forward first.

knee when an individual stands from a sitting, stooping, or bending position.

Because toilets are usually low, these muscles must work especially hard to extend the hips and knees when an individual stands from a toilet. Lack of height and armrests to help the individual push off make standing from a seated position on the toilet difficult.

With Mary's balance problems, she is especially fearful during toilet transfers and tries to stand from an erect sitting posture (Figure 9-11). In the erect position, her center of gravity projects directly through the base of support (toilet) but far behind her transitional base (feet on the floor). Mary must move forward a considerable distance to balance over her transitional base of support and stand. If not, she may begin weight bearing on her feet before she is able to move forward far enough to project her center of gravity through that transitional base, causing her to fall backward.

The OT practitioner convinces Mary to lean forward before attempting to stand (Figure 9-12). Her head moves over her knees so that her body's center of gravity projects closer to her transitional base of support before she begins to stand. This makes standing easier and reduces her risk of falling backward between her feet and the toilet.

Consider the equilibrium torques at Mary's knees. Her upper-body weight produces torque toward knee flexion as soon as she begins standing and weight bearing through her feet. Mary's quadriceps (especially the right) must produce equal torque toward knee extension to balance this effect of gravity. The erect sitting posture (see Figure 9-11) places Mary's center of gravity 33 cm from the axis of motion in her knee (Figure 9-13). The forward-leaning position (see Figure 9-12) places her center of gravity 22 cm from the axis of motion at her knee (Figure 9-14). With this shorter moment arm, Mary's upper-body weight produces less knee flexion torque, and her quadriceps generate less force to extend the knees when she stands.

How much more force do Mary's quadriceps generate when she stands from an erect sitting posture as opposed to a forward-leaning sitting posture? The quadriceps' moment arm is 5 cm when the knee is flexed to 90 degrees. Because only Mary's upper-body weight produces knee-flexion torque, subtract the weight of the lower extremities from her total 70-kg weight (see Appendix B, Table B-1). Each upper leg is 9.7%, each lower leg is 4.5%, and each foot is 1.4% (the product being rounded):

$$2(0.097 + 0.045 + 0.014) \times 70 \text{ kg} = 21.84 \text{ kg}$$

$$70 \text{ kg} - 22 \text{ kg} = 48 \text{ kg} = \text{Weight of body flexing the knee}$$

Converting centimeters to meters and kilograms to newtons, calculate the force Mary's quadriceps must produce when she stands from an erect sitting posture:

$$480 \text{ N} \times 0.33 \text{ m} = 0.05 \text{ m} \times \underline{\qquad} \text{ N}$$

$$\frac{158.4 \text{ Nm}}{0.05 \text{ m}} = \underline{\qquad} \text{ N}$$

$$3168 \text{ N}$$

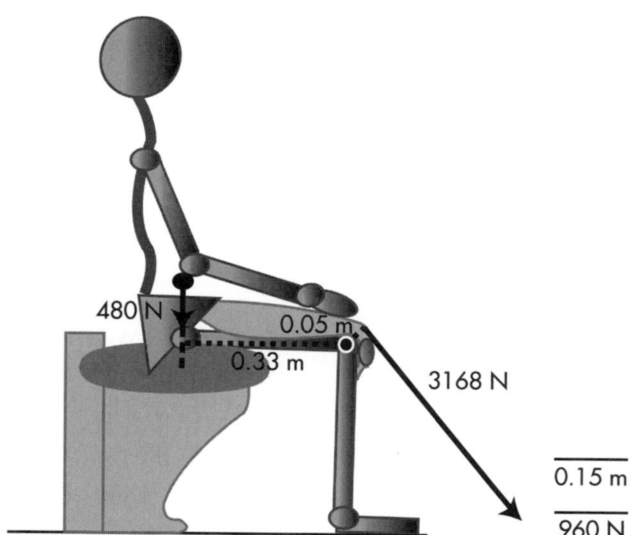

FIGURE **9-13**
Mary's quadriceps muscle must produce 3168 N of force to balance the downward pull of gravity on the upper body when she attempts to stand from an erect sitting posture.

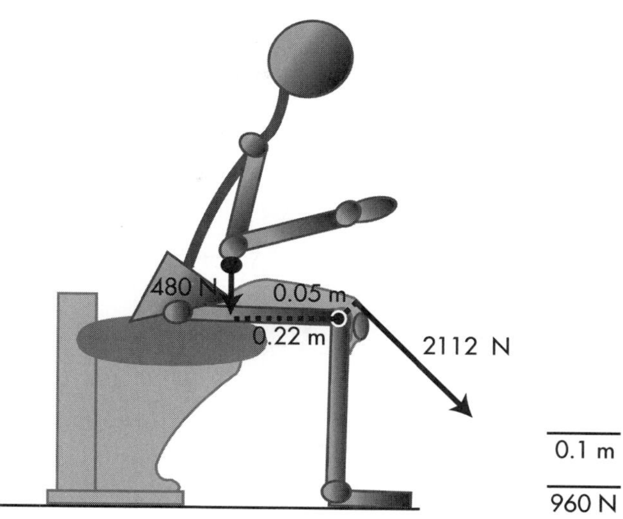

FIGURE **9-14**
Mary's quadriceps must produce 2112 N of force to balance her upper-body weight when she attempts to stand from a forward-leaning position.

Calculate the force Mary's quadriceps must produce when she stands from a forward-leaning sitting posture:

$$480 \text{ N} \times 0.22 \text{ m} = 0.05 \text{ m} \times \_\_\_\_\_\_ \text{ N}$$

$$\frac{105.6 \text{ Nm}}{0.05 \text{ m}} = \_\_\_\_\_\_ \text{ N}$$

$$2112 \text{ N}$$

Mary needs an additional 1000 N of quadriceps force when she stands from an erect as opposed to a forward-leaning sitting posture. The extra force is an unnecessary strain that Mary cannot handle. Leaning forward is clearly a superior technique, but Mary's quadriceps still must exert considerable force for her to stand from a forward-leaning sitting posture.

Individuals with weak quadriceps like Mary benefit from leaning forward and using armrests to push themselves up when they stand from sitting positions (Figure 9-15). Placing the hands on armrests allows the triceps to extend the elbows in a closed-chain motion. Closed-chain elbow extension produces upward trunk movement (A Closer Look Box 9-5).

WHEELCHAIRS

Wheelchairs have large bases of support, substantial weight, relatively low centers of gravity, and centers of gravity projection well within their bases of support. Usually all these factors work together to make them stable. Sometimes, semirecliners have rear bases of sup-

BOX 9-5

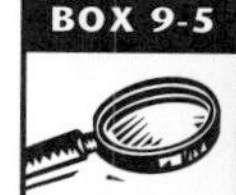

A **CLOSER** LOOK

Benefits of Raised Toilet Seats

Raised toilet seats prevent the erect upper body from developing a longer moment arm when an individual sits on the toilet. When the individual stands, the upper-body weight projects through the knee axis, so no flexion moment exists at the knee. Sitting causes the upper body to move backward in relation to the feet and knees, and the moment arm for knee flexion increases to maximum length in full sitting position (hips and knees flexed to 90 degrees).

The raised toilet seat allows the individual to sit with less than 90 degrees of hip and knee flexion, preventing development of the upper body's long moment arm for knee flexion. Standing from this raised position involves less quadriceps force because upper-body weight pulls down with a shorter moment arm at the knee and produces less knee-flexion torque. Raising sofa and chair legs onto blocks approximates this result, but such efforts often are stymied by soft, sinkable cushions.

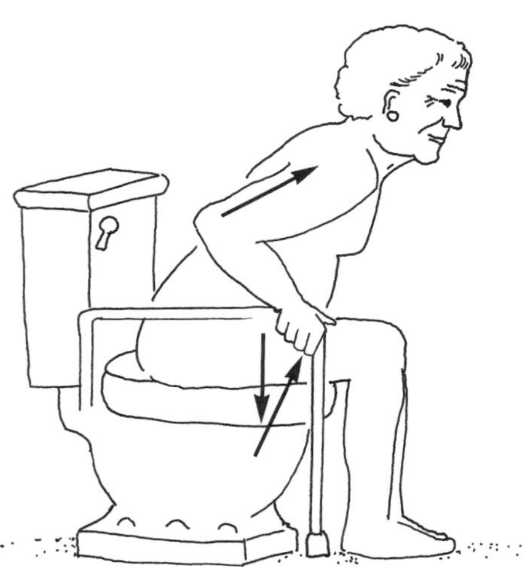

FIGURE **9-15**
Mary pushes herself off armrests to reduce the load on her quadriceps as she stands.

port that are too short when the chair backs are fully reclined. An individual with bilateral lower-extremity amputation who uses a standard wheelchair experiences a backward shift in the center of gravity projection, resulting in instability. Lightweight sport wheelchairs often have built-in rearward centers of gravity projection to ease maneuverability. The sport wheelchair's front wheels pop up easily, making it possible for the user to hop curbs and maneuver stairs. However, these "wheelies" require practice to reduce the risk of backward falls in this unstable position.

Semirecliners

A fully reclined wheelchair back tilts the center of gravity projection backward. Full recliners are built with extended frames to accommodate this projection. Semirecliners allow some degree of recline with shorter wheel bases to improve maneuverability. Because the base of support is shorter than in a full recliner, moving the center of gravity projection backward comes close to the rear limit of the base of support in the "full" semireclined position (Figure 9-16).

As long as the projection stays within the base of support, the semirecliner remains upright. Even a slight forward force, such as a sudden push, can throw the chair off balance enough to cause the user to fall backward. The forward push moves the wheels, which form the base of support, in front of the center of gravity projection, tipping the chair backward (Figure 9-17). The same quick start creates little risk with an upright chair back because the center of gravity projection is farther forward.

Wheels

Changing the positions of the front casters and rear wheels changes the wheelchair's stability. The front casters change positions every time the wheelchair reverses direction, which modifies the depth (front-to-rear dimensions) of the chair's base of support. The front casters point toward the rear when the chair stops moving forward and toward the front when it stops backing up (Figure 9-18). As a result the base of support is shorter as the chair moves forward and longer as it moves backward (Figure 9-19). As the user bends forward to pick up an object from the floor, weight is shifted onto the footrests, moving the center of gravity and its projection forward in the base of support. As the user reaches too far forward, the projection is pushed in front of the base, causing the chair to fall forward (Figure 9-20).

Xavier Morales is a 50-year-old salesman who lost both his legs during a tour of duty in Vietnam. He often wears prostheses to stand for presentations and uses a standard wheelchair at work. When Xavier reaches for his briefcase and other objects on the floor, he pivots to place objects to his side between his casters and wheels and leans to the side rather than forward. If he needs to get something in a corner or tight place, Xavier automatically pushes his chair slightly backward to pivot his casters backward. Sometimes he uses the shorter casters-backward base motion to tip his chair onto its footrests but only when he can use his desk or wall as a brace to regain an upright position.

Individuals who use lightweight wheelchairs can adjust their chairs easily. Adjusting the base of support involves moving the wheels forward or backward. Normally the center of gravity projects near the rear edge of the base, so moving the wheels forward brings this projection closer to the rear edge. Xavier intentionally adjusts his wheelchair this way so that he can pop up the front casters in a wheelie. Xavier maintains his balance by keeping the center of gravity projection through the axle of the rear wheels. His base of support is only as deep as the portion of rear wheels touching the ground, directly under the axle (Figure 9-21). Balanced on the two rear wheels, Xavier can hop up or down curbs and some stairs.

Xavier first learned this technique in the veterans' rehabilitation hospital, where he practiced with mats while OT staff members guided him. He tried for months before he learned the proper control. A slightly too forceful forward push moves the projection of gravity too far behind the base. The wheelchair quickly spins backward on the wheels, accelerating the seat and the individual backward until something hits the ground. When this happened, Xavier's push handles usually hit the ground and his quick reflexes and strong neck flexors saved him from injury. A couple times Xavier hit his head hard enough to "see stars," but he continued to practice on his

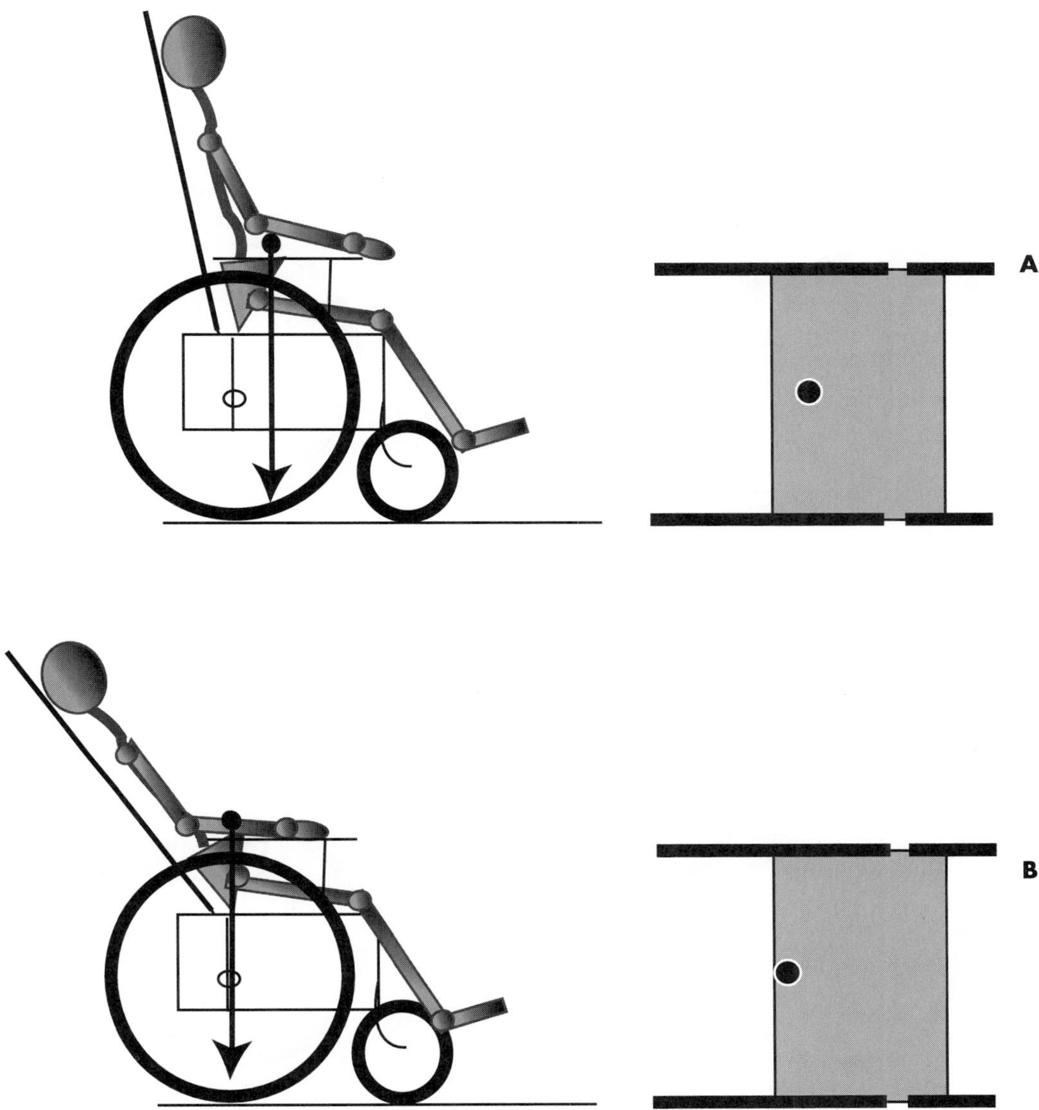

FIGURE **9-16**
A, Side view of a semirecliner and top view of the base of support and projected center of gravity when the chair back is upright. **B,** Same two views when the chair back is fully reclined.

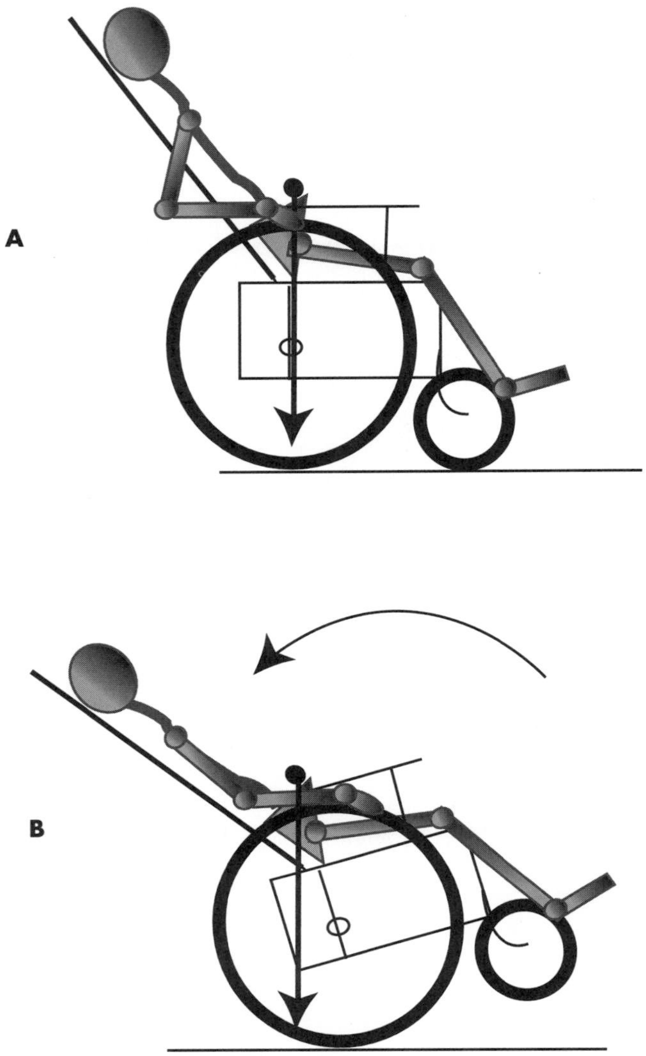

FIGURE **9-17**
A, The reclined position moves the center of gravity projection toward the back of the base of support. **B,** The quick start moves the base of support from under the center of gravity projection, and the chair falls backward.

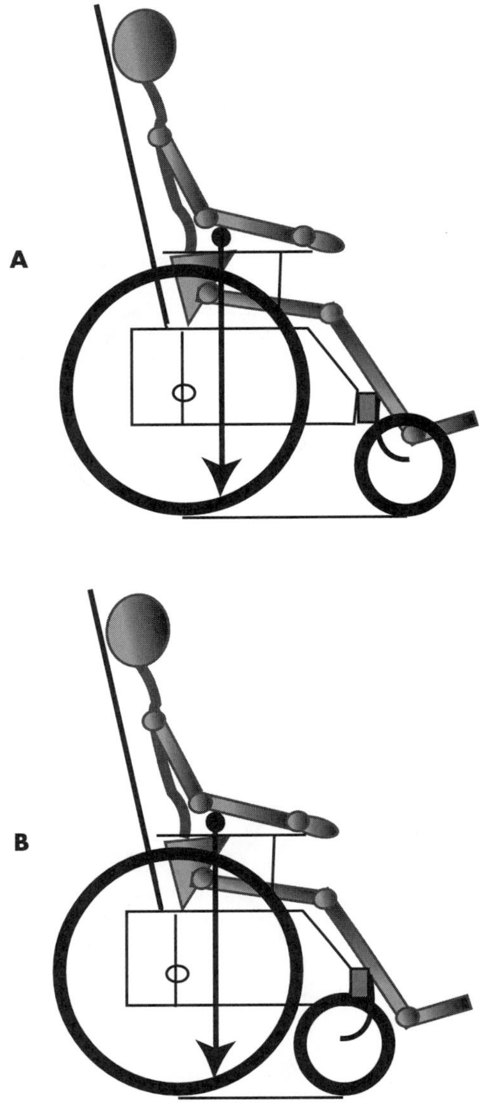

FIGURE **9-18**
The front casters swivel to point to the front when the chair stops backing up **(A)** and to the rear when it stops moving forward **(B).**

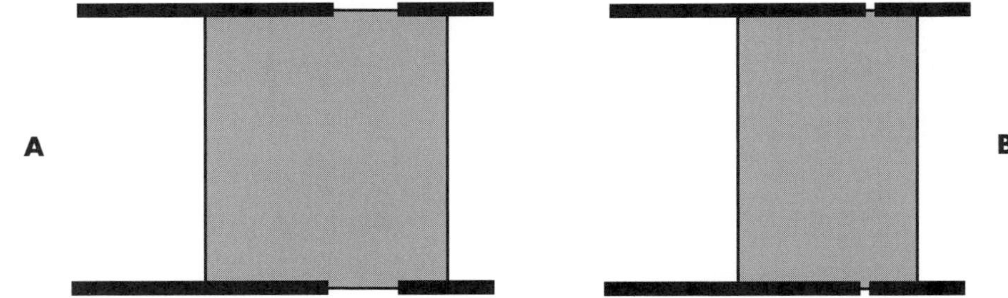

FIGURE **9-19**
Top view of the base of support as affected by the position of the front casters. As the chair backs up, it has a longer base of support **(A)** than as it moves forward **(B).**

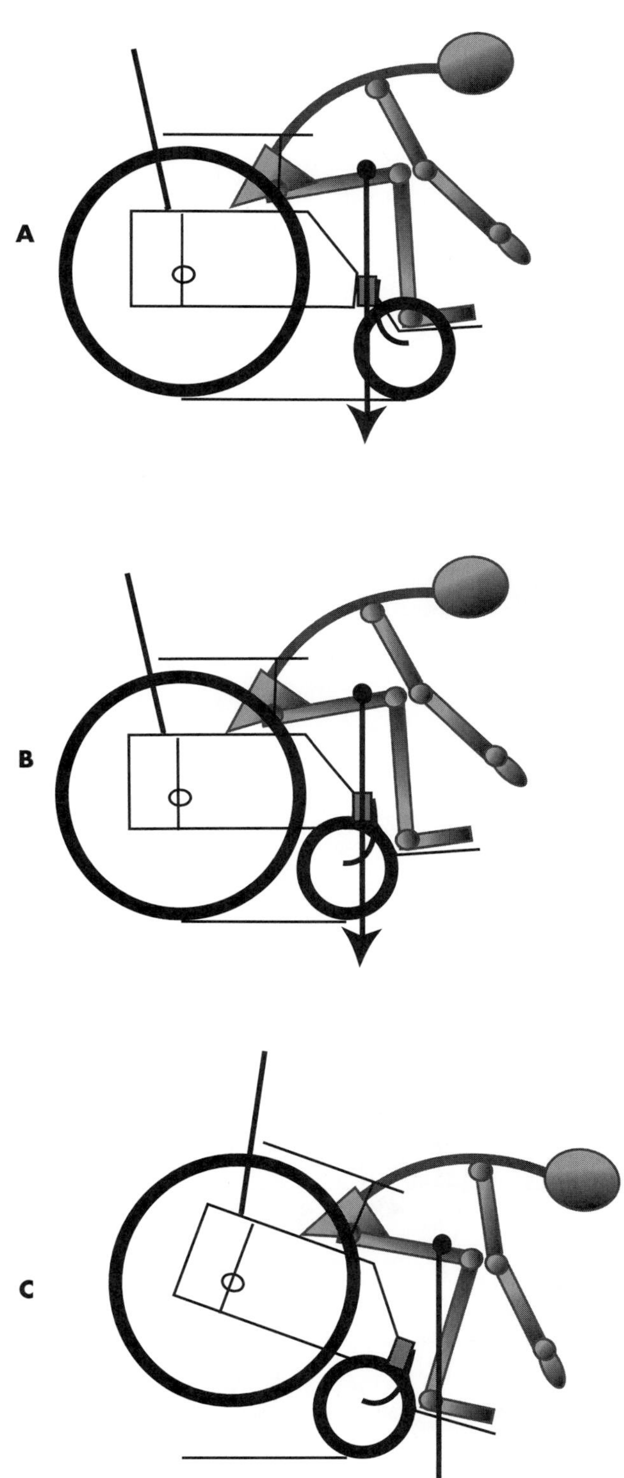

FIGURE **9-20**
Forward leaning moves the center of gravity projection forward. **A,** It remains inside the base of support when the casters point forward. **B,** It moves outside the base of support when the casters point to the rear. **C,** This causes the chair to fall forward.

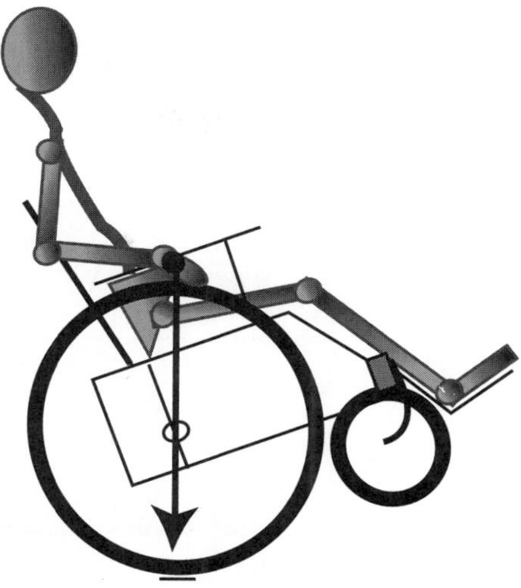

FIGURE **9-21**
Xavier balances his chair in a wheelie.

own in wheelchair athletics. Although difficult at first, eventually wheelies become natural and their advantage in overcoming architectural barriers makes them worth the practice.

Rear wheels on sport chairs can be tilted so that the bottoms of the rims are farther apart than the tops. This tilt, or **camber,** makes maneuvering the chair easier (Figure 9-22). Because the tops of the wheels are closer to the body than the bottoms, the shoulders can push from a more relaxed position (less shoulder abduction). Slight abduction of the arms and hands as they follow the rims makes the forward stroke more natural.

Camber also widens the base of support and increases the chair's stability. Cambered wheels provide a base that used to be available only in extra-wide chairs. More sideways stability combines with greater maneuverability to make camber an essential feature in all sport wheelchairs.

Instability after amputation

Because an individual's center of gravity is the sum of the segmental centers of gravity, Xavier's center of gravity shifts substantially when he does not wear his prostheses. Without this weight, Xavier loses much of the body weight that projects forward in sitting and his center of gravity projects more toward the rear than normal (Figure 9-23). Like the person in the semirecliner wheelchair, Xavier's risk of falling backward is greater than normal. In his case the posterior center of gravity projection is due to loss of mass in front, not to the chair's reclined position. Quick starts move this projection behind his base of support, and the front of his chair tips

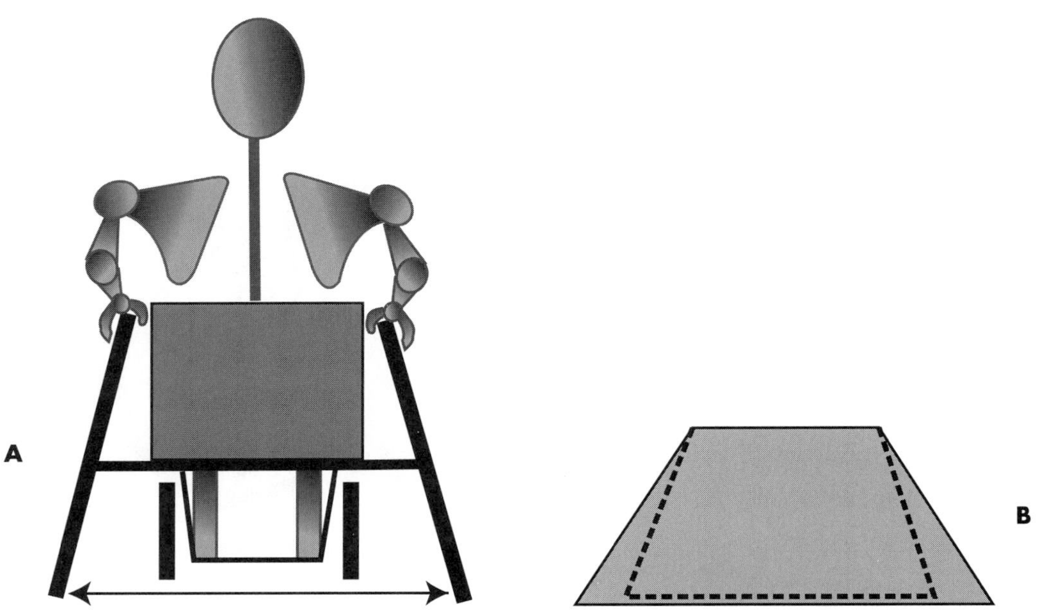

FIGURE **9-22**
Rear-wheel camber **(A)** and its effect on the width of the base of support **(B).**

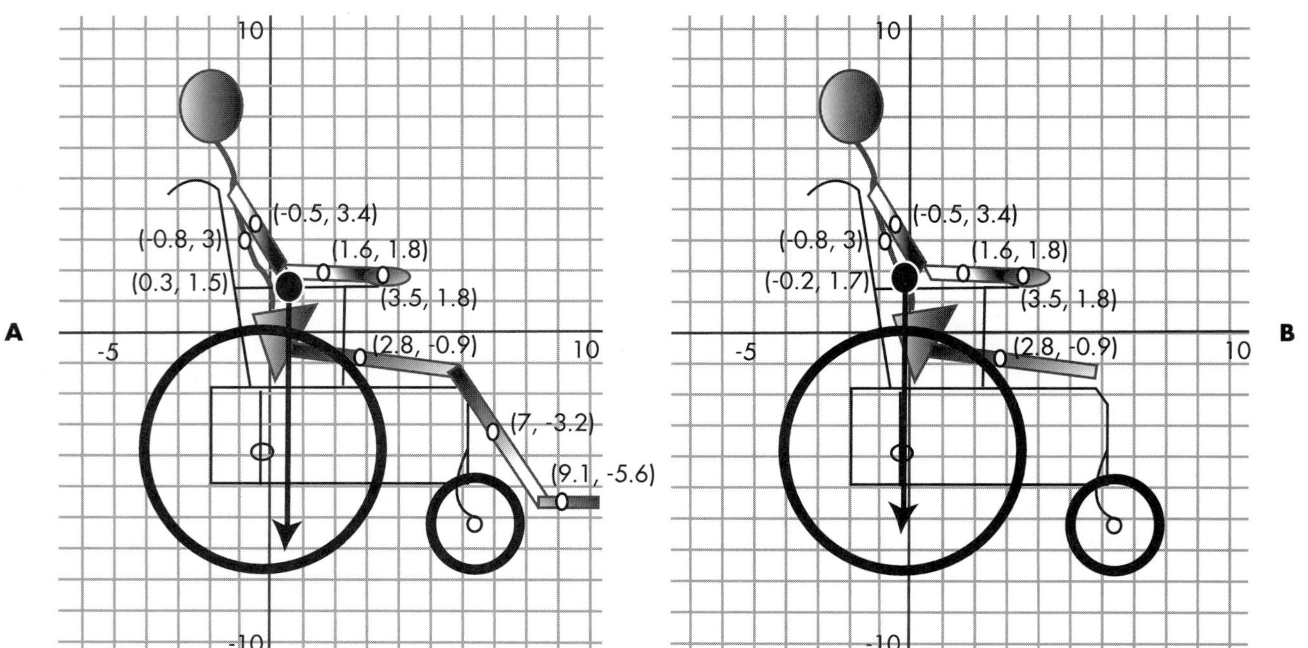

FIGURE **9-23**
A, The segmental centers of gravity are determined using the process described in Chapter 3. **B,** The center of gravity projection shifts toward the rear when an individual whose lower extremities have been amputated sits in a wheelchair.

up. Before Xavier entered the rehab hospital, the degree of instability in his standard chair frightened him. Xavier could not adjust his balance in time, and the fear of falling kept him rooted in one spot, dependent on others for mobility.

As soon as Xavier got to the rehab hospital, OT practitioners placed sandbag weights on his footrests. The added weight anterior to his center of gravity adjusted his center of gravity projection and gave him immediate relief. As a longer-term adaptation, OT staff members ordered him a rear-axle extender, a piece of wheelchair frame that bolts onto the original frame. They removed his rear wheels from their original positions and reattached them more toward the rear on the extender. This adjustment extended his base of support, and Xavier's center of gravity projection fell more toward the center of the new base. Xavier became more mobile and moved into his lightweight wheelchair to pursue a more active lifestyle.

Adjustments affecting stability and pressure

Footrests are probably the most neglected adjustments in wheelchairs. Many individuals in long-term care facilities, hospitals, and rehab centers rest their feet at two different heights and degrees of internal or external rotation. Footrest adjustment is critical for pressure distribution, stability in positioning, and comfort. Neglecting adjustment is puzzling, however, because adjusting footrests requires the use of only one wrench and a little effort.

Footrests that are too low put too much pressure on the posterior thighs, threatening venous return from the leg and foot, and promote posterior pelvic tilt as the buttocks slide forward. Posterior pelvic tilt leads to sacral sitting posture, reversed lumbar curve, and pressure sores on the sacrum and lumbar spines.

On the other hand, footrests that are too high shift pressure distribution from the posterior thighs to the ischial tuberosities and promote posterior pelvic tilt as increased hip flexion pulls the ischial tuberosities forward through the hamstring link. Recall that hip flexion stretches the hamstrings. If the hamstrings are short, additional hip flexion caused by high footrests pulls the pelvis into posterior tilt, leading to sacral sitting posture and a rounded lower back. Both effects promote the development of pressure sores.

Rotating footrests so that the feet are in a neutral forward position can be done at the same time the footrest height is adjusted. Toes rotated inward or outward usually cause discomfort and appear awkward. However, if rotation is far enough from alignment, the individual often opts to cease using the footrests, creating the same problems associated with low footrests.

Normal Gait and Variations

Gait cycle is the term used to describe normal walking patterns. A full gait cycle encompasses the series of motions occurring between the time one lower extremity makes contact with the floor until it makes contact again. The gait cycle consists of two phases. The first, the stance phase, includes initial contact of the heel with the ground, loading of the body's weight onto the lower extremity for midstance and terminal stance, and lifting of the heel off the ground into preswing. The swing phase begins as the toe leaves the ground, continues as it accelerates into midswing, and ends after it decelerates into terminal swing.

During initial contact and loading in stance, the knee and hip extensors stabilize the supporting lower extremity to carry the weight of the body. Dorsiflexors eccentrically contract to prevent the foot and toes of the supporting extremity from slapping the ground. Hip stabilizers (abductors) like the gluteus medius maintain the body's alignment over the supporting leg to balance gravity's pull toward closed-chain hip adduction. Weight shifts medially onto the inside of the supporting foot via closed-chain action of the supinators.

By midstance the plantar flexors prevent the body from falling forward at the ankles. Hip stabilizers, including the tensor fasciae latae and iliotibial band, control the knee while maintaining balance over the supporting extremity. Weight rolls onto the inside of the foot and over the arch, which absorbs the shock of impact.

In terminal stance the plantar flexors support the body weight while the momentum of the swinging leg helps propel the body forward. Hip stabilizers maintain balance over the supporting extremity, and weight remains on the inside of the foot for added stability. The flexor of the great toe provides the individual the power to push. As weight shifts during preswing, the erector spinae, lower abdominals, and hip abductors contract to stabilize the trunk and counterbalance pelvic movement. Plantar flexors and toe flexors provide the final push before the stance leg leaves the ground.

Hip flexors pull the swinging leg off the ground to initiate a forward progression and continue that activity throughout the swing. In initial swing the dorsiflexors concentrically contract to raise the toes and foot off the ground. They continue into midswing while the erector spinae counterbalance the trunk's lateral flexion tendency and the pelvis progresses forward toward initial contact. The iliopsoas brings the leg forward into terminal swing while the hip extensors eccentrically contract to control the swing's momentum. Knee extensors keep the leg straight in preparation for initial contact, and dorsiflexors keep the foot from slapping the ground on contact.

RUNNING

Running follows a sequence similar to normal gait except that both feet come off the ground immediately after terminal stance on one side and before initial contact on the other. More muscle force is necessary to raise the body off the ground and propel it with greater speed. Consequently, the lower extremity and spine must absorb greater impact forces.

JUMPING AND HOPPING

Jumping and hopping require greater muscle force from the knee and hip extensors and the plantar and toe flexors to propel the body into the air. Strong hip stabilizers maintain balance over one leg in hops and minimize the impact in jumps. The adductor longus and brevis also flex the hip in jumps.

CRAWLING AND CLIMBING

The sartorius runs diagonally from the ilium to the medial epicondyle of the knee. It flexes the hip and knee while rotating the knee away from the body, as in cross-legged sitting or highland dancing. The sartorius is active in normal gait movements, but simultaneous hip and knee flexion are especially useful in crawling, marching, and climbing stairs. In crawling or climbing the sartorius positions the legs so that the quadriceps and gluteus maximus are ideally situated for propulsion of the body forward or upward.

Biomechanical Analysis

Every time we consider movements and the muscles used we analyze the actions with biomechanical analysis. Our recent discussion on gait, for example, used information obtained from biomechanical analysis. Often, computer analysis uses sophisticated equipment to provide multiple views of an activity. Electromyographic recordings can monitor muscle activity by recording the actual electrical event of muscle activation.

OT practitioners generally use visual analysis to determine the joints, their movements, and the muscles used in these movements. Thus they can identify problematic links in ineffective function. For example, when an individual has difficulty in self-feeding, the OT practitioner may determine that the extreme supination typically necessary for this task is a barrier to independence. Identifying limited supination is then the first step in helping the individual regain function. Use of a different grip pattern may remove the need for supination in the hand-to-mouth movement and restore the individual's independence in self-feeding.

Initial attempts at biomechanical analysis often seem overwhelming. Identifying all the movements at all the joints is a formidable task, but using guesswork to determine muscle activity is the most difficult aspect. Undertaking such a task may seem futile because muscle use in activity can be confirmed through electromyographic analysis only.

Nonetheless, clinically relevant biomechanical analysis must be a part of OT practice. Determining muscle activation in the context of activity performance requires consideration of each movement of the activity in relation to the resistance encountered. Does the movement occur against or with gravity? Does the movement occur against some resistance greater than gravity's pull? Does the movement occur rapidly? Each question helps the OT practitioner make an educated guess about the muscle groups responsible for movement.[2]

Figure 9-24 is a form for biomechanical analysis. Appendix G is a copy of the referenced article that gives a thorough presentation of the process used to complete the form. We use this process to analyze daily activities such as donning shoes and socks.

George O'Hara lives in a group home. He crosses one leg over the other to reach his foot when he dons his shoes and socks. To analyze this activity, determine which lower-extremity movements he uses and identify hip flexion and hip external rotation (Table 9-1). Analyze hip flexion from left to right across the form. Move back to the left of the form, and begin the process for the next movement observed. Stay focused on one movement to narrow the options. Proceed through all other joints involved, one segment at a time.

Beginning the process with hip flexion, estimate the percentage of full range of motion used to identify any extreme of joint range. In this case, crossing one leg uses more than 50% of hip flexion in the crossed leg (50% or 90 degrees being necessary for sitting). Indicate this percentage by marking *>50%* in the table and placing an asterisk in the box to highlight an extreme. Extreme joint motions are often the aspects of the task that cause difficulty. Identifying extremes helps locate problematic links.

Next, discern the active muscle group by asking several questions. Is the motion (hip flexion) rapid or resisted by an external object or force? It is neither when George dons his socks and shoes. Does the movement (hip flexion) occur with or against gravity? Movements against gravity require concentric activation of the agonist named for the motion. Movements with gravity are controlled by eccentric contraction of the antagonist to the movement observed. George flexes his hip against gravity, so he uses his hip flexors in concentric contraction.

Consider what happens with this same hip flexion when George lies in a supine position in bed to don his socks. Initial hip flexion occurs against gravity, but once

SEGMENT		INITIAL MOTION				HOLDING POSITION			
MOTION/ POSITION OBSERVED	% ROM	RESISTED OR RAPID	GRAVITY ASSISTS/ RESISTS	AGONIST GROUP/ CONTRACTION TYPE (CON OR ECC)	RESISTED	GRAVITY EFFECT	ISOMETRIC AGONIST	REP
V FLEX								
Reaching for foot	*50%*	*No*	*Assists*	*Extensors/ECC*	*No*	*Promotes flexion*	*Extensors*	*No*
V EXT								
Returning from flexion	*N/A*	*No*	*Resists*	*Extensors/CON*	*N/A*			
V L-ROT								
Turning to reach right foot	*<50%*	*No*	*No*	*Left rotators/CON*	*No*	*None*	*Left rotators*	*No*
S PRO								
Reaching forward	*>50%*	*Slight resistance at end*	*Slight assist*	*Protractors/CON*	*Slightly*	*Little if any*	*Protractors*	*No*
S RET								
Pulling sock	*N/A*	*Resisted*	*N/A*	*Retractors/CON*	*N/A*			
GH FLEX								
Reaching forward and placing sock	*<50%*	*No*	*Resists*	*Flexors/CON*	*No*	*Promotes extension*	*Flexors*	*No*
E FLEX								
Positioning-	*<50%*	*No*	*Resists*	*Flexors/CON*	*No*	*Promotes extension*	*Flexors*	*No*
Pulling sock-	*50%*	*Resisted*	*N/A*	*Flexors/CON*	*N/A*			

FIGURE **9-24**
Format for clinical biomechanical analysis. Analysis of motion involving the vertebral joints, scapula, glenohumeral, and elbow joints. *ROM,* Range of motion; *CON,* concentric; *ECC,* eccentric; *REP,* repetition; *V FLEX,* vertebral flexion; *V EXT,* vertebral extension; *V L-ROT,* vertebral left rotation; *S PRO,* scapular protraction; *S RET,* scapular retraction; *GH FLEX,* glenohumeral flexion; *E FLEX,* elbow flexion; and *N/A,* not applicable. (Modified from Greene D: A clinically relevant approach to biomechanical analysis of function, *Occup Ther Pract* 1(4):44-52, 1990.)

TABLE 9-1
Biomechanical Analysis of the Donning of Socks and Shoes

SEGMENT		INITIAL MOTION			HOLDING POSITION			
MOTION/ POSITION OBSERVED	% ROM	RESISTED OR RAPID	GRAVITY ASSISTS/ RESISTS	AGONIST GROUP/ CONTRACTION TYPE (CON OR ECC)	RESISTED	GRAVITY EFFECT	ISOMETRIC AGONIST	REP
H FLEX								
Lifting of one leg to cross over the other	>50%*	Neither	Resists	Hip flexors/CON	N/A	N/A	N/A	No
Holding of position during the donning of socks and shoes	>50%*	N/A	N/A	N/A	No	Hip extension while support of the other lower extremity holds hip flexion	None	No

H FLEX, Hip flexion; *ROM,* range of motion; *CON,* concentric; *ECC,* eccentric; *N/A,* not applicable; *REP,* repetition.
*Indicates extreme joint movement.

the hip flexes past 90 degrees, gravity assists the motion and the hip extensors are the active group in eccentric contraction. If George had weak hip flexors, the supine position would allow them to contract through less range—0 to 90 degrees instead of 0 to more than 90 degrees of flexion. Furthermore, if George donned socks in bed, he could bring his hip up while he lay sideways, never having to contract weak hip flexors against gravity's resistance.

After identifying the motion and active muscle group, analyze the muscle contractions necessary to hold the position. George holds his hip flexed as he manipulates and places the shoe or sock on his foot. Ask the same questions as before to determine the active muscle group. Is the position (hip flexion) held against some external resistance? Is the position (hip flexion) held against gravity?

Gravity causes hip extension, so George's hip flexors may appear to be active. That would be true if George held his foot in the air with isometric contraction of the hip flexors. George, however, crosses one leg and rests it. Gravity pulls his hip into extension, but the thigh of his supporting lower extremity matches that force. We can conclude that a continuous muscle contraction is not needed to hold the hip flexed.

Some movements that occur against gravity via contraction of one muscle group maintain that position with isometric contraction of the opposite group. For example, Xavier works under his car and reaches to pick up a wrench from the floor. Xavier's elbow flexes against gravity. Past 90 degrees, gravity helps flex the elbow. Xavier uses his elbow flexors to bring the wrench into position, but he holds it against gravity's flexion effect with his elbow extensor. Xavier's elbow extensors stay active as long as he uses the wrench. In other words, his extensor maintains his elbow flexion.

Problem solving based on biomechanical analysis of activity is commonplace in OT practice, although formal, written biomechanical analyses seldom are performed in the clinic. Students sometimes wonder why they "have to write it all out" in school. Visual analysis involves a lengthy thought process that requires practice and attention. Writing out the analysis illustrates the steps involved. Step by step, biomechanical analysis becomes as easy as it looks.

Summary

Most individuals think of the lower extremities solely in terms of walking. This association is especially useful after injuries and accidents that impair mobility. However, the lower extremities do more than just transport the body from place to place. Muscles at the hip produce closed-chain actions that move and position the trunk for reach. They also balance the trunk at the hip in sitting and maintain the center of gravity projection through the base of support in standing. The weight shifts required in sitting, standing, and walking involve lateral trunk flexion and extension, forward flexion, and inclination of the trunk through closed-chain abduction, adduction, flexion, and extension of the hip.

The lower extremities provide bases of support in sitting and standing and move the body from one base to the next in wheelchair or mat transfers. When lower-extremity function is impaired, wheelchairs serve as locomotive extensions of the trunk. In wheelchairs, all the same principles of stability apply. However, those principles are altered largely by the presence and position of the lower extremities.

Biomechanical analysis provides a tool for the understanding of function through systematic determination of movement, position, and muscle activation. Biomechanical analysis concentrates on details—components of movement and positioning. Ultimately, biomechanical analysis and a heightened understanding of the musculoskeletal system through kinesiology enrich the clinical perspective. An informed view leads to more effective problem solving. Through adaptation, we, as OT practitioners, can transform or reincorporate impaired function so that the tasks essential for role performance keep individuals actively engaged at home and in their communities.

Applications

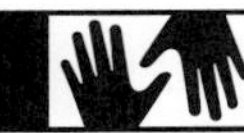

APPLICATION **9-1**

Muscle Shortening During Hip Flexion

Place the heel of your hand on the anterior pelvis (anterior superior iliac spine) and the fingertips just distal to the anterior hip crease. In this position, your hand represents the deep hip flexors (iliopsoas). Lift one foot off the ground using hip and knee flexion. While you flex the hip, keep your fingertips in one place on the anterior thigh and allow the fingers to flex as the proximal thigh approaches the trunk. This simulates the shortening of the hip flexors.

Put the foot down again, allowing your fingers to extend with the moving thigh. With the hand still in place, bend over at the hip with a straight back, as if to stretch the hamstrings. What happens to the fingers in this movement? How do these two movements—lifting the foot versus bending over—compare?

APPLICATION **9-2**

Open- and Closed-Chain Hip Abduction

Use your hand to mark the origin and insertion of the hip abductor. Place your left hand on the lateral aspect of the left hip with the heel of your hand on the iliac crest and your fingertips over the trochanter. Stand on your right foot and raise your left leg into abduction, foot out to the side of the body. Watch the fingers curl as the lateral thigh comes up. Now, stand on the left leg with your left hand still in place, allowing your right foot to leave the ground as you lean and bend to the left. What happens to the fingers in this movement? How do these two movements—abduction of the left leg to the side versus leaning and bending to the left—compare?

APPLICATION 9-3
Wheelchair Instability

Sit in a wheelchair and ask a friend to stand at the back of the chair, hands on the handles ready to catch the chair. Balance the wheelchair with the front casters in the air, as in a wheelie. Do not attempt to push into a wheelie yourself. Let your feet dangle, push up with plantar flexion of your ankles, and have your friend slowly tilt the chair backward, letting go when you feel you can control the wheels. (Your friend must be ready to balance the chair immediately if needed.) What is the single-most unstable aspect of this maneuver? Why do slight forward and backward movements keep the chair balanced on the rear wheels?

See Appendix C for solutions to Applications.

REFERENCES

1. Behrman RE and others: *Textbook of pediatrics,* ed 15, Philadelphia, 1996, WB Saunders (CD-ROM).
2. Greene D: A clinically relevant approach to biomechanical analysis of function, *Occup Ther Pract* 1(4):44-52, 1990.

RELATED READINGS

Calliet R: *Low back pain syndrome,* ed 2, Philadelphia, 1968, FA Davis.

Calliet R: *Understanding your backache: a guide to prevention, treatment, and relief,* Philadelphia, 1984, FA Davis.

Hockenberry J: *Moving violations, war zones, wheelchairs, and declarations of independence,* New York, 1995, Hyperion.

Luttgens K: *Kinesiology: scientific basis of human motion,* ed 9, New York, 1996, McGraw-Hill.

Nordin M and others: *Basic biomechanics of the musculoskeletal system,* ed 2, Philadelphia, 1989, Lea & Febiger.

Pedretti LW: *Occupational therapy practice skills for physical dysfunction,* ed 4, St Louis, 1996, Mosby

Trombly CA: *Occupational therapy for physical dysfunction,* ed 4, Baltimore, 1995, Williams & Wilkins.

Wiktorin CH, Nordin M: *Introduction to problem solving in biomechanics,* Philadelphia, 1986, Lea & Febiger.

Williams PL, Bannister LH: *Gray's anatomy: the anatomical basis of medicine and surgery,* ed 38, New York, 1995, Churchill Livingstone.

Appendixes

APPENDIX **OUTLINE**

English to Metric Conversions

T*hroughout history,* most cultures have required a commonly understood system of weights and measurements that allows for sharing of information and trade goods. Like those of the Babylonians, Egyptians, and Romans, the English system of weights and measures developed from body measurements. The more variable digit, palm, span, and cubit became a more uniform inch, foot, and yard through royal decrees. This system was used wherever English was the language of trade from the seventeenth through nineteenth centuries.

In the early eighteenth century the French attempted to establish a uniform system of measurement that would be used throughout Europe and European territories. The British refused to be involved in developing the new system; therefore it was developed entirely by French academicians. The new system was based on the meter, a measurement that was 1/10,000,000 of the distance from the North Pole to the equator on a line passing through Paris.

A great deal of resistance to the new system emerged, even in France, but by the nineteenth century the system caught on among scientists because units of measurement reliably could be reproduced. The system was revised and modernized by the General Conference of Weights and Measures in 1960. It is called *Le Systeme International d'Unites* (International System of Units), which is abbreviated as SI.

Because this metric system is used by most of the world, it is the system of measurement used throughout this book. Table A-1 gives the most common conversions needed in biomechanical analysis.

TABLE A-1
Common British to Metric Conversions

BRITISH UNIT	×	= SI UNIT	×	= BRITISH UNIT
Length				
Inches (in)	2.54	Centimeters (cm)	0.3937	Inches
Feet (ft)	0.3048	Meters (m)	39.37	Inches
Yard (yd)	0.9144	Meters		
Mile	1.609	Kilometers (km)		
Mass				
Pounds (lb)	0.4536	Kilograms (kg)	2.205	Pounds
Slug	14.594	Kilograms		
Force				
Pound	4.4482	Newtons (N)	0.2248	Pounds

Body Segment Parameters

M*easurements of the human body* are needed to solve most problems in biomechanics. Whenever possible, actual measurements should be taken. However, statistical research data are used for proportional weight and center of gravity in each body segment because actual measurement cannot be made on living subjects.

The primary data for average body weights and centers of gravity were taken from a study done on eight elderly male cadavers.* These data have been revised by other researchers to make allowances for differences in age and gender; however, Dempster's data continue to be widely used. Adaptations of these data, presented in Table B-1 and Figure B-1, give estimates adequate for most problem solving in the OT clinic. More exact data may be obtained by consulting bioengineers or human factors specialists.

Figure B-1 provides the percentage of distance from either end of each body segment to that segment's center of gravity. These measurements are used to determine moment arms in problems involving torque. Table B-1 gives the proportional weight of each body segment, also used to calculate torque.

TABLE B-1

Proportional Percentages of Body Segments to Total Body Weight

BODY SEGMENT	% OF TOTAL BODY WEIGHT
Head and neck	7.9
Trunk with head and neck	56.5
Upper arm	2.7
Forearm	1.5
Hand	0.6
Thigh	9.7
Lower leg	4.5
Foot	1.4

*Dempster WT: *Space requirements of the seated operator,* WADC technical report 55-159, Fairborn, Ohio, 1995, Wright-Patterson Air Force Base.

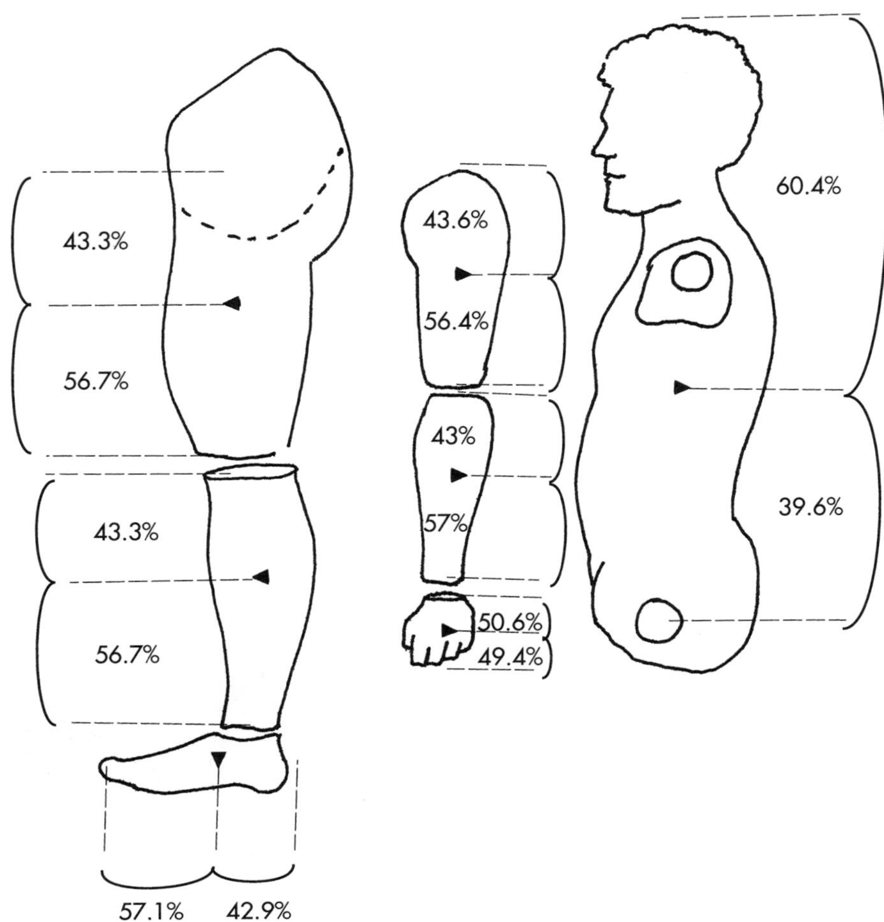

FIGURE **B-1**
Center of gravity for each body segment as a percentage of distance from the end of the segment.

Solutions to Chapter Applications

Chapter 2 Solutions

APPLICATION **2-1**

Appreciating Mass and Gravity

The value of the atomic number for lead is 82 (from the periodic table; the atomic number for aluminum is 13. The difference in weight is proportional to the different atomic numbers. Gravity's effect is to accelerate each to the ground at a rate of roughly 10 kg-m/sec^2. Therefore the difference in the weight is due only to the difference in mass.

APPLICATION **2-2**

Identifying the Active Muscle

1. The triceps should be more stiff than the biceps. If you are unsure, palpate directly on the skin with no clothes interfering with touch.
2. Again the triceps is active. The biceps remains quiet. Be sure to use only the strength necessary to do the task. Unnecessary straining leads to contraction of muscles surrounding the joint, which may skew results.
3. The triceps still is active.
4. The triceps long head origin-to-insertion distance increases as the elbow flexes, and the active muscle already has been identified as the triceps. The triceps is active while the elbow flexes, and the muscle lengthens as it contracts. These actions do not appear to make sense from an anatomical perspective. A muscle contraction that occurs when the muscle elongates is an eccentric contraction. The weight of the book pulls the elbow into flexion, and the contraction of the triceps controls the effect of the book on the elbow. We see eccentric contractions whenever we control the effect of gravity (moving slowly downward).
5. When you hold the book steady, this involves an isometric contraction of the triceps. The length of the triceps (as implied by the unchanged origin-to-insertion distance) is unchanged.
6. When you raise the book up, the origin-to-insertion distance shortens. Because the triceps again is active and shortened, the action is a concentric contraction. We see concentric contractions when we move against the effect of gravity (moving upward).

Regardless of elbow motion, the elbow extensor is active throughout these movements. The situation is the same with a push-up. Which muscle is active throughout the elbow motion in a pull-up?

Chapter 3 Solutions

APPLICATION **3-1**

Creation of a Mobile

The answer depends on the objects used in the mobile. Generally, an object is balanced if it assumes any position in which it is placed.

APPLICATION **3-2**

Scale Drawing of Your Lab Partner

Refer to Appendix B and Table 3-1 to determine this solution.

APPLICATION **3-3**
Vector Indicating Gravity's Effect on a Laundry Basket

Decide on a scale for a drawing of the vector, for example, 50 N equals 1 cm. (Note that only in a scale for a drawing is a measure of weight equal to a measure of distance.) Figure C-1 shows the weight of the basket drawn as a vector. The vector indicating a half-full basket of laundry would be half as long.

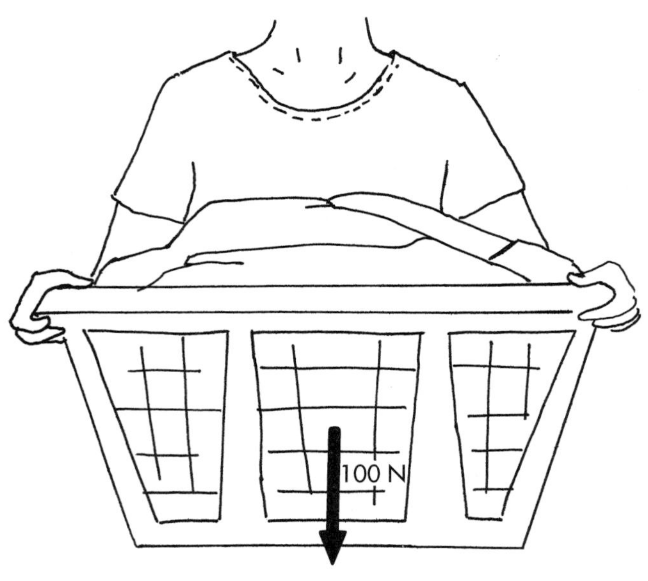

FIGURE **C-1**
A vector representing 100 N points directly downward from the center of this laundry basket.

APPLICATION **3-4**
Force of Gravity Acting on a Spoon

To find the center of gravity for the spoon, balance it on a finger (Figure C-2). The point at which the spoon balances is its center of gravity. Indicate this center with a dot on the drawing.

In Figure C-3 the arrows point directly downward regardless of the angle of the spoon. The center of gravity remains the same no matter how an object is positioned. Gravity always pulls toward the center of the Earth. The vector's length remains the same in each diagram because it indicates the actual force gravity exerts on the spoon.

APPLICATION **3-5**
Force of Gravity Acting on Spoons of Different Weights

Draw a diagram of each spoon. To find each spoon's center of gravity, balance the spoon on a finger as before. The center of gravity, which is affected by weight distribution, may differ by several centimeters from the previous exercise. Individual spoons must be balanced to find each one's center of gravity.

The spoon with the built-up handle weighs 0.02 kg more than the regular spoon. (This is indicated in Figure C-4 by a slightly longer arrow.) Gravity vectors point directly downward regardless of the angle of the object itself. For the best comparison, keep vectors to scale and indicate the proportions on the diagram.

APPLICATION **3-6**
Gravity Operating on the Forearm

Use Appendix B to determine the center of gravity of your forearm. Measure the distance from the olecranon process to the styloid process and multiply this distance by 0.43 because the table indicates the center of gravity for the forearm is located at a distance 43% of the length of the forearm beginning at the olecranon process. (Use

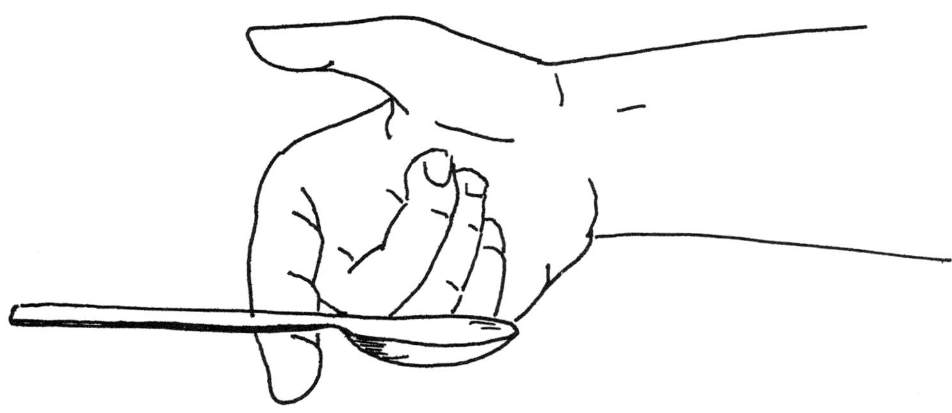

FIGURE **C-2**
Balance a spoon on one finger to find its center of gravity.

0.57 if you measure from the styloid process.) Mark this point on your forearm on the anterior surface in the center of the radioulnar width.

0.43 × Length of the forearm = Distance from the olecranon process to the center of gravity

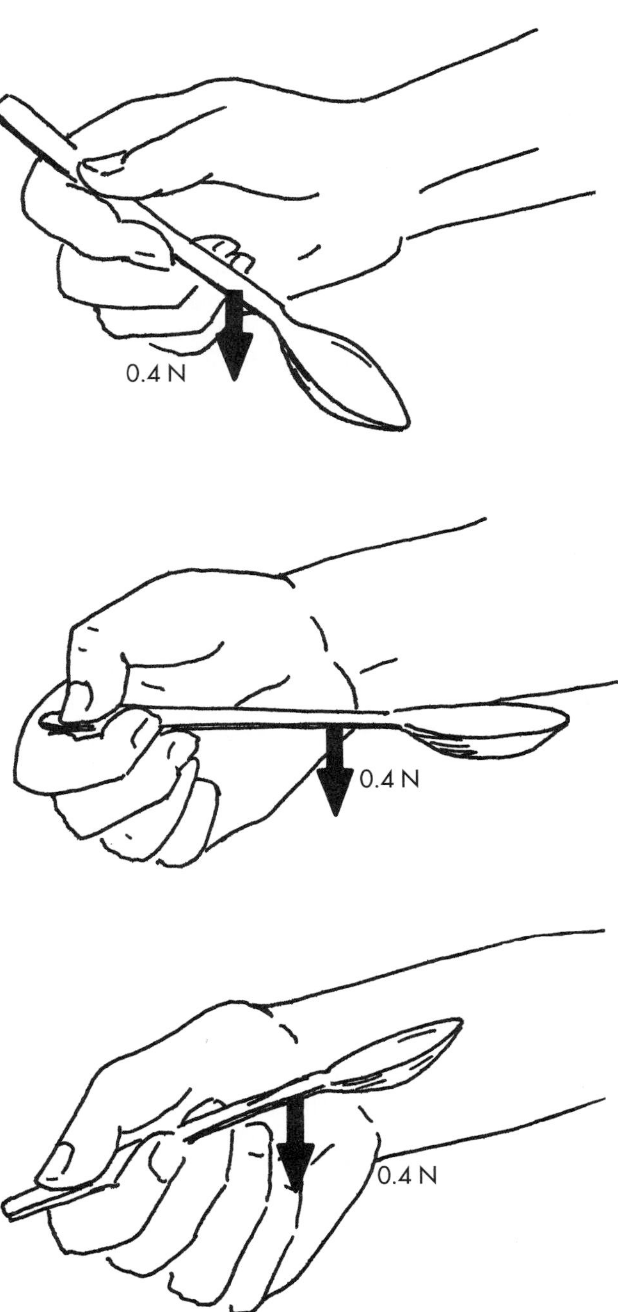

FIGURE **C-3**
Regardless of the spoon's position, the vector representing gravity always points directly downward.

Multiply your total body weight in pounds by 0.021. (One forearm and hand combined are 2.1% of the total body weight and therefore 0.021 times total body weight.) Use pounds since you are more likely to know your weight in pounds than in newtons. (Using pounds makes multiplication by gravity unnecessary because the pound is a unit of weight times gravity (32 ft/sec^2). Remember to keep the measurement scale the same when you draw vectors representing the forearm and the tools.

The spoons has a gravitational force less than that of the forearm (Figure C-5). When the forearm brings the spoon to the mouth, the weight of the forearm is more important than the weight of the spoon. If the weight of the spoon or another object were greater than the weight of the forearm, the focus would shift to the weight of that tool.

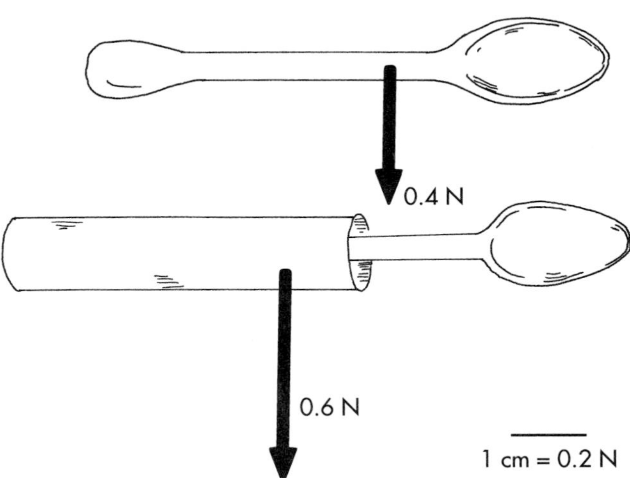

FIGURE **C-4**
The extra weight of the built-up handle shifts the spoon's center of gravity from the bowl of the spoon.

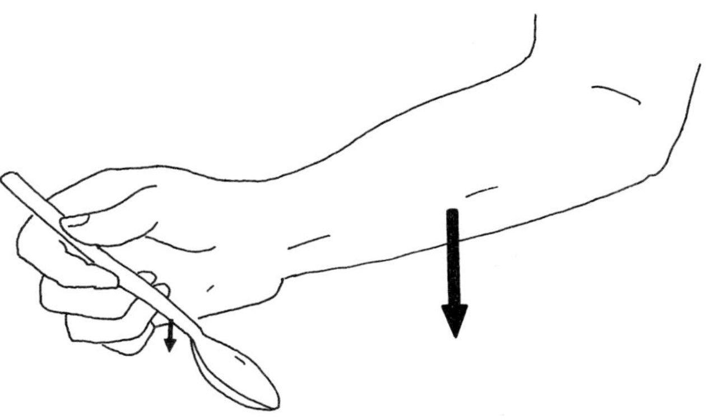

FIGURE **C-5**
The vector representing the weight of the forearm is longer than the vector representing the weight of the spoon.

Chapter 4 Solutions

APPLICATION **4-1**
Adding Forces and Establishing Equilibrium

Determining the amount of force is a simple problem of addition and subtraction based on the idea that downward forces must equal upward forces. The idea is represented as a formula by the equation $\Sigma F = 0$. Thus the summation of forces in each direction (up and down) equals zero. Put another way, $F_{up} = F_{down}$. Set up the equation with values of all the forces involved and solve for the unknown amount:

$$x = 3.5\text{ N} + 5\text{ N} + 3\text{ N}$$
$$x = 11.5\text{ N directed upward}$$

Stated as the summation of forces, assign the positive sign to all forces in one direction and the negative sign to all forces in the opposite direction (see Figure 4-2):

$$\Sigma F = 0 = 3.5\text{ N} + 5\text{ N} + 3\text{ N} - 11.5\text{ N}$$

APPLICATION **4-2**
Adding Forces

Add the 60-N force of the wrist weight to the 70-N force of the bucket of sand for total downward weight:

$$60\text{ N} + 70\text{ N} = 130\text{ N}$$

A graphic representation should show the two vectors drawn in line, one starting where the other ends (see Figure 4-13, *B*). Using a scale of 10 N = 0.5 cm, the resultant force measures 6.5 cm, the combined length of both vectors. Spiros must exert more than 130 N of upward force.

APPLICATION **4-3**
Finding the Resultant Force

Subtract the 40-N upward force from the 60-N downward force of the cast. Henry uses slightly more than 20 N of force to lift his arm.

$$60\text{ N} - 40\text{ N} = 20\text{ N}$$

APPLICATION **4-4**
Analyzing Forces by Direction and Amount

Give right-side players positive values: Zachary pulls with a force of 400 N and Tony with 200 N. Give left-side players negative values: Yasmeen pulls with 300 N, Crystal with 100 N, and Karen with 500 N:

$$400\text{ N} + 200\text{ N} + (-300\text{ N}) + (-100\text{ N}) + (-500\text{ N}) = -300\text{ N}$$

The girls will win the game much faster than the right side won the last game because they use more than twice the force as the last winning team (see Figure 4-15).

APPLICATION **4-5**
Combining Forces

George's vector is 225 N to the right. Raul's vector is oriented upward at right angles to George's so that it meets the diagonal line, representing the 350 N of force it takes to move the cart.

Use the Pythagorean theorem to determine an absolute value for Raul's vector:

$$a^2 + b^2 = c^2$$
$$a^2 + 225^2 = 350^2$$
$$a^2 + 50{,}625 = 122{,}500$$
$$a^2 = 122{,}500 - 50{,}625$$
$$a^2 = 71{,}875$$
$$a = 268\text{ N}$$

Draw the parallelogram with a scale of 50 N = 1 cm (see Figure 4-17). George's vector measures 4.5 cm long oriented to the right. The diagonal vector is 7 cm long oriented upward and to the right at about 45 degrees to George's vector. Raul's vector measures 4.7 cm long oriented upward. Raul must push more than twice as hard this time to move the cart.

APPLICATION **4-6**
Combining Force Vectors to Determine the Resultant Force

To determine the final direction, draw the vectors accurately in orientation and scale (for example, 50 N = 1 cm) and place the vectors end to end (see Figure 4-18). Raul's vector points 45 degrees northeast and is 6 cm long (300 N). George's vector points north and is 3 cm long (150 N). Spiros' vector points east and is 9 cm long (450 N). Eduardo's vector points 45 degrees southwest and is 4.5 cm long (225 N). Fred has no vector. The resultant force connects the last vector with the first vector. Use a scale of 50 N = 1 cm, and the resultant measures 10.75 cm (540 N). This vector should point toward the southwest at approximately 75 degrees.

APPLICATION **4-7**
Determining Force Capability

For a general idea, estimate the bulk of the biceps muscle by palpating it and grasping it between your thumb and index finger. (You may need to give some resistance to make it easier to see and feel.) Remove your hand and hold the contour of the fingers representing the shape of the muscle. Trace this on paper and close the circle with a curved line. Find the cross section by measuring the height and width of the circle and multiplying them. (Use centimeters because centimeters are the units of the constant provided in this example.) Multiply the cross section by the constant for vertebrate skeletal muscle, 100 N/cm^2.

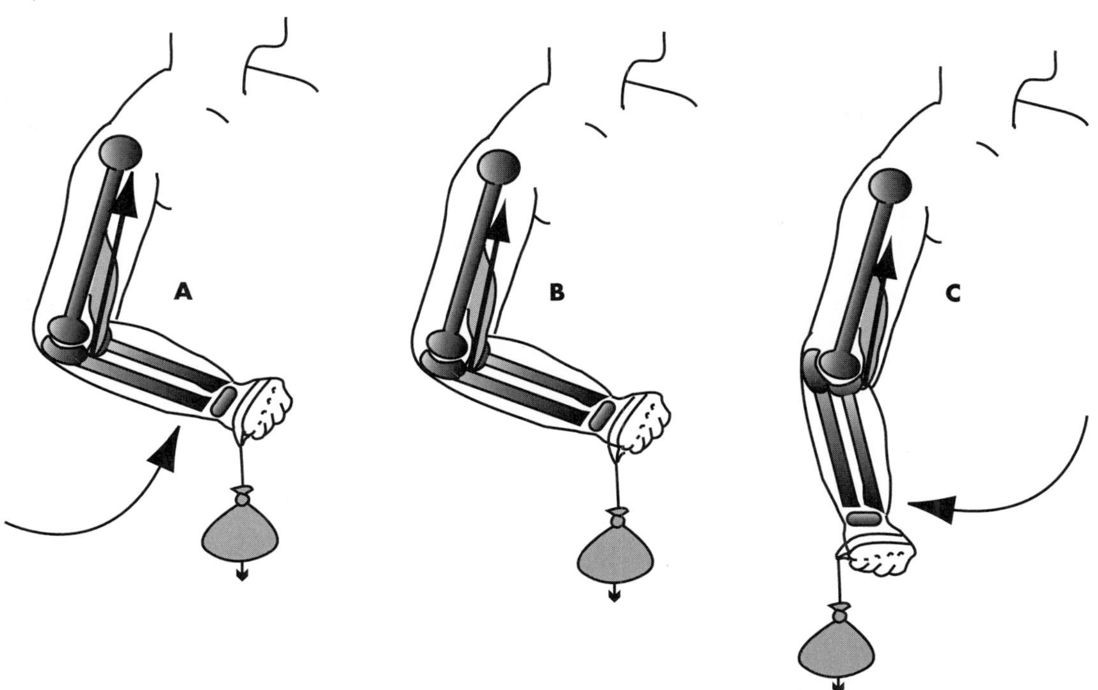

FIGURE **C-6**
Each vector begins at the insertion and demonstrates a force directed proximally in a concentric contraction **(A)**, an isometric contraction **(B)**, and an eccentric contraction **(C)**.

APPLICATION **4-8**
Determining Excursion

Measure the length of the long head of the triceps from the infraglenoid tubercle to the olecranon with the upper extremity in full shoulder and elbow flexion. Divide this number by two to find the muscle's approximate maximal excursion.

APPLICATION **4-9**
Drawing Vectors Indicating Contractions

Figure C-6 shows the three vectors drawn correctly. Each begins at the insertion and demonstrates a force directed proximally because in each case, it is the insertion that moves. In all three conditions the same weight is used, and all three forces differ in amount. The three magnitudes indicate overcoming the weight in a concentric contraction (see Figure C-6, *A*), holding the weight in an isometric contraction (see Figure C-6, *B*), and lowering the weight in an eccentric contraction (see Figure C-6, *C*). Therefore the longest vector indicates the concentric contraction.

Chapter 5 Solutions

APPLICATION **5-1**
Effort Needed to Open and Close a Valve

You probably noticed more effort was needed to turn on the water when you held the lever closer to the connecting screw than when you held it toward the end of the lever. The connecting screw is the center of rotation, the axis. The placement of your fingers determines the distance of the force from the axis; thus the lever length from the screw to your finger placement is the moment arm.

APPLICATION **5-2**
External Torque Produced by a Barbell

Figure C-7 shows an elbow flexed in four positions—30, 60, 90, and 120 degrees. All the segments and force vectors are drawn to scale. Draw the moment arms using the method described in this chapter. Notice that for many of the elbow positions, you move the T square along the force and never reach a point at which you can draw a

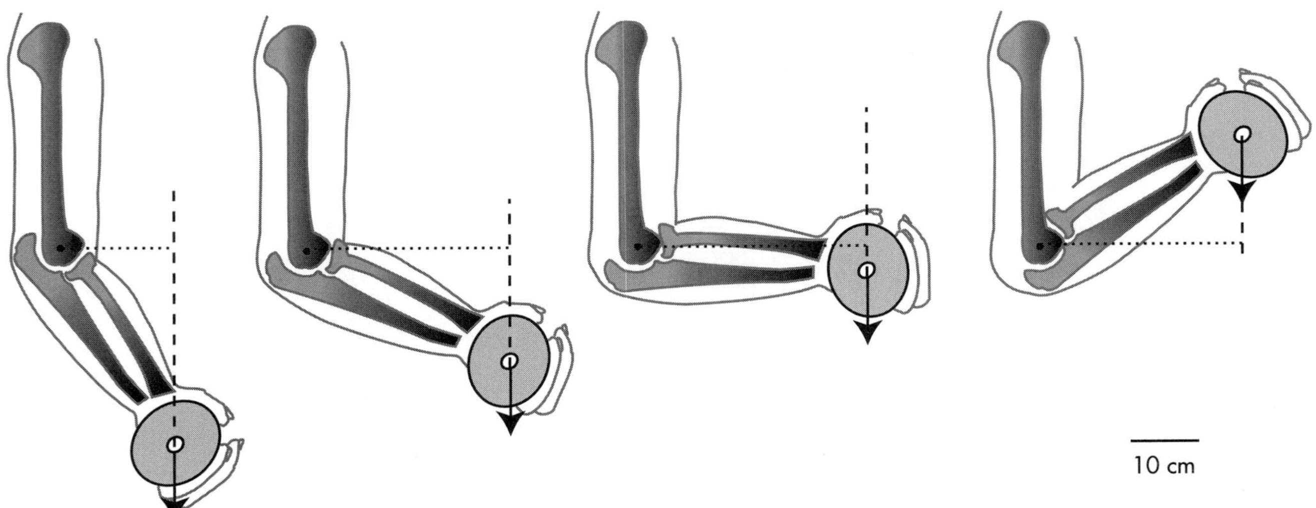

FIGURE **C-7**
The factors involved in external torque. Vectors and moment arms are drawn to scale.

perpendicular between the force and the axis. When this occurs, use a dotted line to extend the force in the direction needed to draw the perpendicular distance. To estimate the length of the moment arm, measure with a ruler and convert to the scale shown. (A more accurate measurement requires the use of trigonometry, as shown in the solution to Application 5-4).

Converting kilograms to newtons, multiply the length of the moment arm by the force of the barbell to obtain the value of the torque produced by the barbell. The following equations demonstrate the torque present at elbow positions of 30, 60, 90, and 120 degrees of flexion, respectively:

$$50 \text{ N} \times 17 \text{ cm} = 850 \text{ N-cm}$$
$$50 \text{ N} \times 30 \text{ cm} = 1500 \text{ N-cm}$$
$$50 \text{ N} \times 34 \text{ cm} = 1700 \text{ N-cm}$$
$$50 \text{ N} \times 30 \text{ cm} = 1500 \text{ N-cm}$$

External torque changes throughout the range of motion as the length of the moment arm changes.

APPLICATION 5-3
Force Produced by the Biceps

Figure C-8 shows four figures representing the four ranges of motion. Lines representing the distance to the biceps tendon and the force of the biceps are to scale. The biceps pulls directly upward and parallel to the humerus. Each elbow position can be set up as an equilibrium equation because we know from the previous application how much torque is created by the 5-kg weight. The following equations illustrate the torque present at elbow positions of 30, 60, 90, and 120 degrees of flexion, respectively. Answers to these equations have been rounded:

$$141.7 \text{ N} \times 6 \text{ cm} = 850 \text{ N-cm}$$
$$187.5 \text{ N} \times 8 \text{ cm} = 1500 \text{ N-cm}$$
$$200 \text{ N} \times 8.5 \text{ cm} = 1700 \text{ N-cm}$$
$$250 \text{ N} \times 6 \text{ cm} = 1500 \text{ N-cm}$$

The biceps moment arm changes throughout the range of motion. The biceps force changes to match the torque created in the opposite direction by the barbell. Internal torque usually operates in response to external torque. Supporting a weight held in the hand translates into creating enough torque internally to match the effect of the external torque operating at the same joint, the elbow.

APPLICATION 5-4
Effort Needed to Lift a Rock With a Crowbar

In Figure C-9 the crowbar/lever is drawn to scale. The small rock used as a fulcrum (axis) lies one fourth of the distance from the end of the lever and between the effort and the resistance forces. This is a first-class lever.

To solve this problem with trigonometry, the lever is viewed as the hypotenuse of a right triangle oriented 30 degrees to the base of the triangle. The base is a line drawn parallel to the ground from the pivot point (axis) to the resistance-force extension line. Another right triangle is formed with the remaining length of the lever from the pivot to the effort force serving as the hypotenuse and the base from the pivot to the effort-force extension line.

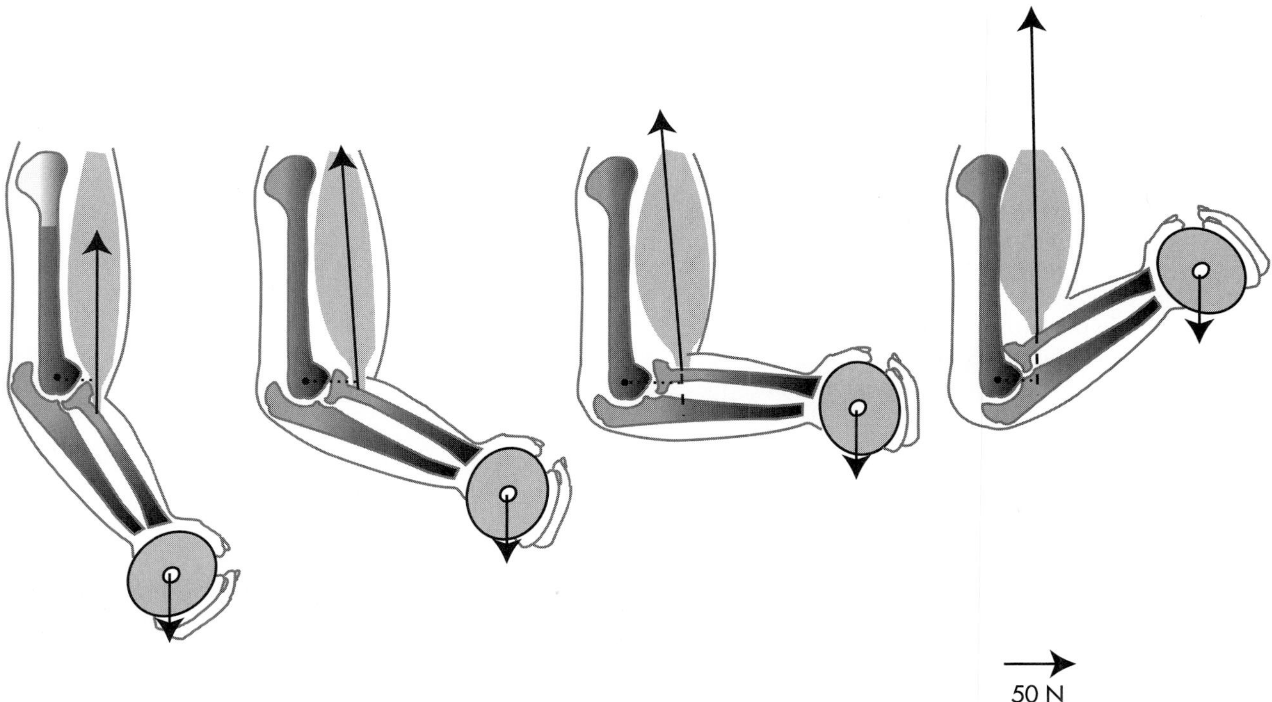

FIGURE **C-8**
The factors involved in internal torque. Vectors and moment arms are drawn to scale.

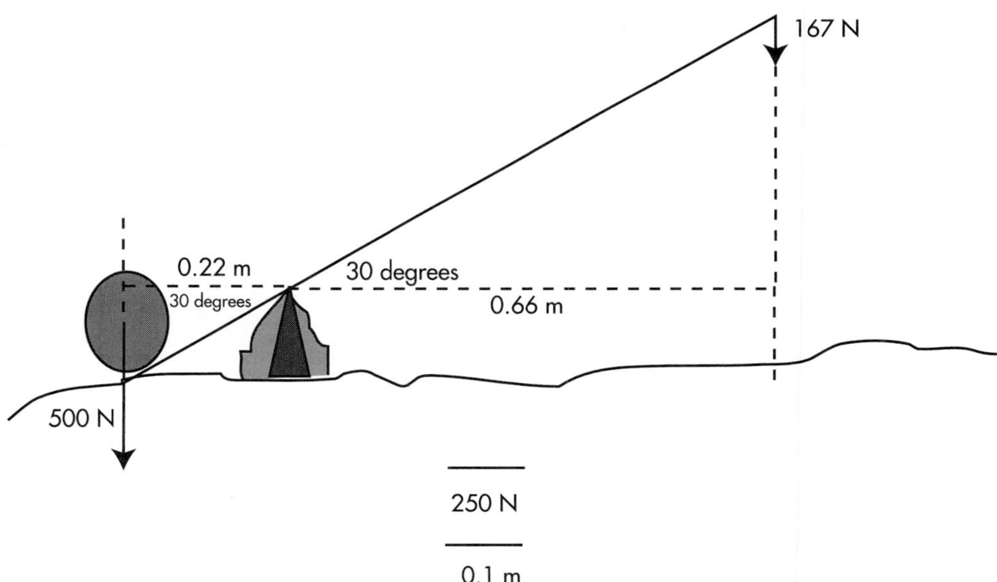

FIGURE **C-9**
An effort force of 167 N is needed to counteract the torque produced by the 500-N force of the rock.

This is an equilibrium problem. To determine the amount of force Spiros needs to lift the large rock, use the formula $\Sigma M = 0$, in which *M* stands for moments. In the following equation, *MA* is the moment arm:

$$0 = (\text{Resistance} \times \text{Resistance MA}) - (\text{Effort} \times \text{Effort MA})$$

Put known values into the formula:

$$0 = (500\text{ N} \times \text{Resistance MA}) - (\text{Effort} \times \text{Effort MA})$$

Use the cosine function, or cosine equals the adjacent side divided by the hypotenuse, to determine moment arms. From the table of functions in Appendix E, cosine 30 degrees is 0.87. The following answers are rounded:

$$\cos 30 \text{ degrees} = \frac{\text{Adjacent side}}{0.25\text{ m}}$$

$$0.87 = \frac{\text{Adjacent side}}{0.25\text{ m}}$$

$$0.87 \times 0.25\text{ m} = \text{Adjacent side} = \text{Resistance moment arm}$$

$$0.22\text{ m} = \text{Resistance moment arm}$$

Effort moment arm is determined in the same way:

$$\cos 30 \text{ degrees} = \frac{\text{Adjacent side}}{0.75\text{ m}}$$

$$0.87 = \frac{\text{Adjacent side}}{0.75\text{ m}}$$

$$0.87 \times 0.75 = \text{Effort moment arm}$$

$$0.66\text{ m} = \text{Effort moment arm}$$

Substitute the values for moment arms into the original equilibrium equation:

$$0 = (\text{Resistance} \times \text{Resistance MA}) - (\text{Effort} \times \text{Effort MA})$$

$$0 = (500\text{ N} \times 0.22\text{ m}) - (\text{E} \times 0.66\text{ m})$$

$$0 = 110\text{ Nm} - 0.66 \times \text{Effort}$$

$$\text{Effort} \times 0.66 = 110\text{ Nm}$$

$$\text{Effort} = 167\text{ N}$$

The advantage of using the crowbar is one of leverage. Spiros can lift the rock by applying less force (167 N) than if he were to lift it straight up by hand without a lever (500 N).

APPLICATION 5-5
Balance Needed to Hold a Tray of Food

First, convert centimeters to meters and kilograms to newtons. In Figure C-10 the torque produced by the sandwich must equal the torque produced by the soft drink. Again, use the equilibrium formula, in which *MA* is moment arm:

$$(5\text{ N} \times 0.06\text{ m}) - (3.5\text{ N} \times \text{Sandwich MA}) = 0$$

$$0.3\text{ Nm} = 3.5\text{ N} \times \text{Sandwich MA}$$

$$\text{Sandwich MA} = 0.1\text{ m}$$

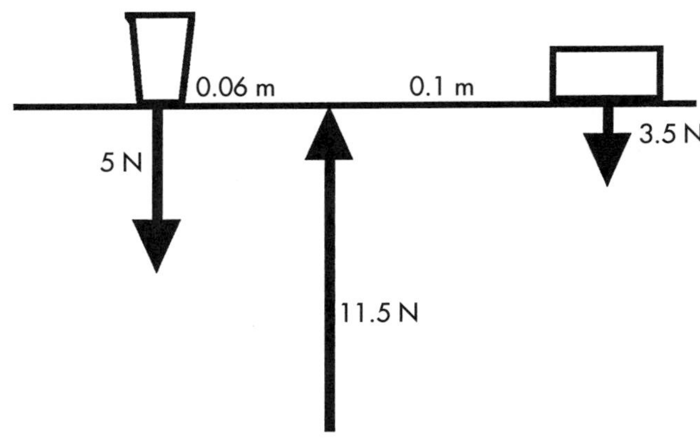

FIGURE **C-10**
The sandwich must rest 0.1 m from the center of the tray to balance the torque produced by the soft drink.

Chapter 6 Solutions

APPLICATION 6-1
Upper-Extremity Reach

Reaching forward with both hands involves forward trunk flexion, a movement initiated by the trunk flexors, controlled by eccentric contraction of the extensors, and assisted by gravity. Holding the position while reaching requires an isometric contraction of the extensors. In each case, bilateral contractions are involved.

Reaching to one side involves lateral flexion. As in the previous case, the movement is initiated by one side and controlled and maintained by the opposite side.

Reaching straight up requires that the trunk extensors extend in a bilateral contraction. This is such a common position that we overlook its contribution to reach. Try reaching up with trunk flexion to feel the difference.

Reaching the right upper extremity across to the left side of the body involves rotation of the anterior trunk to the left. Remember that turning involves a unilateral contraction of the transversospinalis, in this case the right transversospinalis.

APPLICATION 6-2
Open- and Closed-Chain Hip Movements

Long sitting is usually less comfortable than crossed-legged sitting because long sitting maximally stretches the hamstrings (passive insufficiency).

Moving into a crossed-legged position involves open-chain hip flexion because the distal end of the chain (the foot) moves freely in space as the hip flexes and externally rotates with knee flexion. Moving into long sitting is a closed-chain movement because the distal end of the

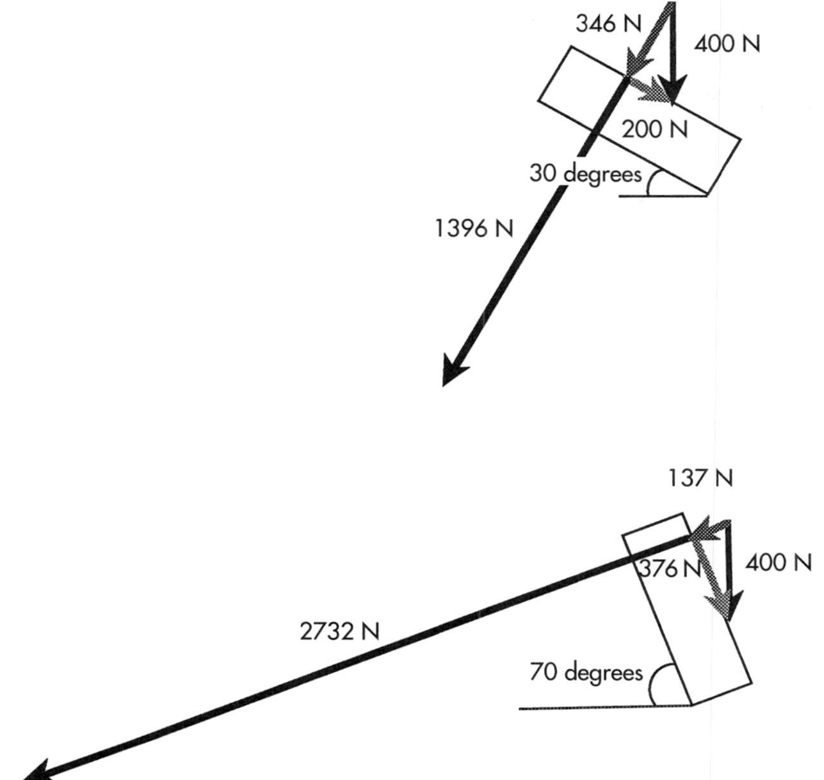

FIGURE **C-11**
The parallelogram method of adding forces provides a graphic solution in attempts to determine compressive and shear forces operating on a disk.

lower-extremity chain is stabilized. Achieving the position involves hip flexion, but movement of the proximal attachments (origins) of the hip flexors causes the trunk to flex over the lower extremity.

Reaching for the toes in long sitting brings the hip extensors (hamstrings) to the end of their excursion. At some point even the longest hamstrings find their limit and prevent further hip flexion by pulling distally on the ischial tuberosities. (Distal is in the opposite direction from which the ischial tuberosities move in closed-chain hip flexion.) Once pelvic motion ceases, hip flexion stops. Continued forward motion to touch the toes involves vertebral flexion in the lumbar area. If the hamstrings are short, hip flexion stops even sooner in this effort and a greater degree of lumbar flexion is necessary.

APPLICATION **6-3**
Stance

When Paul bends over his treatment table, it produces the same types of forces as when Nancy bends over the sink. Paul's erector spinae must work twice as hard as when he stands erect. Placing his foot on a step stool changes the dynamics of posture. The stool introduces a counter force with a vector that operates at a greater distance from the L5 disk than from Paul's center of gravity. Even a small amount of force can produce a sizable countertorque because of its longer moment arm. The same principle was at play when Nancy placed her hand on the side of the sink to support her upper body.

L5 DISK PROBLEM **(p. 73)**

In Figure C-11 the compressive and shear forces can be calculated with graphics and mathematics.

Graphic Solution

Draw the L5 disks at 30 degrees and 70 degrees to the horizontal plane. The force of the weight of the body (400 N) lies 90 degrees to the horizontal plane. This weight line forms the hypotenuse of a right triangle that has the disk surface as its base. The right triangle has an angle that corresponds to the angle of the disk on the horizontal plane, that is, 30 degrees or 70 degrees. The vector lying perpendicular to the base of the triangle represents the compressive forces operating on the disk surface from the weight of the body. The vector connecting these first two vectors lies along the base of the disk surface and represents the shear forces operating on the disk. Draw the diagram to scale so that the measurements estimate the compressive and shear forces operating on the disk. Remember that the compressive weight of the body must be added to the compressive force of the erector spinae. Through this addition the total compressive force that acts on the intervertebral L5 disk may be obtained.

Mathematical Solution

A right triangle representing the upright position has a hypotenuse of 400 N and one angle of 30 degrees. A second right triangle representing the bent position has a hypotenuse of 400 N and one angle of 70 degrees. The compressive force (C_W) of the weight of the body lies adjacent to this angle, and the shear force (*S*) lies opposite this known angle. Use sines to determine sides opposite the angles and cosines to determine sides adjacent to the angles:

$$S = 400\text{ N} \times \sin 30\text{ degrees}$$
$$S = 200\text{ N standing}$$
$$S = 400\text{ N} \times \sin 70\text{ degrees}$$
$$S = 376\text{ N bending}$$
$$C_W = 400\text{ N} \times \cos 30\text{ degrees}$$
$$C_W = 346\text{ N standing}$$
$$\text{Total compression} = 1396\text{ N} + 346\text{ N}$$
$$\text{Total compression} = 1742\text{ N standing}$$
$$C_W = 400\text{ N} \times \cos 70\text{ degrees}$$
$$C_W = 137\text{ N bending}$$
$$\text{Total compression} = 2732\text{ N} + 137\text{ N}$$
$$\text{Total compression} = 2869\text{ N bending}$$

Chapter 7 Solutions

APPLICATION **7-1**

Muscle Function Simulations

1. Pulling from the deltoid tubercle toward the acromion lateral to the front-to-back axis simulates contraction of the middle deltoid and produces humeral abduction at the glenohumeral joint.
2. Pulling toward the distal clavicle anterior to the side-to-side axis simulates contraction of the anterior deltoid and biceps long head, which together flex the humerus at the glenohumeral joint.
3. Pulling toward the midspine of the scapula posterior to the side-to-side axis simulates extension of the humerus by the posterior deltoid at the glenohumeral joint.
4. Pulling inferiorly and posteriorly toward the sacrum simulates extension of the humerus by the latissimus dorsi at the glenohumeral joint. The string pull differs from the actual pull of the latissimus because the string fails to show the latissimus' rotational effect on the humerus. The latissimus runs medial to the humerus and inserts on its anterior side. This medial relationship to the rotation axis and posterior pull of the latissimus results in internal humeral rotation. The string used in this application, like the latissimus, originates on the posterior side. Unlike the latissimus, the string moves to the lateral side of the humerus, placing it on the opposite side of the latissimus' rotation axis. A posterior pull lateral to the rotation axis results in external rotation of the humerus.

Notice that it takes considerable force to produce upper-extremity movement with the pull of a string. The string has a very short moment arm, and gravity acts on the upper extremity with a long moment arm. The muscles simulated must generate great magnitudes of force against even small amounts of resistance.

APPLICATION **7-2**

Muscle Function Drawings

Refer to Figure C-12. Notice that the segments are drawn as simple rectangles; no fancy artwork is necessary. Also notice that the force vector of the reattached brachialis (*B*) continues straight, even though the muscle curves around the elbow. Its new inferior and posterior relationship to the elbow's side-to-side axis extends the elbow.

APPLICATION **7-3**

Limited Shoulder Strength

Solve this problem by determining the amount of force available in the anterior and middle deltoid fibers. Combine these forces using the parallelogram method. The resultant force is the amount of power available for operation of the switch.

7-3A: Fair Muscle Grades. Calculate the force of the anterior and middle fibers of the deltoid muscle by using equilibrium of torques. In Figure C-13 the force from the anterior and middle deltoid fibers (*D*) is angled up and to the right. The force of gravity acting on the arm is valued at 30 N (*R*). The formula, in which *MA* stands for moment arm, is as follows:

$$(R \times RMA) = (D \times DMA)$$

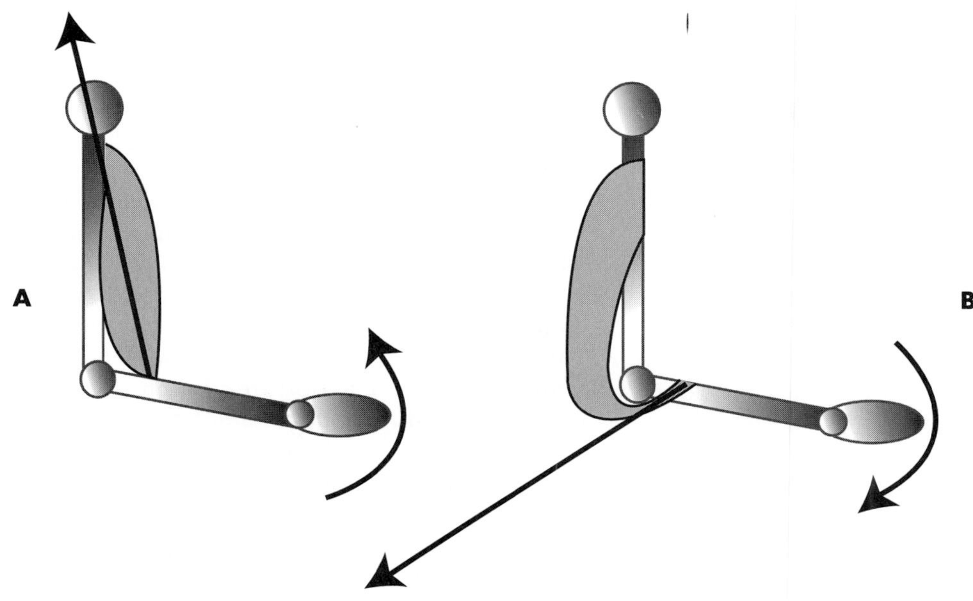

FIGURE **C-12**
The brachialis in its anatomical **(A)** and surgically transferred **(B)** positions.

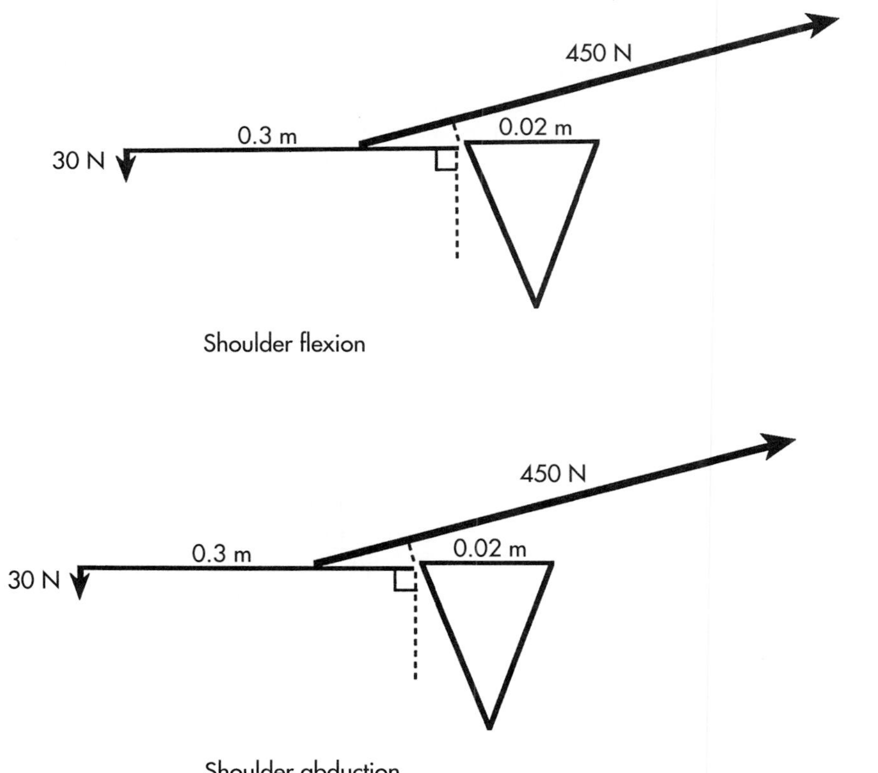

FIGURE **C-13**
Fair muscle grades in the anterior and middle deltoid fibers indicate 450 N of force available for this individual in shoulder flexion or abduction.

The arm's approximate weight (2.88 kg) is derived from 4.8% of 70 kg. At 90 degrees the arm's center of gravity lies 30 cm from the axis of motion. Remember to convert centimeters to meters and kilograms to newtons:

$$(30 \text{ N} \times 0.30 \text{ m}) = (\text{D} \times 0.02 \text{ m})$$
$$9.0 \text{ Nm} = \text{D} \times 0.02 \text{ m}$$
$$\text{D} = 450 \text{ N}$$

Fair-strength anterior and middle deltoid muscles each can produce 450 N of force.

7-3B: Poor Muscle Grades. In Figure C-14, moment arms (MA) for 50 degrees of shoulder abduction by the middle deltoid and for 70 degrees of flexion by the anterior deltoid are drawn, respectively, as the sides of a right triangle opposite the angle of the joint. The lengths of these sides are calculated through the use of sines:

$$\sin 50 \text{ degrees} = \frac{\text{Opposite side}}{30 \text{ cm}}$$
$$\text{Opposite side} = 30 \text{ cm} \times 0.7660 = 23 \text{ cm}$$
$$\sin 70 \text{ degrees} = \frac{\text{Opposite side}}{30 \text{ cm}}$$
$$\text{Opposite side} = 30 \text{ cm} \times 0.9397 = 28 \text{ cm}$$

The force of the anterior deltoid is determined based on equilibrium of torques—gravity producing extension torque and the anterior deltoid producing flexion torque. In the following equation, $D_{anterior}$ stands for the force of the anterior deltoid. Remember to convert centimeters to meters and kilograms to newtons:

$$30 \text{ N} \times 0.28 \text{ m} = \text{D}_{\text{anterior}} \times 0.02 \text{ m}$$
$$8.4 \text{ Nm} = \text{D}_{\text{anterior}} \times 0.02 \text{ m}$$
$$\text{D}_{\text{anterior}} = 420 \text{ N}$$

The force of the middle deltoid is determined based on equilibrium of torques—gravity producing adduction torque and the middle deltoid producing abduction torque. In the following equation, D_{middle} stands for the force of the middle deltoid. Again, remember to convert centimeters to meters and kilograms to newtons:

$$30 \text{ N} \times 0.23 \text{ m} = \text{D}_{\text{middle}} \times 0.02 \text{ m}$$
$$6.9 \text{ Nm} = \text{D}_{\text{middle}} \times 0.02 \text{ m}$$
$$\text{D}_{\text{middle}} = 345 \text{ N}$$

7-3C: Combined Muscle Fibers. The fair-grade anterior and middle deltoid fibers each pull with a force of about 450 N at an angle of approximately 30 degrees from each other measured at the insertion. In Figure C-15 these forces make up two sides of a parallelogram. The resultant force is a diagonal connecting the opposite corners. Calculate the resultant force by drawing a graphic representation or using mathematics. A drawing of the parallelogram is essential for a graphic solution and helpful for a mathematical one.

Graphic Solution. Figure C-15 illustrates the vectors representing the forces of the anterior and middle deltoid fibers at a 30-degree angle from each other. Complete the parallelogram by drawing the remaining two sides as dotted lines. The line that runs between the deltoid forces and extends to the opposite corner is the resultant force of the two portions of the deltoid that hold the arm in the position between flexion and abduction. Draw the vectors to scale and use the same scale to measure the resultant force and approximate the force available to operate a switch.

Mathematical Solution. When both sets of muscle fibers pull with equal force, the resultant force divides the parallelogram into two equal triangles. Connecting the ends of the two 450-N forces forms a line that bisects the resultant force and produces two right triangles, each with a hypotenuse of 450 N and one angle of 15 degrees (see Figure C-15, *A*). The base of each triangle is the side adjacent to the 15-degree angle and has a value of one-half the resultant force (*R*). Use cosine to determine the value of the adjacent side, the combined forces of the anterior and middle deltoids with fair muscle strength producing flexion and abduction:

$$\cos 15 \text{ degrees} = \frac{\text{Adjacent side}}{\text{Hypotenuse}}$$
$$\cos 15 \text{ degrees} = \frac{\text{R}/2}{450 \text{ N}}$$
$$\text{R}/2 = 450 \text{ N} \times \text{Cos } 15 \text{ degrees}$$
$$\text{R}/2 = 450 \text{ N} \times 0.9659$$
$$\text{R}/2 = 435 \text{ N}$$
$$\text{R} = 870 \text{ N}$$

When an individual has poor muscle strength, the two portions of the deltoid are pulled with different amounts of force. Again the resultant force divides the parallelogram into two equal triangles (see Figure C-15, *B*). Draw a line from the end of each force to form a 90-degree angle with the resultant force. This forms two unequal right triangles with respective hypotenuses of 345 N and 420 N. In the following equation, $R_{anterior}$ is the resultant force of the anterior deltoid and R_{middle} is the resultant force of the middle deltoid. Determine the combined forces producing flexion and abduction:

$$\cos 15 \text{ degrees} = \frac{\text{R}_{\text{anterior}}}{420 \text{ N}}$$
$$\text{R}_{\text{anterior}} = 420 \text{ N} \times 0.9659$$
$$\text{R}_{\text{anterior}} = 406 \text{ N}$$
$$\cos 15 \text{ degrees} = \frac{\text{R}_{\text{middle}}}{345 \text{ N}}$$
$$\text{R}_{\text{middle}} = 345 \text{ N} \times 0.9659$$

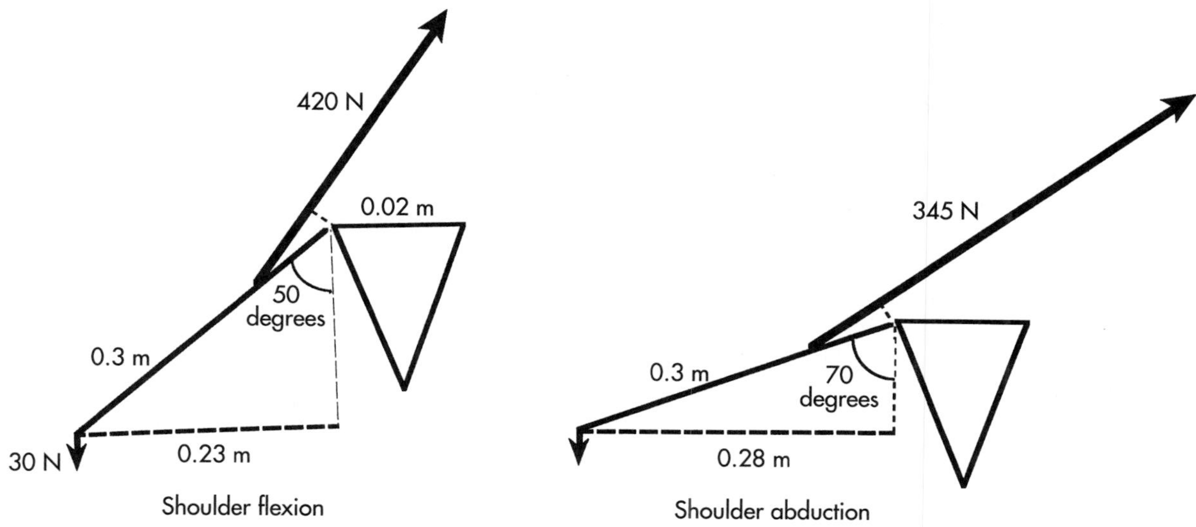

FIGURE **C-14**
For this individual, poor muscle grades indicate 420 N of force available in the anterior deltoid for shoulder flexion and 345 N of force available in the middle deltoid for abduction.

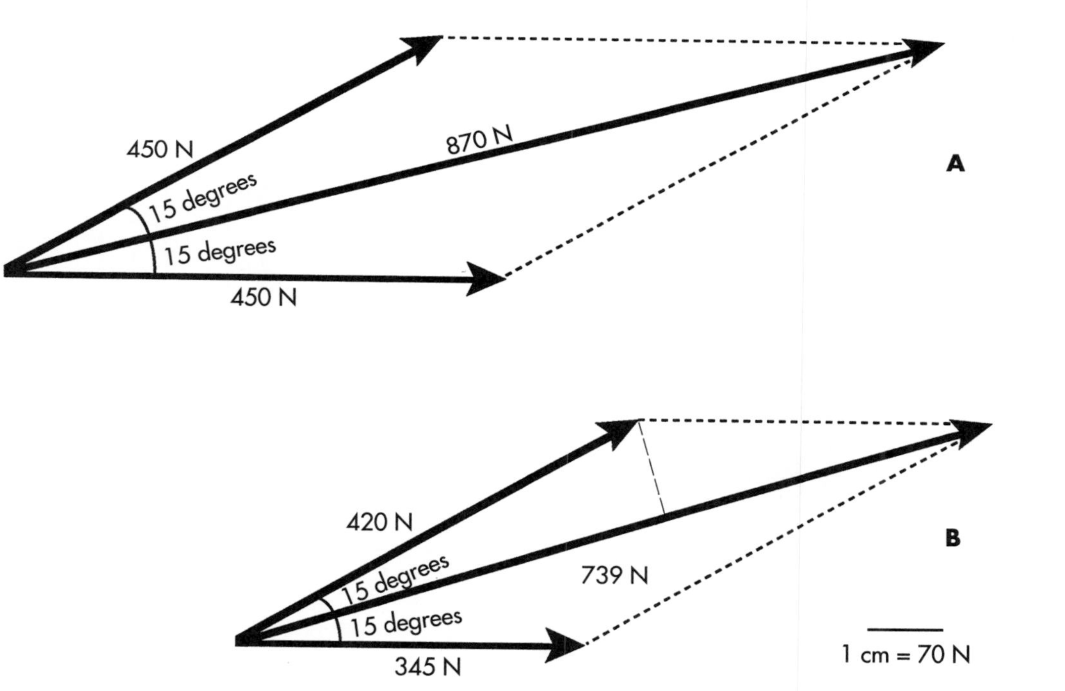

FIGURE **C-15**
A parallelogram is used to find the amount of force available for midrange shoulder flexion and abduction in individuals with fair **(A)** and poor **(B)** muscle grades.

$$R_{middle} = 333\ N$$
$$R = 406\ N + 333\ N$$
$$R = 739\ N$$

Discussion. Both poor and fair muscle grades produce nearly double the amount of force available in the midrange position between shoulder flexion and abduction. Placing a switch in this midrange position maximizes an individual's available muscle strength. Generally, individuals use motions that combine muscle groups to increase their power in activity. In muscle testing, combination motions often are referred to as "substitutions" because they use the strength of two or more muscles or muscle groups and do not give a true picture of individual muscle strength. Awkward or unusual movements in activity are often the result of the combination of muscle groups to assist weaker muscles.

In designing adaptive equipment, calculate approximate values of muscle force by using manual muscle testing and joint range through goniometry. Calculate force for fair muscle grades using the body weight to estimate the weight of the body part being lifted. Calculate force for poor muscle grades by measuring the available range of motion, then measuring or calculating the distance of the body part's center of gravity from the axis of motion. For good and normal muscle grades, add extra weight at the center of gravity for the body part being lifted and calculate the maximum amount of force available for movement. These estimates and calculations help us as OT practitioners design and solve problems involving adaptive equipment.

APPLICATION 7-4
Loads on Upper-Extremity Joints

First, determine the combined centers of gravity for the humerus, forearm, and hand, which create extension torque at the shoulder, and the forearm and hand, which create extension torque at the elbow (Figure C-16). Find the center of gravity for the hand where it creates flexion torque at the wrist. Draw the upper extremity on a grid, determine the coordinates, and plot them as shown in Chapter 3 (Figure C-17).

Torques created at each joint are calculated with the standard torque formula, weight times moment arm. Multiply the weight of the upper extremity (the arm, forearm, and hand) by the moment arm for the combined effect of the center of gravity at the shoulder axis. Then multiply the weight of the forearm and hand by their combined moment arm. Finally, multiply the weight

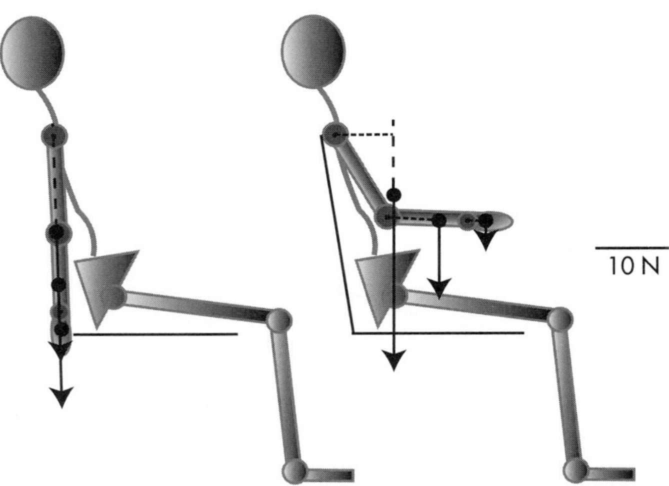

FIGURE **C-16**
No torques exist with the arm at the side because all the weight pulls through the shoulder, elbow, and wrist axes. When the upper extremity is suspended forward to type, various torques are created—extension by weight of the upper extremity at the shoulder, extension by weight of the forearm and hand at the elbow, and flexion by weight of the hand at the wrist. All must be balanced by muscle contractions producing equal torques of flexion at the shoulder and elbow and extension at the wrist.

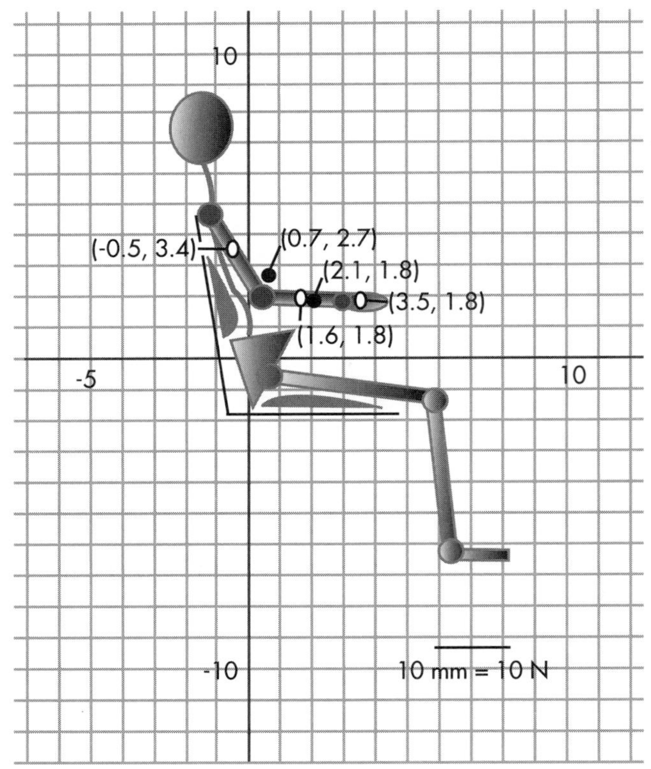

FIGURE **C-17**
Coordinates show the various centers of gravity affecting the shoulder, elbow, and wrist.

of the hand by its moment arm. Remember to convert kilograms to newtons:

24 N × 7.7 cm = 184.8 N-cm of extension torque at the shoulder

10.5 N × 6.8 cm = 71.4 N-cm of extension torque at the elbow

3 N × 2.3 cm = 6.9 N-cm of flexion at the wrist

Each tendency created by gravity must be matched, exactly and in the opposite direction, by a muscle force at each joint. A series of equilibrium formulas yields exact amounts of force required. (Remember that muscle contractions are constant as long as the arm holds its position.) The solution is simple: Provide supports, such as arms on desk chairs and keyboard pads. If the chair is adjustable and lined up so that it supports the forearm at the level of the keyboard, expensive solutions may be unnecessary. If the computer operator uses the supports, less muscle activation is necessary.

Chapter 8 Solutions

APPLICATION **8-1**

Balanced Wrist Function

As you move from straight wrist flexion toward ulnar deviation, notice that the flexor carpi radialis tendon softens a bit. This tendon, a radial deviator, must relax as it is pulled distally to allow ulnar deviation. Meanwhile, a contraction begins in the extensor carpi ulnaris to balance ulnar deviation. The opposite reaction occurs as you move into flexion and then radial deviation. The flexor carpi radialis and ulnaris tendons work together in pure flexion to balance each other's deviation effects. Radial deviation requires that the ulnaris yields as the radialis deviates. Activity picks up in the extensor carpi radialis longus to hold the wrist in radial deviation. As the two deviators work together, they cancel their opposite effects as flexors and extensors. (Note that if you try too hard, the muscles may go into static contraction. Try to think only of the movement. If necessary, have another person move a hand in the same direction and observe.)

APPLICATION **8-2**

Shorter Longitudinal Arch

If you drew your hand parallel to the edge of the paper, you should uncover the radial marking (proximal palmar crease) first. Because the palmar creases line up with the MCP joints, this action locates the second MCP distal to the fifth. The distal border of a volar splint should follow a line that connects these two creases. Any splint extending beyond this line interferes with MCP flexion as rigid splint material distal to the MCP joints blocks the proximal phalanges in their flexion arc.

Chapter 9 Solutions

APPLICATION **9-1**

Muscle Shortening During Hip Flexion

The fingers of the hand should curl (flex) as the movements occur. Both movements have the same effect on the fingers because both are hip flexion. In the open-chain movement, the thigh moves closer to the pelvis. The approximation of the insertion to the origin causes the fingers to flex, representing the shortening of the muscle fibers. In the closed-chain motion, the pelvis (origin) approaches the thigh (insertion). This indicates slackening of the hip flexors because eccentric contraction of the hip extensors (hamstrings and gluteus maximus) controls closed-chain hip flexion with gravity.

APPLICATION **9-2**

Open- and Closed-Chain Hip Abduction

This activity mimics the hip flexion application in a different plane. Closed-chain hip abduction on the weight-bearing side usually is accompanied by lateral flexion of the trunk, which also occurs in the frontal plane. Distinguish vertebral movement from hip movement and realize that both occur.

APPLICATION **9-3**

Wheelchair Instability

The most unstable aspect of this maneuver is the almost nonexistent base of support. The wheelchair can only be balanced when its center of gravity projection falls within this base of support, and the base of support is only as deep as the contact surface of the rear wheels with the floor. Slight forward and backward movements keep the chair balanced because these movements adjust the base of support. When the projection of gravity falls behind the base, you move the chair backward to "catch" the projection. When it falls in front, you push the wheels of the chair slightly forward. Balancing a vertical broomstick in the palm of the hand is a similar act.

Review of Mathematics

Working with Variables in an Equation

When an equation contains an undetermined value, isolate this variable on one side of the equals sign. Add, subtract, divide, or multiply equally on both sides of the equation so that the numbers on one side cancel and leave the variable to stand alone:

PROBLEM 1

$$8x = 48$$

$$x = \frac{48}{8}$$

$$x = 6$$

When numbers and values in an equation involve addition and subtraction and multiplication and division, isolate these different functions with parentheses and move the values within parentheses as a whole:

PROBLEM 2

$$0.3x + 0.25 \times 4 - 16 = 0$$

$$0.3x + (0.25 \times 4) - 16 = 0$$

$$0.3x = 16 - (0.25 \times 4)$$

$$0.3x = 16 - 1$$

$$x = \frac{15}{0.3}$$

$$x = 50$$

When numbers and values in an equation are isolated by parentheses, solve the functions to remove the parentheses:

PROBLEM 3

$$5\,(x - 4) + 10 = 45$$

$$5x - 20 + 10 = 45$$

$$5x = 45 + 10$$

$$5x = 55$$

$$x = 11$$

PROBLEM 4

$$12x - 6 - 2(4x \times 8) = 0$$

$$12x - 6 - 8x - 16 = 0$$

$$4x = 6 + 16$$

$$4x = 22$$

$$x = 5.5$$

Find a common denominator to solve fractions:

PROBLEM 5

$$\frac{x}{3} + \frac{1}{2} = \frac{3}{4}$$

$$\frac{x}{3} = \frac{3}{4} - \frac{1}{2}$$

$$\frac{x}{3} = \frac{(2 \times 3) - (4 \times 1)}{8}$$

$$\frac{x}{3} = \frac{6 - 4}{8}$$

$$\frac{x}{3} = \frac{1}{4}$$

$$x = \frac{3}{4}$$

Simple Geometry

The following formulas and concepts are used to solve simple problems in geometry. They are used frequently in biomechanics:

Supplementary angles. A line intersected by another line forms two angles that equal 180 degrees when added together:

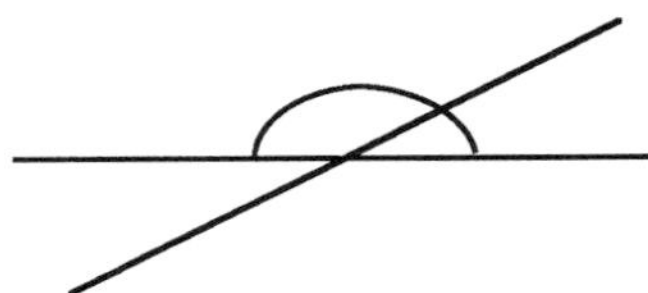

Alternate angle. When two parallel lines are intersected by a third line, the angles on opposite sides of the intersecting line are equal:

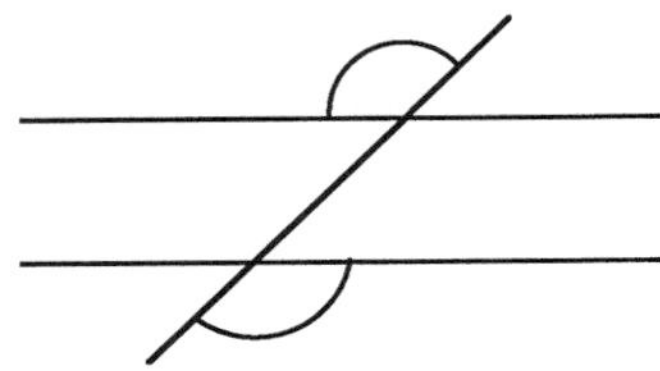

Sum of the angles. All the angles of a triangle added together equal 180 degrees.

Outer angle. An angle outside a triangle equals the two opposite inside angles:

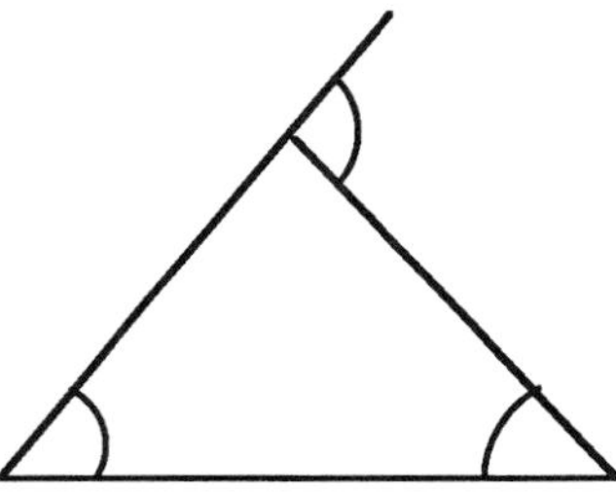

Right triangle. A right triangle has one angle of 90 degrees. This designation is specified by a boxlike marking in the 90-degree right angle.

Pythagorean theorem. In a right triangle, the horizontal and vertical sides are multiplied by themselves and when added together equal the diagonal hypotenuse multiplied by itself. The hypotenuse is generally assigned the letter *c*:

$$c^2 = a^2 + b^2$$

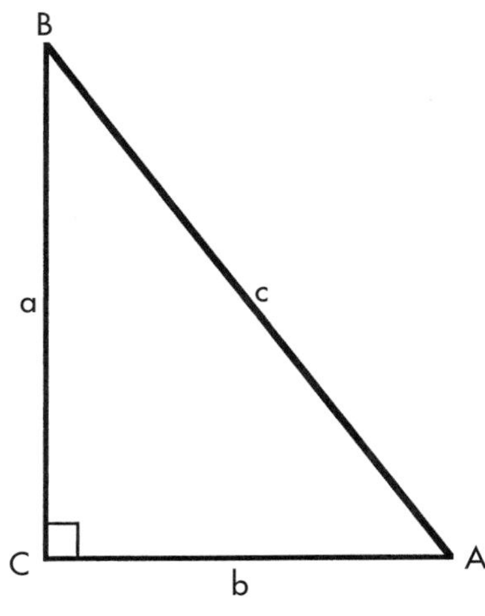

PROBLEM 6

In the following parallelogram, ABCD, side a is 5 cm and side b is 8.5 cm. Angle A is 40 degrees. Line e divides the parallelogram into two equal triangles. Line f divides ABC into two right triangles. The values of the angles in each right triangle include the following:

Angle A (intervening angle) = 40 degrees
Angle A (bisected) = 20 degrees
Angle B (alternate angle) = 140 degrees
Angle B (bisected) = 70 degrees
20 + 70 + 90 = 180 degrees

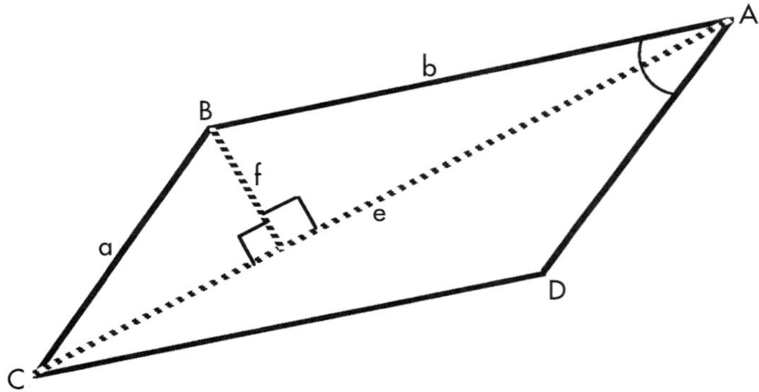

PROBLEM 7

In the right triangle on the following page, ABC, side a is 4 cm and side b is 3 cm. The following solution determines the length of side c:

$$c^2 = a^2 + b^2$$
$$c^2 = 4^2 \text{ cm} + 3^2 \text{ cm}$$
$$c^2 = 16 \text{ cm} + 9 \text{ cm}$$
$$c^2 = 25 \text{ cm}$$
$$c = 5 \text{ cm}$$

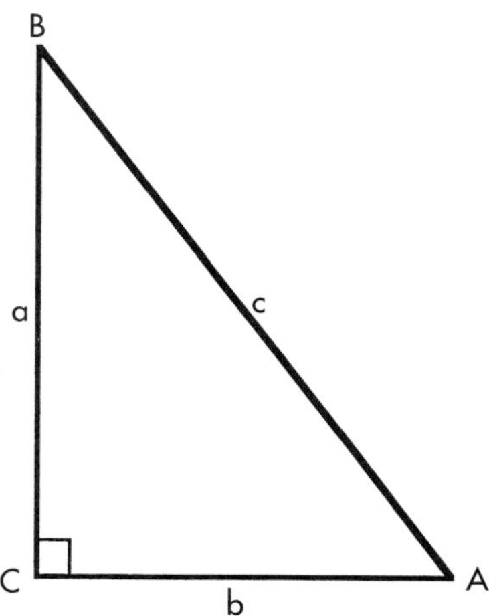

Basic Trigonometry

Trigonometry uses the ratio of known angles to known sides in triangles to determine the values of unknown sides and angles. Through the use of trigonometric functions these values can be determined with very little information. Imaginary triangles in space, on land, or between body parts can produce numerical values for distances and forces that often cannot be measured.

Trigonometric functions were determined by ancient civilizations and were used in the building of pyramids. They are used today to compute the distances of stars and other astronomic objects. Understanding their derivations is a complex mathematical feat. As with the pyramids themselves, they are easier to accept as wonders of nature; understanding why they work is a difficult process.

Sines, cosines, and *tangents* are names given to fixed ratios of angles to sides in right triangles. Use sines and cosines when given the value of the hypotenuse and a side or a side and an angle of a right triangle. Use tangents and cotangents when given the value of two sides or a side and an angle of a right triangle. Scientific calculators have these ratios built into their memory chips. A table of sines, cosines, tangents, and cotangents can be found in Appendix E.

Sine. In a right triangle the sine of an angle is the ratio of the opposite side to the hypotenuse:

$$\sin A = \frac{a}{c}$$

Cosine. In a right triangle the cosine of an angle is the ratio of the adjacent side to the hypotenuse:

$$\cos A = \frac{b}{c}$$

Tangent. In a right triangle the tangent of an angle is the ratio of the opposite side to the adjacent side:

$$\tan A = \frac{a}{b}$$

Cotangent. In a right triangle the cotangent of an angle is the ratio of the adjacent side to the opposite side:

$$\cot A = \frac{b}{a}$$

PROBLEM 8

In the following right triangle, ABC, side a is 4 cm, and side c is 8 cm. How large is angle A:

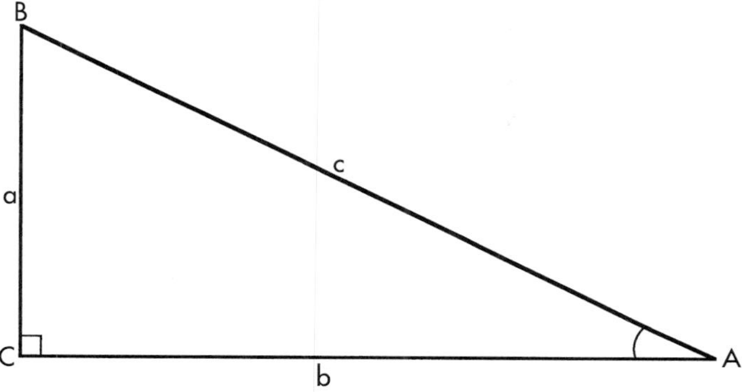

Because the value of side a and the hypotenuse are given, use sines to solve this problem:

$$\sin A = \frac{a}{c}$$

$$\sin A = \frac{4 \text{ cm}}{8 \text{ cm}}$$

$$\sin A = 0.5$$

$$A = 30 \text{ degrees}$$

PROBLEM 9

In the following right triangle, ABC, the hypotenuse is 12 cm and angle A is 15 degrees. How long are the sides?

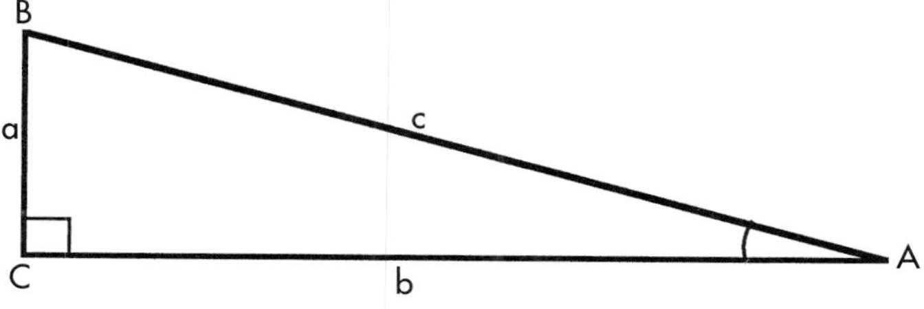

Because the hypotenuse is given and the values of both sides are needed, use sines and cosines to solve this problem:

$$\sin A = \frac{a}{c}$$

$$\sin 15 \text{ degrees} = \frac{a}{12 \text{ cm}}$$

$$a = 12 \text{ cm} \times \sin 15 \text{ degrees}$$

$$a = 12 \text{ cm} \times 0.259$$

$$a = 3.11 \text{ cm}$$

$$\cos A = \frac{b}{c}$$

$$\cos 15 \text{ degrees} = \frac{b}{12 \text{ cm}}$$

$$b = 0.966 \times 12 \text{ cm}$$

$$b = 11.59 \text{ cm}$$

Supplementary angle. When one line intersects another, two supplementary angles are formed. The sines of both supplementary angles are equal to each other:

$$\sin A = \sin (180 \text{ degrees} - A)$$

The cosine of one angle is equal to the negative cosine of the other angle:

$$\cos A = -\cos (180 \text{ degrees} - A)$$

Sines and cosines can be used when working with triangles that are not right triangles:

Sine theorem. Two angles and an opposite side or two sides and an opposite angle can yield the values for the rest of any triangle because sides are proportional to the sines of their angles:

$$\frac{a}{\sin A} = \frac{b}{\sin B} = \frac{c}{\sin C}$$

Cosine theorem. Three sides or two sides and an adjacent angle can yield the values of the rest of the triangle because of the relationships between them:

$$a^2 = b^2 + c^2 - (2 \text{ bc} \times \cos A)$$

PROBLEM 10

In the following triangle, ABC, side b is 6.0 cm, side c is 9.0 cm, and angle A is 60 degrees. From this information, side a can be determined:

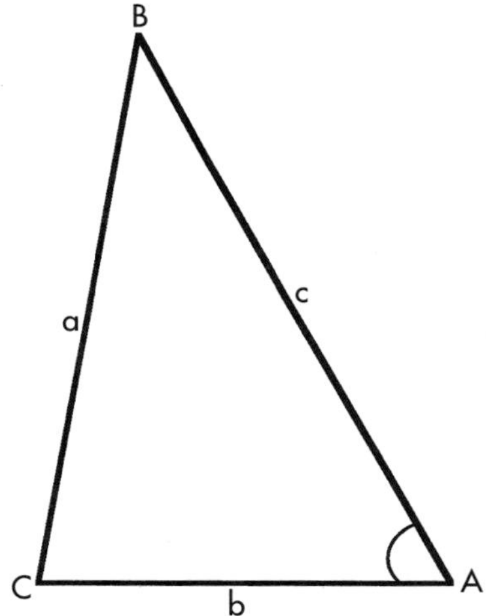

Because two sides and an adjacent angle are given, use the cosine theorem to solve this problem:

$$a^2 = b^2 + c^2 - (2 \text{ bc} \times \cos A)$$

$$a^2 = 6^2 \text{ cm} + 9^2 \text{ cm} - [2(6 \text{ cm} \times 9 \text{ cm}) \times \cos A]$$

$$a^2 = 36 \text{ cm} + 81 \text{ cm} - (108 \text{ cm} \times 0.5)$$

$$a^2 = 63 \text{ cm}$$

$$a = 7.9 \text{ cm}$$

Trigonometric Functions

DEGREES*	SINES	COSINES	TANGENTS	COTANGENTS	
0	.0000	1.0000	.0000		90
1	.0175	.9998	.0175	57.290	89
2	.0349	.9994	.0349	28.636	88
3	.0523	.9986	.0524	19.081	87
4	.0698	.9976	.0699	14.301	86
5	.0872	.9962	.0875	11.430	85
6	.1045	.9945	.1051	9.5144	84
7	.1219	.9925	.1228	8.1443	83
8	.1392	.9903	.1405	7.1154	82
9	.1564	.9877	.1584	6.3138	81
10	.1736	.9848	.1763	5.6713	80
11	.1908	.9816	.1944	5.1446	79
12	.2079	.9781	.2126	4.7046	78
13	.2250	.9744	.2309	4.3315	77
14	.2419	.9703	.2493	4.0108	76
15	.2588	.9659	.2679	3.7321	75
16	.2756	.9613	.2867	3.4874	74
17	.2924	.9563	.3057	3.2709	73
18	.3090	.9511	.3249	3.0777	72
19	.3256	.9455	.3443	2.9042	71
20	.3420	.9397	.3640	2.7475	70
21	.3584	.9336	.3839	2.6051	69
22	.3746	.9272	.4040	2.4751	68
23	.3907	.9205	.4245	2.3559	67
24	.4067	.9135	.4452	2.2460	66
25	.4226	.9063	.4663	2.1445	65
26	.4384	.8988	.4877	2.0503	64
27	.4540	.8910	.5095	1.9626	63
28	.4695	.8829	.5317	1.8807	62
29	.4848	.8746	.5543	1.8040	61
30	.5000	.8660	.5774	1.7321	60
31	.5150	.8572	.6009	1.6643	59
32	.5299	.8480	.6249	1.6003	58
33	.5446	.8387	.6494	1.5399	57
34	.5592	.8290	.6745	1.4826	56
35	.5736	.8192	.7002	1.4281	55
36	.5878	.8090	.7265	1.3765	54
37	.6018	.7986	.7536	1.3270	53
38	.6157	.7880	.7813	1.2799	52
39	.6293	.7771	.8098	1.2349	51
40	.6428	.7660	.8391	1.1918	50
41	.6561	.7547	.8693	1.1504	49
42	.6691	.7431	.9004	1.1106	48
43	.6820	.7314	.9325	1.0724	47
44	.6947	.7193	.9657	1.0355	46
45	.7071	.7071	1.0000	1.0000	45
	COSINES	SINES	COTANGENTS	TANGENTS	DEGREES

*Note: With angles above 45 degrees, use the headings that appear at the bottom of the columns.

Commonly Used Formulas in Biomechanics

Length (Unmeasurable Elements)

When one angle and one side are known or when the hypotenuse of a right triangle is known, the following equations can be used to determine the unknown value:

$\sin A = \frac{a}{c}$ for an angle and an opposite side

$\cos A = \frac{b}{c}$ for an angle and an adjacent side

When two sides of a right triangle are known, the following equations can be used to determine the unknown value:

$$\tan A = \frac{a}{b}$$

$$\cot A = \frac{b}{a}$$

When two angles and an opposite angle or two angles and an opposite side of any triangle are known, the following equation can be used to determine the unknown value:

$$\frac{a}{\sin A} = \frac{b}{\sin B} = \frac{c}{\sin C}$$

When three sides or two sides and an adjacent angle of any triangle are known, the following equation can be used to determine the unknown value:

$$a^2 = b^2 + c^2 - (2\,bc \times \cos A)$$

Force (Linear Motion)

$$\underset{\text{Force}}{F} = \underset{\text{Mass}}{m} \times \underset{\text{Acceleration (Gravity)}}{a}$$

Force Equilibrium

$\Sigma F = 0$ (The sum of all forces equals 0.)

or

$\Sigma F_x = 0$ (All horizontal forces equal 0.)

and

$\Sigma F_y = 0$ (All vertical forces equal 0.)

TORQUE (ROTARY MOTION)

$$\underset{\text{Torque}}{T} = \underset{\text{Force}}{f} \times \underset{\text{Moment arm}}{ma}$$

MOMENT EQUILIBRIUM

$\Sigma M = 0$ (The sum of clockwise and counterclockwise torque equals 0.)

or

$$\underset{\text{Effort force}}{EFA} \times \underset{\text{Effort moment arm}}{EMA} = \underset{\text{Resistance force}}{RFA} \times \underset{\text{Resistance moment arm}}{RMA}$$

STRESS (PRESSURE)

S	=	f	÷	t	×	w
Stress		Force		Tissue length		Tissue width

WORK

Lifting work can be determined with the following formula:

L	=	mg	×	h	×	r
Lifting work		(Mass × gravity)		Height lifted		Number of repetitions

Carrying work can be determined with the following formula:

C	=	mg	×	d	×	r
Carrying work		(Mass × gravity)		Distance		Number of repetitions

Biomechanical Analysis of Function

T ***he philosophical basis*** of OT practice states that "Man is an active being whose development is influenced by the use of purposeful activity."[4] This is a short statement, but every OT student learns quickly that the words *purposeful activity* evoke lengthy discussion. Activity analysis helps OT practitioners understand whether an activity is purposeful and has therapeutic value. Through activity analysis the practitioner gains an appreciation of the activity's components and characteristics, which differentiate the therapeutic value of one activity from another. This begins the process that ultimately leads to the therapeutic use of occupation.[1]

An important consideration in the therapeutic use of activity is the determination of the need for adaptation to facilitate task performance. A full understanding of the individual's abilities and limitations is needed. This is possible only through comprehensive biomechanical analysis, which ensures identification of the real problems to be addressed in the adaptive process. Thus the subsequent problem-solving process is correctly focused. As Parham[5] suggested in her discussion of problem setting, inadequate time spent identifying the appropriate problem to solve can render even brilliant problem solving useless.

Successful adaptation that facilitates an individual's involvement in purposeful activity requires problem setting first. Problem setting includes the identification of priority aspects of a patient's need to receive intervention. Not only must the specific focus of intervention be sorted out from various presenting problems, but the problem-setting process also must occur at a deeper level—specification of the musculoskeletal segment most responsible for activity dysfunction. In this process, which is the essence of biomechanical analysis, the dysfunctional link is tagged, and problem solving leading to adaptation begins.

*Modified from Greene D, A clinically relevant approach to biomechanical analysis of function, *Occup Ther Pract* 1(4):44-52, 1990.

Background of Biomechanical Analysis

Let us review the basic models from which biomechanical analysis was developed. Reed[7] describes three different biomechanical models—reconstruction, orthopedic, and kinetic. Each model adheres to the assumption that function resulting from voluntary muscle contraction and control (and dysfunction resulting from a lack of the same) depends on muscle strength, joint range of motion, and physical endurance. Although the reconstruction model suggests the use of voluntary movements in academic and vocational activities, the orthopedic approach more specifically addresses differential treatment of pathological conditions. The kinetic model differs from both in its attention to the analysis of motion during activities and the adjustment of strategies on the basis of the analysis. This model suggests a specific methodology for analysis of motion. The kinetic model is elaborated in the text *Occupational Therapy Principles and Practice*,[3] which was written in collaboration with our profession's founder, William Rush Dunton, Jr.

As our professional emphasis has moved toward greater accountability through the quantification of information, observation analysis has been refined and augmented by methods employing electromyographic (EMG) measurements. Basmajian and De Luca[2] and Trombly and Cole[11] have used EMG measurements to describe specific muscle activity in the hand. These studies have provided valuable information to help the practitioner better understand motion and the agonists responsible for motion in activity performance.

Analyses such as these represent the most accurate methods for absolute determination of muscle activity during function. OT practitioners should use documented studies based on these technical methods whenever possible. However, not every movement in every activity used in the clinic has been studied; studies of normal individuals cannot be directly applied to injured individuals who, in adjusting to their pathological conditions, have developed compensatory movements. Even in its less than absolute nature, biomechanical analysis through activity observation remains a necessary practice.

As a result of time constraints or the belief that analysis can be done intuitively and briefly while setting up the activity, many OT practitioners do not routinely perform biomechanical analysis. The examples that follow suggest that prior biomechanical analysis in each task would have yielded better judgment by the OT practitioner and more effective treatment for the client.

In the use of a deltoid assist in a tabletop activity, the goal is to strengthen the external shoulder rotators to facilitate greater ease in self-feeding. The upper extremities are positioned in 90 degrees of shoulder abduction, and the weights of the assist are moved up and down as internal and external rotation bring the hands to and from the table. However, this arrangement actually resists internal rotation and assists external rotation and therefore does not strengthen the intended motion.

Another example is in the use of a mobile arm support to allow self-feeding for an individual who exhibits an inability to bring the hand to the mouth. This individual has adequate shoulder external rotation and elbow flexion but an absence of shoulder abduction and weak wrist extension. Because of the weakness in wrist extension, the individual is unable to maintain grasp and, because of wrist drop, cannot fully elevate the hand to the mouth through external shoulder rotation.

When the arm is placed in the mobile arm support, the individual still cannot self-feed because the real problem—weak wrist extension—is ignored. Meanwhile, external shoulder rotation is possible without the device. With the identification of the real problem, intervention with a simple wrist cock-up splint proves a more successful strategy.

Thus even some of the simplest solutions require reasoning skills beyond simple matching of equipment with common problems. Schön[9] suggests that as the emphasis of intervention shifts more toward technical skills, we may find that problem solving is made more difficult by a narrow application of theory. We, as OT practitioners, must strengthen our ability to reason out solutions based on the uniqueness of a patient's symptoms, which is fully illustrated through biomechanical analysis.

Review of Terms

Biomechanical analysis leads to ideas and terms that require definition. The terms associated with biomechanical analysis are used frequently in daily practice, but a clear definition is necessary for universal application.

Force, as defined by Soderberg,[10] is the action or effect of one body on another (for example, a skeletal muscle acting on a bony segment). The muscle that produces the force responsible for the motion is known as the *agonist,* or *prime mover.* Although muscles often generate force affecting the skeletal system, gravity[6] is a force not produced by a muscle. Gravity is unique in its constant effect, which is to pull a body or bony segment toward the center of the Earth, or straight down in general terms. A gravity-assisted motion is one that occurs even in the absence of muscle contraction. Yet muscular forces are important even in this type of motion because gravity-assisted motions usually are controlled by contractions of muscles that typically perform the motion opposite the one observed. Thus for example, the elbow flexors are the active group in gravity-assisted elbow extension, as in the controlled lowering of the hand from the mouth to the table.

However, elbow flexors that contract to extend the elbow make sense only in the context of muscle contraction. Although a muscle typically shortens during contraction (concentric contraction), contraction performed against an external force of adequate magnitude to prevent motion results in a contraction with no appreciable change in muscle length (isometric contraction). If the external force exerted on a segment overcomes the muscular force attempting to move the segment in the opposite direction, a lengthening (eccentric) contraction occurs. This is the case in the previous example, in which gravity-assisted elbow extension is controlled by eccentric contraction of the elbow flexors.

A Usable Methodology

Biomechanical analysis has widespread application in the various specialties of OT practice, from handling and positioning of the infant to adaptation and activity design of the adult population. We can use a universally familiar task to demonstrate biomechanical analysis. (Figures G-1 and G-2 are examples of the

SEGMENT		INITIAL MOTION			HOLDING POSITION			
MOTION/ POSITION OBSERVED	% ROM	RESISTED OR RAPID	GRAVITY ASSISTS/ RESISTS	AGONIST GROUP/ CONTRACTION TYPE (CON OR ECC)	RESISTED	GRAVITY EFFECT	ISOMETRIC AGONIST	REP
V FLEX								
Reaching for foot	*50%*	*No*	*Assists*	*Extensors/ECC*	*No*	*Promotes flexion*	*Extensors*	*No*
V EXT								
Returning from flexion	*N/A*	*No*	*Resists*	*Extensors/CON*	*N/A*			
V L-ROT								
Turning to reach right foot	*<50%*	*No*	*No*	*Left rotators/CON*	*No*	*None*	*Left rotators*	*No*
S PRO								
Reaching forward	*>50%*	*Slight resistance at end*	*Slight assist*	*Protractors/CON*	*Slightly*	*Little if any*	*Protractors*	*No*
S RET								
Pulling sock	*N/A*	*Resisted*	*N/A*	*Retractors/CON*	*N/A*			
GH FLEX								
Reaching forward and placing sock	*<50%*	*No*	*Resists*	*Flexors/CON*	*No*	*Promotes extension*	*Flexors*	*No*
E FLEX								
Positioning-	*<50%*	*No*	*Resists*	*Flexors/CON*	*No*	*Promotes extension*	*Flexors*	*No*
Pulling sock-	*50%*	*Resisted*	*N/A*	*Flexors/CON*	*N/A*			

FIGURE **G-1**
Analysis of motion involving the vertebral joints, scapula, and glenohumeral and elbow joints. *ROM,* Range of motion; *CON,* concentric; *ECC,* eccentric; *REP,* repetition; *V FLEX,* vertebral flexion; *V EXT,* vertebral extension; *V L-ROT,* vertebral left rotation; *S PRO,* scapular protraction; *S RET,* scapular retraction; *GH FLEX,* glenohumeral flexion; *E FLEX,* elbow flexion; *N/A,* not applicable.

method used to record the observations made during the task's performance.)

The task is donning socks in a seated position, crossing the lower extremities to allow easier access to the foot. This task can be difficult, especially in the older population. Careful analysis that considers the common problems associated with the older client reveals specific steps of great difficulty that can be made easier.

This analysis begins as the OT practitioner observes one joint at a time to establish whether the joint moves into and is held in a position other than its anatomical position. The OT practitioner then develops questions regarding this motion and position. If the motion is cyclic and returns the segment to the original anatomical position, as in shoulder flexion and extension in moving the hand to place an object on a tabletop, only the motion is considered because no position is held. Finally, the practitioner determines whether the motion involved (and any resulting position held) is repetitive or occurs only once in the total performance of the activity. All entries on the form (see Figures G-1 and G-2) are brief, often composed of one-word answers. They are designed to mimic an actual practitioner's notations.

For the purposes of the present discussion, only the analysis of specific segments that present problems is described in detail on the sample forms. The segments discussed include the intervertebral joints, glenohumeral joint, joints of the hand, and hip joint. In the actual clinical setting, the choice can be made as to whether all musculoskeletal segments or only specific ones are analyzed.

INTERVERTEBRAL JOINTS

As the subject reaches to place the sock on the foot, the OT practitioner observes flexion. This description is

SEGMENT		INITIAL MOTION			HOLDING POSITION			
MOTION/ POSITION OBSERVED	% ROM	RESISTED OR RAPID	GRAVITY ASSISTS/ RESISTS	AGONIST GROUP/ CONTRACTION TYPE (CON OR ECC)	RESISTED	GRAVITY EFFECT	ISOMETRIC AGONIST	REP
MCP FLEX								
Holding sock	50%	No	N/A	Flexors/CON	Yes	N/A	Flexors	No
MCP EXT								
Opening hand	>50%	No	N/A	Extensors/CON	N/A			
IP FLEX								
Holding sock	<50%	No	N/A	Flexors/CON	Yes	N/A	Flexors	No
IP EXT								
Opening hand	50%	No	N/A	Extensors/CON	N/A			
CM#1 ABD								
Opening hand	50%	No	N/A	Abductors/CON	N/A			
CM#1 ADD								
Holding sock	<50%	No	N/A	Adductors/CON	Yes	N/A	Adductors	No
OPP								
Opening hand; holding sock	100%	No	N/A	Abductors, flexors, opponens/CON	Yes	N/A	Adductors, flexors, opponens	No
H FLEX								
Crossing legs	>50%	No	Resists	Flexors/CON	N/A →	Legs are crossed	N/A	
Leaning forward	>50%	No	Assists	Extensors/ECC	No	Promotes flexion	Extensors	No
H E-ROT								
Crossing legs	>50%	No	Resists	External rotators/CON	N/A →	Legs are crossed	N/A	

FIGURE **G-2**
Analysis of motion involving the metacarpophalangeal and interphalangeal joints, thumb carpometacarpal joint, and hip joint. *ROM,* Range of motion; *CON,* concentric; *ECC,* eccentric, *REP,* repetition; *MCP FLEX,* metacarpophalangeal flexion; *MCP EXT,* metacarpophalangeal extension; *IP FLEX,* interphalangeal flexion; *IP EXT,* interphalangeal extension; *CM#1 ABD,* thumb carpometacarpal abduction; *CM#1 ADD,* thumb carpometacarpal adduction; *OPP,* opposition; *H FLEX,* hip flexion; *H E-ROT,* hip external rotation; *N/A,* not applicable.

briefly stated on the form (see Figure G-1). Nothing else concerning placement of the sock on the foot (for example, the wrist position) is addressed at this time. Also, no other vertebral position is recognized.

As the practitioner considers next the percentage range of motion, the extent of flexion is approximately 50%. (An estimate is sufficient.) The anatomical position is assumed to be 0% and the full extent of flexion normally possible, 100%.

Next, the OT practitioner considers the nature of the flexion to determine whether the movement is performed rapidly or against resistance. (Resistance is external resistance directed in the opposite direction of the movement and in addition to the effect of gravity.) A motion performed rapidly or against resistance is generally a result of a contraction of the anatomical agonist. Vertebral flexion does not occur rapidly or against resistance. However, with enlargement of the abdomen or decrease in vertebral flexibility, the individual may encounter resistance to vertebral flexion. The agonist (flexors) is thus identified on the basis of this determination regardless of the effect of gravity. In this case the question regarding the effect of gravity is preempted.

If the individual does not encounter resistance, the vertebral flexion observed is assisted by gravity. In fact, gravity may be considered the prime mover after a slight initial burst of flexor activity. As stated clearly by Rosse and Clawson,[8] "When the prime moving force is generated not by muscle but by gravity, the movement will be controlled, paradoxically, by muscles capable of producing the converse movement, that is, by the antagonists." Therefore the flexion is the result of eccentric contraction of the vertebral extensors. Identification of the vertebral extensors as agonists provides the basis for the understanding that an individual's inability to move slowly into vertebral flexion may be the result of dysfunction in the vertebral extensors.

Identification and characterization of the movement are not enough if the movement leads to a position the individual must hold during the activity. In the example of the donning of socks, the individual holds vertebral flexion as the sock is positioned and put on the foot. The effect of gravity is to attempt to continue the flexion. Therefore the isometric agonist is the extensor group, which contracts to resist gravity's flexion tendency.

Finally, as the individual dons the sock, the OT practitioner observes only one flexion motion of the vertebral column for each sock donned.

With identification and analysis of vertebral flexion completed, the OT practitioner views each possible movement in each segment in order. Vertebral extension is observed when the subject returns from the flexed position. Percentage range of motion is not applicable because this motion is considered a return motion (from flexion to the anatomical position). If a fixed deformity prevents an individual from returning to full vertebral extension, the limitation is documented on the left side of the form with a descriptor such as "lacking 20%" if desired.

Extension is not resisted (by any force in addition to gravity) or performed rapidly, but gravity resists the motion. Therefore the movement is a result of the concentric contraction of the extensor group. Because extension results in the assumption of the anatomical position, no further characterization is necessary other than documentation that this movement, like vertebral flexion, is not repetitive.

The OT practitioner observes slight rotation to the left and right in donning the right and left socks, respectively. Only left rotation is considered in this discussion because the same discussion applies to the right side.

Left rotation is less than 50%. It is not performed rapidly, nor is it usually a movement against resistance in this activity. As in vertebral flexion, however, decreased vertebral flexibility may result in at least some resistance. Although difficult to assess, the ease with which the individual performs the motion is a good indication of the degree of resistance.

Rotation is performed in the gravity-eliminated plane in the anatomical position, but in this activity it is performed in a forward-flexed position. Nevertheless, the counterbalancing effect of the two upper extremities neutralizes the effect of gravity. Without gravity's influence, the left rotator group performs and holds left rotation. Increased resistance resulting from decreased flexibility results in a stronger contraction of the same group; in either case a concentric contraction moves into position and an isometric contraction of the same group holds the position.

GLENOHUMERAL JOINT

Glenohumeral function flexion is apparent as the individual moves the sock toward the foot and places it on the foot. It is less than 50% and occurs slowly against gravity only. The agonist group is the flexor group, which contracts concentrically. As the individual holds the position, again only gravity resists and the isometric agonist is the flexor group. This segment and movement (shoulder flexion) often limits the older population as they dress the lower extremities. Biomechanical analysis can help OT practitioners determine whether this is the weak link in the chain.

METACARPOPHALANGEAL, INTERPHALANGEAL, AND CARPOMETACARPAL JOINTS

Because of their relatively small mass, the digits are negligibly affected by gravity, yet the percentage of time they move and hold positions against resistance is great. Therefore in the consideration of joints distal to the wrist, gravity's effect is ignored and performance against resistance and rapidity of motion receive greater emphasis.

The position of the hand in holding the sock requires partial metacarpophalangeal and interphalangeal flexion (see Figure G-2). In this case, metacarpophalangeal and interphalangeal flexion initially occur against little resistance as the individual flexes the digits into position to hold the sock. The flexor group contracts concentrically. Flexion does occur against resistance because some strength of grip is required to hold the sock and pull it onto the foot. The isometric agonist is the digit flexor group. The motion is not repetitive.

The carpometacarpal thumb joint is abducted as the individual moves the thumb into position to receive the sock. Abduction is not held, however, because on receiving the sock, the adductors contract concentrically and thus the thumb grasps the sock through a slight adduction movement. A slightly adducted position is maintained in part through an isometric contraction of the adductors as the individual pulls the thumb into a pinch, holding the sock between the thumb and the stable post provided by digits 2 through 5.

The description of the thumb as it grasps the sock is confusing. The thumb has moved into a partially adducted position but remains slightly abducted from the palm. Nevertheless, this position is maintained as a consequence of the powerful thumb adductors' contraction against a stable post, the semiflexed, statically positioned fingers. Imagine what would happen if the abductors were activated to hold the desired degree of abduction. The sock would fall because contraction of the abductors generates thumb motion from the palm, a direction in which no stable post is present. Thumb abduction would obliterate grasp.

HIP JOINT

Limitation in hip function (specifically flexion, adduction, and external rotation) often solely prohibits independent function in donning of the socks. An extreme amount of hip flexion is required (for example, nearly 100% in the right lower extremity when donning the right sock) in the combination of sitting, forward bending, and crossing one lower extremity over the other. This extreme often may be responsible for the difficulty many individuals experience. Any lack in hip flexibility is resistance to the individual's attempt to flex the hip when trying to gain access to the foot. Thus many individuals fail to don socks if they do not first stretch to warm the muscles.

Summary

To facilitate function, we, as OT practitioners, must make comparisons between an individual's ability or disability and the demands of an activity through biomechanical analysis. As we become more skillful in performance observation and analysis, we can better interpret and apply the specific and accurate measurements we make, heightening the quality of OT intervention.

In the previous method, the OT practitioner skillfully observes movement using an organized worksheet to characterize performance one joint at a time. Planning of strategies for rehabilitation and adaptation allows the practitioner to use this analysis to develop a more contextual knowledge. Additionally, more objective documentation paves the way for more meaningful and accountable communication with clients, professionals, and third-party payors.

REFERENCES

1. American Occupational Therapy Association: Minutes of the representative assembly, *Am J Occup Ther* 33:785, 1979.
2. Basmajian JV, De Luca CJ. *Muscles alive: their functions revealed by electromyography,* ed 5, Baltimore, 1985, Williams & Wilkins.
3. Dunton WR Jr, Licht S: *Occupational therapy principles and practice,* ed 2, Springfield, Ill, 1957, Charles C Thomas.
4. Hopkins HL, Smith HD: *Willard and Spackman's occupational therapy,* ed 6, New York, 1983, JB Lippincott.
5. Parham D: Toward professionalism, *Am J Occup Ther* 41:555-561, 1987.
6. Rasch PJ, Burke RK: *Kinesiology and applied anatomy,* ed 6, Philadelphia, 1978, Lea & Febiger.
7. Reed KL: *Models of practice in occupational therapy,* Baltimore, 1984, Williams & Wilkins.
8. Rosse C, Clawson DK: *The musculoskeletal system in health and disease,* New York, 1980, Harper & Row.
9. Schön D: *The reflective practitioner,* New York, 1983, Basic Books.
10. Soderberg GL: *Kinesiology: application to pathological motion,* Baltimore, 1986, Williams & Wilkins.
11. Trombly CA, Cole JM: Electromyographic study of four hand muscles during selected activities, *Am J Occup Ther* 33:440-449, 1979.

Synopsis of Characters

T*his appendix contains brief descriptions* of each character in alphabetical order by first name. The characters are based on compilations of many individuals the authors have known. Any similarities to real people, living or dead, are purely coincidental.

Alex Fecteau was recommended for an OT evaluation by his first-grade teacher, who reported that he walked "funny," generally was fatigued, and did not participate on the playground. The school therapist discovered that Alex suffered from generalized muscle weakness, with an increased severity in the proximal muscle groups. The therapist urged his family to seek further medical help. Because Alex's family did not have medical insurance, the school social worker helped them locate a clinic, where a pediatrician diagnosed Alex with Duchenne-type muscular dystrophy.

The school therapist developed alternative playground activities to accommodate Alex's needs and explained the progressive course of Duchenne's dystrophy to the school's staff members. Alex was excused from running laps, which could cause him debilitating fatigue rather than help him build muscle strength.

Bernice Richards is a nightclub singer with C5 quadriplegia, a result of a motor vehicle accident. Fortunately, she has some sparing of left wrist extensor muscles. Bernice stayed in the spinal cord unit of the rehabilitation center for 5 months. She left the hospital driving her own van. Bernice's former employer and loyal fans raised money to make modifications to the stage and restrooms so that she was able to resume her singing career. As a performer, Bernice always cared deeply about her appearance and insisted on relearning to apply her eyeliner before she left rehab.

Crystal Turner is a 4-year-old girl with Down syndrome who came to the outpatient clinic with her parents to learn some activities that would stimulate her gross and fine-motor development. Despite her low muscle tone, she was eager to try most activities and attempted to keep up with the older children.

Donna Nelson is a college student who works in the city's most popular Italian restaurant. During her sophomore year, Donna had to take a leave of absence to learn how to manage her recently diagnosed bipolar disorder. Because her job provides much-needed tip money, maintaining upper-body strength was an important component of her psychiatric hospitalization. She was able to resume college after a semester off and currently is applying to master's degree programs in occupational therapy.

Eduardo Ybarra was an outpatient in the hand therapy clinic after sustaining a radial nerve injury from a power saw. Eduardo was working as a cabinetmaker before his injury and could not return to work. His injury occurred at home while he was making his son a Christmas present, so he received no industrial compensation from the furniture factory. Fortunately, Eduardo had health insurance and underwent surgery and therapy to restore some function in his hand. Vocational rehabilitation has enabled him to take some courses at the local community college. Eduardo is depressed and uncertain about his job possibilities but continues to do some woodworking at home and plans to teach his sons this craft.

Fred Jackson has had rheumatoid arthritis for about 20 years. He came to the hand clinic after undergoing surgery to replace the metacarpophalangeal joints in his hand. The aerospace engineering company where he worked for 30 years recently underwent a merger, and the employees were forced to change medical insurance plans. In the ensuing confusion, Fred's hand rehabilitation was disrupted and the result of the surgery was less than he had expected.

Fred's disappointment and anger sometimes have made him seem difficult in the clinic. As part of his job, Fred has designed many tools for use in the weightlessness of space. Once the OT staff got to know him, they found him to be a great source of information about biomechanics. He often kept staff and clients enthralled with his stories.

George O'Hara is a middle-aged man with mental retardation of unknown etiology. He came to the outpatient clinic for some general reconditioning after he was hospitalized with pneumonia. George lives in a group home and works in a workshop that recycles metal scraps. The generalized weakness that followed his 2-week hospital stay caused him to refuse to dress himself or push the carts of metal scraps at work. He was able to resume both these activities with a little coaching after he regained strength and endurance.

Henry Isaacs is a 70 year-old man who broke his wrist and hip when he slipped on the ice while shoveling the sidewalk in front of his grocery store. Henry's hip had to be replaced, and he spent a short time at Maple Grove Skilled Care Facility. While there, he beat all the OT staff members at checkers. Henry took classes in joint protection principles to reduce his risk of developing carpal tunnel syndrome on his return to the grocery store.

Iris Clark is a housewife and mother of three children under age 6. She cut her hand on a broken glass while washing dishes and severed the A1 and A2 tendon sheaths. Her hand injury and its surgical repair was straightforward and required minimal rehabilitation. Because cooking was an essential job function for her, the OT staff included a kitchen evaluation as part of her treatment. During the time it took for her right hand to fully recover function, they made sure that she could do all the necessary tasks at home.

Jason Black is a third grader with cerebral palsy. The OT practitioners who saw Jason at school communicated his needs to the OT staff members treating him in the community clinic so that his new wheelchair would enable him to sit comfortably all day in the classroom. The OT practitioners in his school also coordinated his other needs for adaptive equipment, and he became much more successful in self-feeding and using his augmentative communication device.

When OT staff members explained that Jason became fatigued halfway through the cafeteria lunch, the school staff began feeding him the rest of his meal. This increased his energy level, which led to better attention and participation in the afternoon. Jason no longer needed an afternoon nap, cried less often, and was better able to respond to his classmates' attentions. Last month, Jason was voted the best student in his class and took home the class mascot, a plush toy wildcat.

Karen Wu fractured her right third metacarpal bone while attempting a maneuver she had seen in a televised ice-skating competition. Although Karen was proud that her subsequent efforts and practice helped her to complete the stunt, she avoided telling her mother about the injury and did not get prompt medical attention. By the time Karen was referred to the hand clinic, tendon adhesions had resulted in limited motion in her right middle finger.

At first, Karen was reluctant to wear the recommended extension splint, but the OT staff members finally convinced her that serious athletes always listen to their trainers. Karen decided to approach hand rehabilitation with the same determination as she approached skating, explaining to her classmates that she was an athlete receiving sports medicine, not just a girl with a splint.

Linda Valdez is a middle-aged woman who visited the OT clinic after she was diagnosed with rheumatoid arthritis. Linda worked as a secretary in a law office and was active in her church as an organizer of the clothing and food banks that served the city in which she lived. On weekends, extended family members gathered at her house to eat and provide each other with material and social support.

The OT staff members taught Linda important joint protection and energy conservation principles and helped her fit them into her busy life. Despite her abilities to delegate and organize, Linda still experienced some of the joint destruction that accompanies rheumatoid arthritis. Over the years, the OT staff members supported Linda through some losses and assisted her in finding creative ways to continue her roles as matriarch and community organizer.

Mary Smith spent her whole life taking care of her family and house until she had a right-side cerebral vascular accident at age 67. Her family described her as a cheerful lady who always put up seasonal decorations and loved to putter around in her garden. They were dismayed that she had changed into a weepy, fearful "old woman" and found it difficult to spend time with her after the cerebral vascular accident. Depression complicated Mary's recovery process, and she required maximal assistance with almost all activities on her arrival at Maple Grove Skilled Care Facility. OT staff members used some gentle rocking and swinging motions to stimulate her vestibular system and concentrated on reducing her fear of falling during transfers.

As she regained more confidence in her sitting balance, Mary took a more active part in self-care and some gardening and cooking groups at the facility. The OT staff members encouraged her family members to learn some transfer techniques, after which her family decided they could safely take Mary out on some day trips.

Nancy Grant works as a computer operator in a small manufacturing firm. Her employer had several employees complain that their aches and pains were due to work-related tasks, so the firm's owner contracted with a company that did job-site analysis and injury-prevention education. Nancy's workstation needed few modifications, but during the injury-prevention education sessions, she learned that her body mechanics at home were contributing to her lower-back pain. She was able to implement a number of the OT practitioners' recommendations and reduce her level of discomfort at work.

Oliver Xiong is a computer operator at the same company as Nancy. Although the company's computer workstations were ideal for Nancy, Oliver's height caused him to assume postures that contributed to upper-back pain. The OT practitioner helped the company make a number of modifications to Oliver's workstation, which eliminated his pain.

Paul Zimmerman is a dermatologist with chronic lower-back pain aggravated by positions he had to assume during medical procedures. The OT practitioner gave him a number of suggestions to modify his workstations and equipment. He incorporated these suggestions when his office and clinic were remodeled. The modifications reduced Paul's discomfort and allowed him to stand longer so that he could make several new surgical procedures available to his clients.

Quentin Keller is a retired farmer who was placed in Maple Grove Skilled Care Facility after a left-side cerebral vascular accident made it impossible for him to live at home alone. Quentin led an independent and active lifestyle before his cerebral vascular accident and had a great deal of difficulty adjusting to his speech and mobility losses. He came to the attention of the OT staff after several falls. Nursing staff had identified several areas over his sacrum as high risk for the development of decubitus ulcers. Nursing staff hoped that the OT department might give him a cushion and lap tray to solve both these problems.

Instead the OT staffers placed Quentin in a shorter wheelchair with an easy-release, 45-degree seat belt and spent several sessions showing him how to transfer from his wheelchair. Quentin was able to move around the facility more easily and stop falling. A firm seat and cushion added to Quentin's comfort, and the skin over his sacrum regained its former integrity. He continued to visit the OT department, particularly when he smelled cookies baking.

Raul Estrada is a young man with a developmental disability who recently began working in the same metal-recycling facility as George O'Hara. Raul complained of back pain and refused to go to work. The OT practitioners consulting with Raul's caregivers decided to visit the job site to determine the root of his problem. They made a number of suggestions to modify the work site to reduce the employees' risk of injury. Raul was given some alternative job tasks and back-strengthening exercises while the job site was modified. Eventually, he took pride in the amount of metal he could move around the facility with ease.

Spiros Prasso is a construction worker who was injured on the job. His rehabilitation program included several weeks in the work-hardening clinic. Spiros spent time in general strength training and learned proper body mechanics to do his job safely. Spiros returned to work on modified duty but eventually resumed full-duty work on construction sites.

Tony Adams is a 7-year-old boy whose left scapular muscles were partially paralyzed after a stray bullet pierced the wall of his family's trailer. The bullet entered his back, piercing the C4 and C5 ventral rami. Tony had difficulty lifting anything with his left hand and tended to neglect using the left arm, causing overall atrophy. Tony's mother was more concerned about his nightmares, recent bad grades, and bad-behavior reports from school.

Tony's mother took a second job to try to earn enough money so that she and her son could move from the trailer park. As a result, Tony was left in the care of a 12-year-old cousin. OT staff tried to show Tony's mother and his cousin some games they could play to strengthen Tony's trapezius and other compensatory muscles, but little follow-up care took place at home. The OT staff contacted the OT practitioner who worked in Tony's school in an effort to maintain some continuity of care after his discharge from the clinic.

Vincent Pearson is a retired postal worker who recovered from Guillain-Barré syndrome with some residual loss of intrinsic hand muscles. He learned many compensatory movements and was fortunate to have a wife who took care of all the household chores. Vincent continued to read the newspaper and explore the Internet, two of his favorite activities.

Wendy Dabdoub packs fruit in a large mail-order company. Her job involves repetitive movements, and the winter holiday season means longer hours and incentives to increase the amount of boxes packed each day. Wendy started the new year with tingling and paresthesia in both hands. Friends urged Wendy to undergo surgery for her carpal tunnel syndrome and leave work on disability. Her employer urged her to give therapy a chance before jumping into surgery.

Wendy's fear of hospitals gave her the extra motivation to try therapy. She learned about the causes of carpal tunnel syndrome and found that rest and antiinflammatory medications helped ease her symptoms. OT practitioners performed a job-site analysis and gave the mail-order company an inservice on the prevention of carpal tunnel syndrome. Wendy's employer instituted warm-up and stretch breaks as part of each employee's work day. Wendy returned to work symptom-free without surgery. The company achieved a 25% reduction in disability costs related to carpal tunnel syndrome in those departments using regular stretch breaks.

Xavier Morales had both legs amputated above the knee during a tour of duty in Vietnam. He was fitted with prostheses and was able to learn to walk using a cane. However, Xavier preferred his wheelchair for mobility and became active in local wheelchair athletics. Xavier continued to use his prostheses when making sales presentations for his auto parts company. Over the years, Xavier developed quite a wheelchair collection—one for work, one for basketball, and a third for tennis. Xavier was recognized for his community work with the Paralympics and for his counseling of Vietnam veterans. His collection of spare chairs and parts helped other men and women with disabilities get started in the wheelchair sports that he says "saved his life."

Yasmeen Harris is a 10-year-old girl who severed her right median nerve when she crashed through a glass storm door while playing tag with the neighborhood children. The nerve healed well, but she had residual paralysis for about 4 months while the nerve regenerated. During that time, she used a thumb spica splint decorated with flower decals to give her a functional hand grip.

Zachary Larson is a 12-year-old boy who crushed his right ulnar nerve when he fractured his elbow while skateboarding. The surgeon had to cut damaged tissue and stretch the nerve to reattach it. Zachary had a lot of discomfort and resented having to wear the bivalve splint for almost a year after his injury. He developed passably legible handwriting with his left hand and learned to hit a baseball using his left hand only. After his recovery, Zachary became an asset as a switch hitter for his high school baseball team.

Overview of Muscle Anatomy

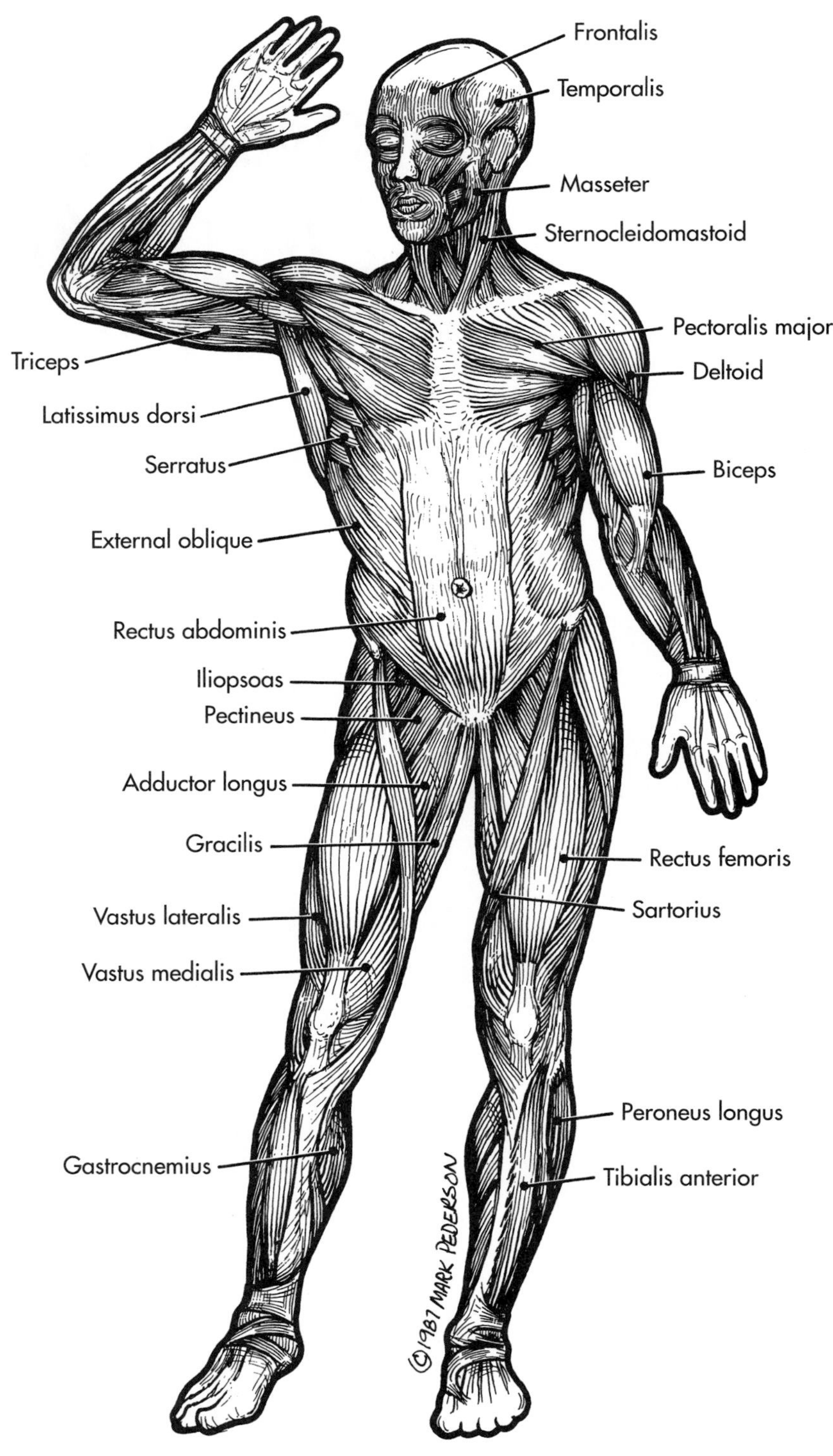
Frontalis
Temporalis
Masseter
Sternocleidomastoid
Pectoralis major
Triceps
Deltoid
Latissimus dorsi
Serratus
Biceps
External oblique
Rectus abdominis
Iliopsoas
Pectineus
Adductor longus
Gracilis
Rectus femoris
Sartorius
Vastus lateralis
Vastus medialis
Peroneus longus
Tibialis anterior
Gastrocnemius
©1987 MARK PEDERSON

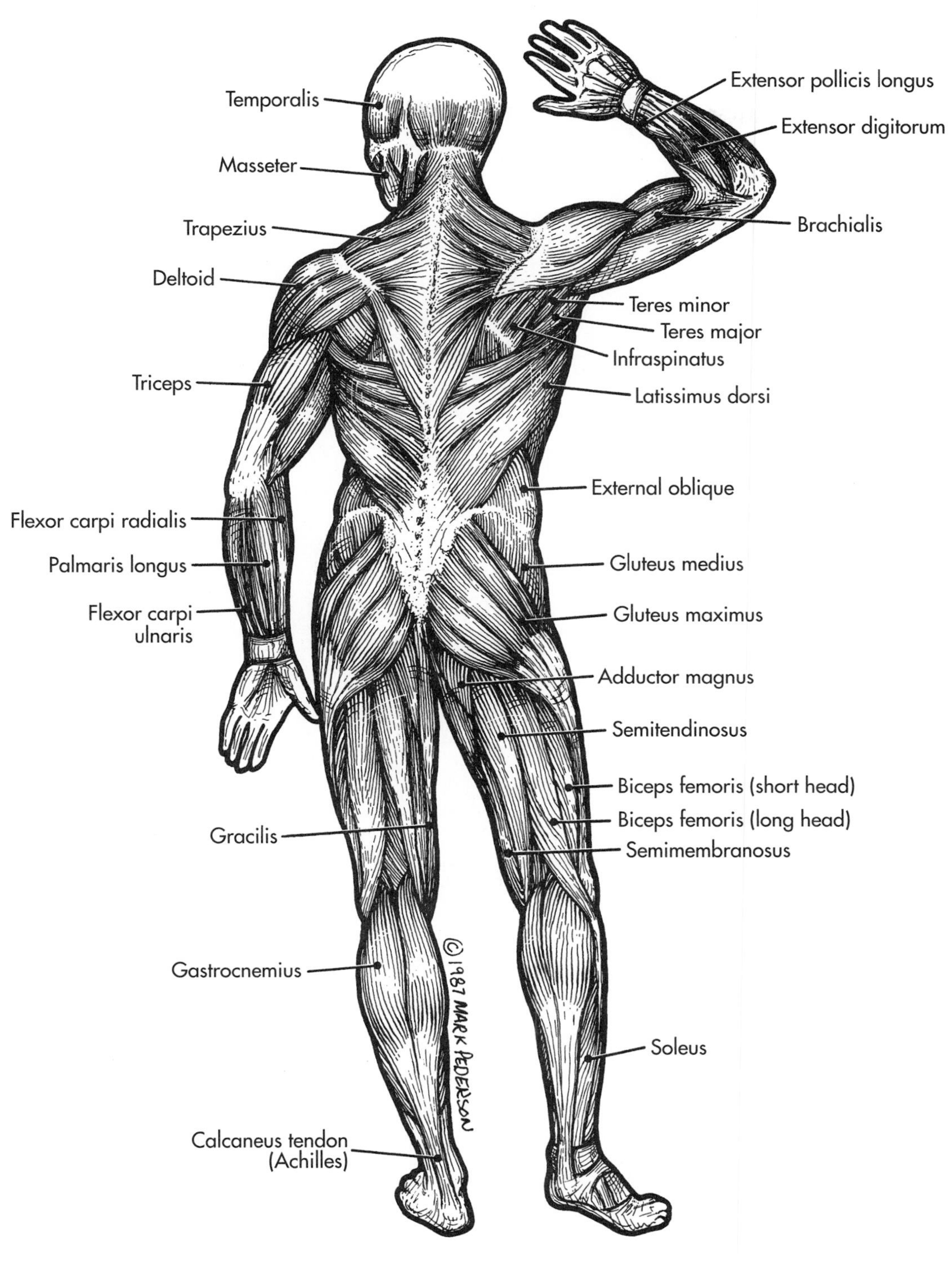
Temporalis
Masseter
Trapezius
Deltoid
Triceps
Flexor carpi radialis
Palmaris longus
Flexor carpi ulnaris
Gracilis
Gastrocnemius
Calcaneus tendon (Achilles)
Extensor pollicis longus
Extensor digitorum
Brachialis
Teres minor
Teres major
Infraspinatus
Latissimus dorsi
External oblique
Gluteus medius
Gluteus maximus
Adductor magnus
Semitendinosus
Biceps femoris (short head)
Biceps femoris (long head)
Semimembranosus
Soleus
©1987 MARK PEDERSON

Working Models of the Fingers and Wrist

B*iomechanical models can be valuable tools* for teachers and students. They present opportunities for hands-on manipulation. Creating those models provides teachers and students alternative ways to learn. The two models in this appendix have been used in class laboratory settings and hospital teaching programs.

Please keep the following points in mind as you create these models:

- The models are designed to demonstrate mechanical principles and are not intended to be anatomically accurate. For example, the finger model includes metacarpophalangeal (MCP) and interphalangeal (IP) joints. In the model, all three joints appear as simple hinge joints to demonstrate movement in one plane only.
- Follow the plans but avoid becoming consumed with measurements. Cut the bony segments generally proportional to the anatomical structures they represent. (For example, the metacarpal bone is longer than the proximal phalanx, which is slightly longer than the middle phalanx, and so on.)
- Be prepared to revise the model. Models often do not "work" the first time. Problem solving around these design details is valuable. For example, place the eyelet pulleys in the approximate positions shown in the diagram at the end of the appendix. After working with the finger model, you may need to move one or two of these eyelets to adjust the relationship of the force (string) with respect to the joint axis.

Please keep the following few items in mind as you use the completed model:

- Orient yourself with the anatomical aspects of the model. For example, the finger model includes the following structures, all of which should be identified before you try to operate the model:
  - Metacarpal shaft and MCP joint
  - Proximal, middle, and distal phalanges and proximal and distal interphalangeal joints
  - Flexor digitorum profundus, extensor digitorum communis, and lumbrical
- As part of your orientation, pull one tendon (string) at a time. Identify what it represents by function and position. For example, if you pull on a string and it flexes the finger, identify this string as the flexor digitorum profundus according to (1) its function in flexing *all* the finger joints, (2) its insertion on the distal phalanx, and (3) its anterior relationship to the side-to-side axes of the MCP and IP joints.
- The model is intended to demonstrate biomechanics; anatomical details have been simplified.

Finger Model

The finger model is a single finger unit including the metacarpal and phalanges. The metacarpal shaft is anchored to the mounting board, and the proximal, middle, and distal phalanges are free to flex and extend. The model is constructed to allow movement (flexion and extension) in one plane only—the plane of the mounting board.

SUPPLIES

You need the following tools and equipment to build the finger model:

1. 12 to 15 small (½-inch) screws to attach the leather hinges to the metacarpal and phalanges
2. 8 to 10 small eyelet screws to serve as pulleys for tendons
3. 3 ½-inch × ½-inch squares of leather for hinges (heavier than suede, about 1⁄16-inch to ⅛-inch thick)
4. 24 inches of soft but strong flexible nylon cord to make tendons
5. Small scrap of ⅛-inch or thinner thermoplastic material
6. A ½-inch × ½-inch board for bony segments (3-, 2.5-, 2-, and 1-inch long pieces for the metacarpal, proximal, middle, and distal phalanges, respectively)
7. A 10-inch × 10-inch piece of ¼-inch-thick plywood for the mounting board
8. 2 screws (about ¾ inch long) to anchor the metacarpal bone onto the mounting board

CONSTRUCTION

Follow these directions, using the diagram of the finger model in this appendix as a guide:

Drill the proper-size holes for the ½-inch screws and attach the bony segments end to end (in order) using the leather hinges and ½-inch screws. Note that the closer together you attach the wood pieces, the less hyperextension of these segments is possible. If you want to show hyperextension (for example, at the MCP joint to demonstrate MCP hyperextension accompanying intrinsic minus hand), attach the leather hinge so that a ⅛-inch gap remains between the metacarpal and the proximal phalanx.

After "articulating" the segments, drill holes and place the eyelet pulleys according to the illustration. Next, attach the metacarpal bone to the mounting board as shown. Finally, attach the strings. (Use three different colors to demonstrate the different functions.) Tie strings to the most distal eyelet on the volar side and on the dorsal side, representing the flexor digitorum profundus and extensor digitorum, respectively. Pass each string through the eyelets as shown. Attach the lumbrical string as shown in the inset illustration.

Try it a few times. Remember, the lessons involved in fine-tuning of the model are as valuable as any. Students must remember that the best thing about models is that they seldom work correctly in the beginning. They demonstrate all the things that can go wrong, things we often take for granted in normal function.

USE OF THE FINGER MODEL

You can demonstrate a normal digital sweep into extension or flexion by pulling on the appropriate strings. Remember, only with the combination of the lumbrical and flexor digitorum profundus does normal flexion occur. You also may need some lumbrical pull at the end of extension depending on how the MCP joint is constructed.

Pathological processes

You also can demonstrate a number of pathological conditions with the finger model. A shallow digital sweep, as in the case of intrinsic paralysis, can be shown as follows:

1. Place an empty soda can directly in front of the metacarpal shaft so that it touches the shaft.
2. Pull on the flexor digitorum profundus only and notice the shallow sweep. The tip of the distal phalanx pushes the can from its position (what would be the palm) instead of flexing around the diameter of the can. (You may have to shift the can slightly proximally or distally to ensure the finger demonstrates the effect described.)
3. Extend the digit again and move the can back into place. This time, exert the initial pull on the lumbrical to begin the sweep with the MCP joint (instead of the more distal joints). As the finger begins flexing around the can, initiate a pull in the flexor digitorum profundus simultaneously with the lumbrical. As flexion continues, you must give the lumbrical some slack to allow the flexor digitorum profundus to flex the IP joints. The end result of this combined effort is to produce a deeper digital sweep around the can, allowing the finger to grasp the can.

You also can demonstrate joint contractures by placing sticky-back, hook-and-loop Velcro across any joint. Attach sticky-back hook Velcro to the bony segments (wood) on either side of the leather hinge. Bridge the gap with loop Velcro. Velcro on the flexor side simulates a flexion contracture and limits joint extension. Notice that the joint is limited in active and passive extension, but you can still actively flex the joint.

Using the model, you also can differentiate joint contraction from tendon adhesion. Set another finger model up with sticky-back hook Velcro wrapped around the flexor tendon in front of the metacarpal shaft. Place sticky-back loop Velcro along the front side of the metacarpal shaft in a place where the flexor tendon can be attached via the Velcro. Partially flex the finger using the flexor digitorum profundus. While holding it flexed, push the tendon against the metacarpal shaft to "form"

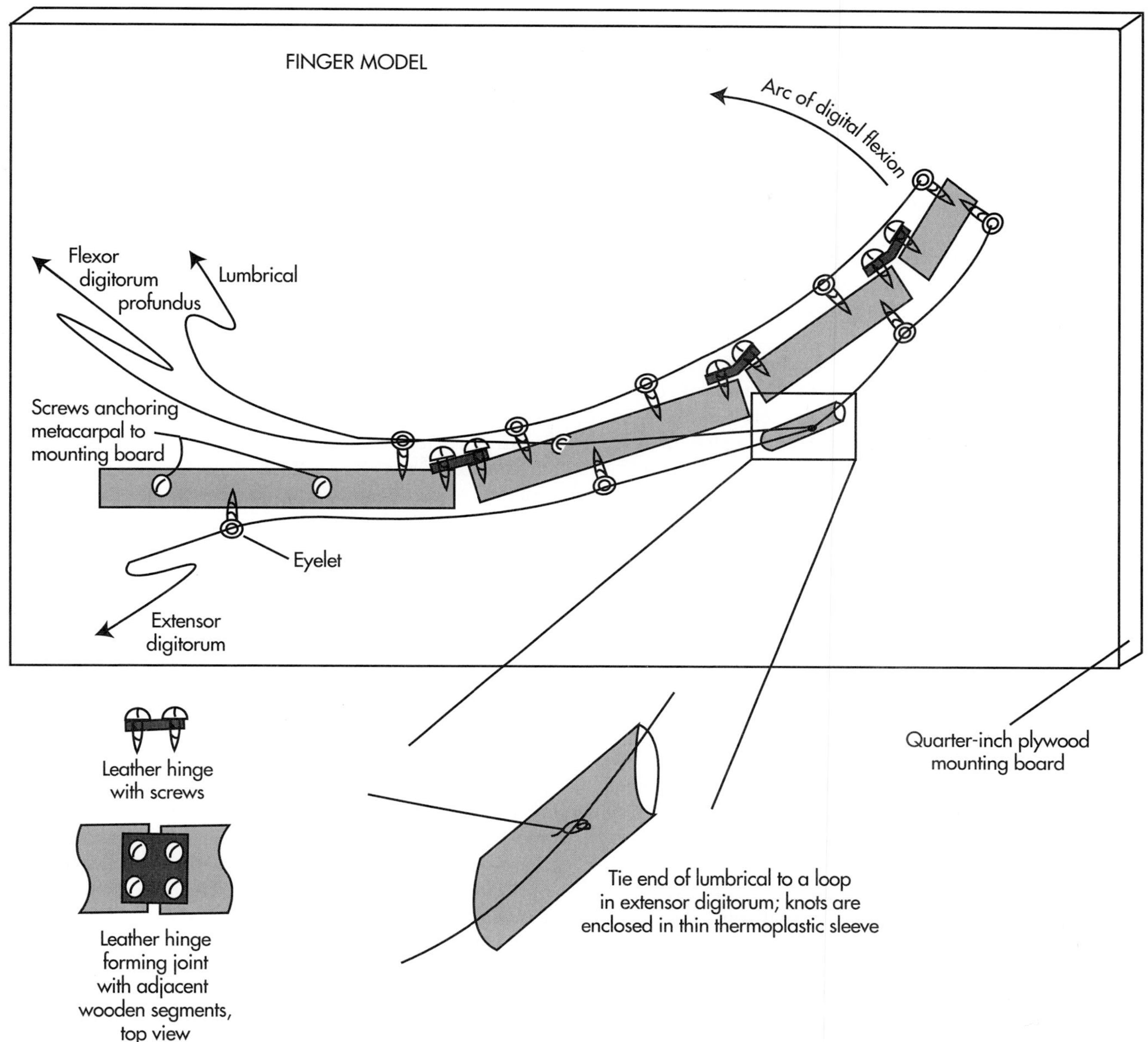

the adhesion. Notice that simultaneous extension of the MCP and IP joints is limited. Passively flexing any joint distal to the adhesion creates slack in the flexor tendon, allowing previously limited joints to be passively extended. Notice also that adhesion prevents active flexion.

Remember that tendon adhesion, unlike joint contracture, demonstrates (1) lack of active motion in the same direction as the tendon adhesion (for example, flexion movement for a flexor tendon adhesion) and (2) limited simultaneous passive motion in the opposite direction of the adhesion in joints distal to the adhesion (for example, extension movement for a flexor tendon adhesion). Joint contracture exhibits limited passive motion in the opposite direction (for example, MCP extension limited by MCP flexion contracture) but no limitation in active motion in the same direction (for example, active MCP flexion with MCP flexion contracture).

Wrist and Finger Model

The wrist and finger model is a model with a wrist, a single working finger similar to the finger model, and a stable thumb post onto which the finger can pinch. Like the finger model, all movements are limited to one plane. The one forearm bone represented is anchored to the mounting board, and the wrist and proximal, middle, and distal phalanges are free to flex and extend.

SUPPLIES

You need all the supplies previously listed for the finger model (minus the lumbrical parts) and the following additional supplies to construct the wrist and finger model:

1. 8 small (½-inch) screws to attach the leather hinges at the wrist
2. 2 to 4 small eyelet screws to serve as pulleys for tendons
3. 2 ½-inch × ½-inch squares of leather for wrist hinges
4. 24 inches of soft but strong flexible nylon cord to use as wrist flexor and extensor tendons
5. A ½-inch × ½-inch board 8 inches long for the forearm bone
6. A ½-inch × ½-inch board 1 inch long for the carpal bone of the wrist
7. A 10-inch × 20-inch piece of ¼-inch plywood for the mounting board
8. 2 screws (about ¾ inch long) to anchor the forearm bone onto the mounting board

CONSTRUCTION

Follow these directions, using the diagram of the wrist and finger model in this appendix as a guide:

Drill the proper-size holes for the ½-inch screws and attach the bony segments end to end (in order) using the leather hinges and ½-inch screws. Note that the closer together you attach the wood pieces, the less hyperextension of these segments is possible. If you want to show hyperextension (for example, at the MCP joint to demonstrate MCP hyperextension accompanying intrinsic minus hand), attach the leather hinge so that a ⅛-inch gap exists between the bony segments. For the wrist, follow the illustration and place one hinge dorsally and the other volarly. This allows the wrist to both flex and extend.

After "articulating" the segments, drill holes and place the eyelet pulleys according to the illustration. Next, attach the forearm bone to the mounting board as shown. Finally, attach the strings. (Use four different colors to demonstrate the different functions.) Tie strings to the most distal eyelet on the volar side and the dorsal side, representing the flexor digitorum profundus and extensor digitorum, respectively. Tie strings to the eyelets on the volar side and the dorsal side of the metacarpal, representing the wrist flexor and extensor. Pass each string through the eyelets as shown.

Try it a few times. Again, anticipate some fine-tuning. The lessons involved here are valuable, just like those of the finger model.

USE OF THE WRIST AND FINGER MODEL

You can demonstrate normal wrist extension and flexion by pulling on the appropriate strings. You also can differentiate wrist and finger muscle functions. Most important, you can demonstrate the need for wrist extensors to stabilize the wrist when the long finger flexors such as the flexor digitorum profundus contract to perform grasp. Pulling the flexor digitorum profundus without the wrist extensor results in simultaneous wrist and finger flexion, which creates active insufficiency of the finger flexors and failed grip. This occurs in radial nerve damage.

Active insufficiency is demonstrated on this model. Measure the excursion necessary for the flexor digitorum profundus to flex the three finger joints from full extension to full flexion. (You must hold the wrist in a neutral position manually to prevent the finger flexor from flexing the wrist.) Record this number as the excursion of the finger flexor. Return all the finger joints into extension, and while stabilizing the fingers in extension with one hand, pull the wrist into flexion via the flexor digitorum profundus. Measure the excursion required for the finger flexor tendon to flex the wrist only. Now free the finger and continue pulling on the flexor tendon only through the distance of the remaining excursion. After exhausting the excursion of the flexor digitorum profundus, you should see the wrist in flexion and the fingers partially flexed. No firm grip or pinch to the thumb post is possible unless the flexor tendon is pulled through more excursion.

The model also can demonstrate passive insufficiency. Passively extend the finger of the model, holding the wrist in a neutral position. Hold the finger fully extended and pull the slack from the flexor digitorum profundus. Place a marker or tie a knot in the flexor tendon to prevent it from passing through the most proximal pulley, which would simulate that this muscle has been stretched to its maximum length. Now attempt passive simultaneous finger and wrist extension and notice how the tightness in the flexor tendon prevents full simultaneous finger and wrist extension.

Tenodesis grasp is probably the most important demonstration this model provides. Passively place the wrist and fingers in partial flexion. Take up the slack in the flexor digitorum profundus and hold the flexor down on the mounting board to prevent it from being pulled distally. Pull the wrist extensor while holding down the flexor tendon and watch the wrist extend and the finger flex. (The finger flexes without pulling the flexor tendon proximally.) Holding down the flexor simulates a shortened finger flexor from either lack of stretch or tenodesis surgery. If you attempt wrist extension without holding the flexor onto the board, wrist extension occurs with very little finger flexion.

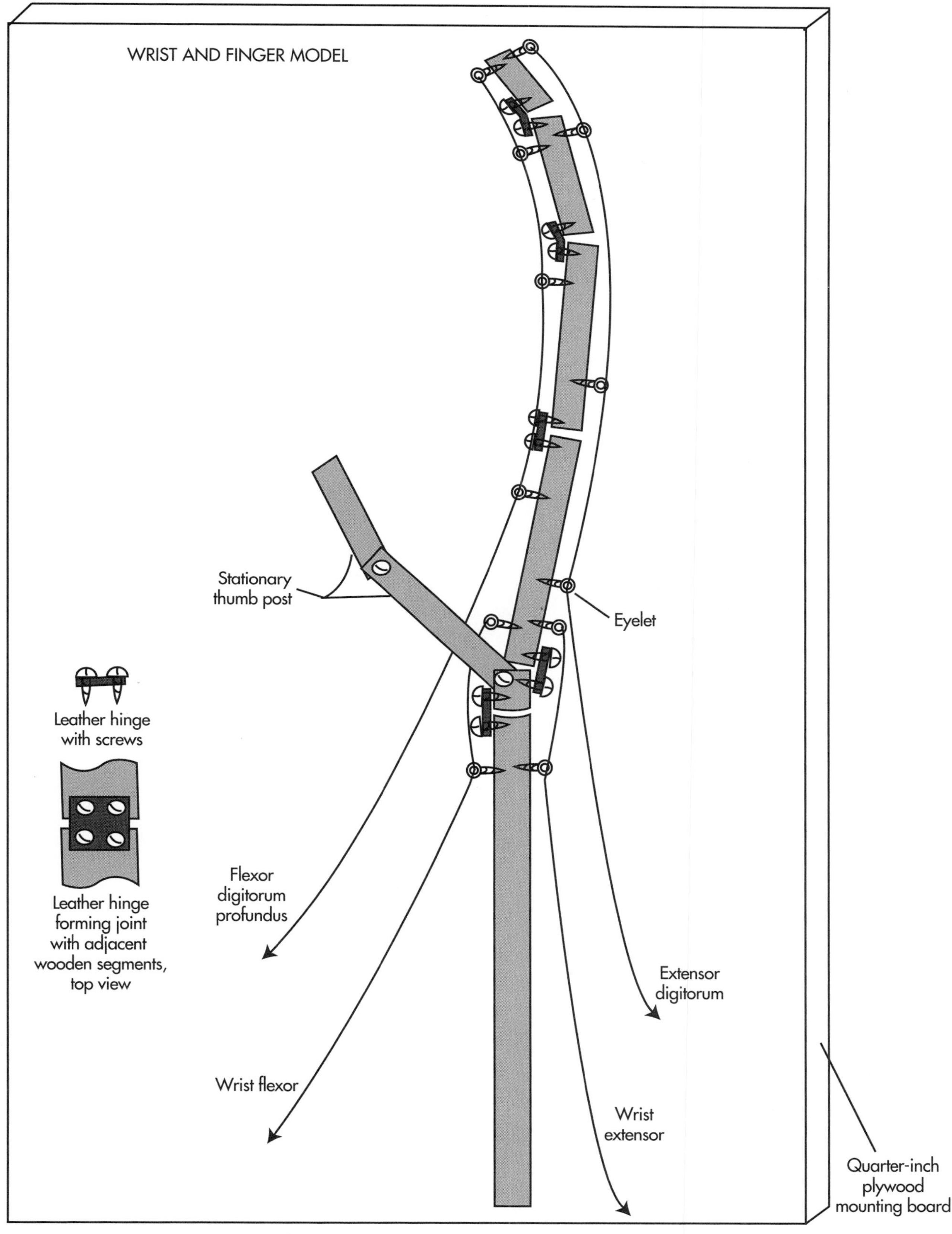
WRIST AND FINGER MODEL
Stationary thumb post
Eyelet
Leather hinge with screws
Leather hinge forming joint with adjacent wooden segments, top view
Flexor digitorum profundus
Extensor digitorum
Wrist flexor
Wrist extensor
Quarter-inch plywood mounting board

Learning Objectives

Many ***students rely on old test questions*** to study for exams. (In some medical and graduate programs, students become collectors and actually make deals about these tests. You hear statements like, "I have the 1967 edition, but I'm missing the last page. Would you trade my compete 1985 Exam II for the last page of the 1967?") Although we do not advocate studying from available exam questions to the exclusion of studying the original text material and course lecture notes, asking and answering one another's questions can be a helpful study tool.

The learning objectives in this appendix serve as study guides for each chapter in the book. In many cases, instructors develop multiple-choice test questions directly reflecting the content emphasized in a course's learning objectives. More directly, students can change each objective into a question when they study for essay or short-answer exam formats.

Chapter 1

- Define *kinesiology* and identify the three physical sciences that contribute to it.
- Describe why kinesiology is considered a narrow approach to movement.
- Identify the basic belief on which OT practice is based.
- Identify the factors influencing individual performance that become clear when movement is viewed within the context of activity.
- Briefly describe and differentiate the mechanistic and transformative philosophies.
- Briefly describe and differentiate the reconstructive, orthopedic, and kinetic models of practice.
- Describe the value of the rehabilitation model as a guide to kinesiologic thinking.

Chapter 2

- Describe the major skeletal movements in terms of planes (surfaces on which the movements occur) and axes (around which the movements are centered).
- Demonstrate the three types of muscle contraction and describe how the two muscle attachments move in each.
- Define *excursion* and describe its effect on muscle length.
- Differentiate the agonist, antagonist, and synergist in a description of muscle action.
- Demonstrate correct use of the terms used to communicate various muscle grades (words and numbers).
- Describe the use of a goniometer to measure joint range of motion and differentiate active and passive joint ranges of motion.
- Provide one-line definitions of the various italicized terms under the section titled "Medical Diagnoses Affecting Movement."
- Differentiate scalar and vector quantities in terms of their measurements.
- Differentiate mass and weight and identify which of the two also is described as force.
- Describe normal force and compare it with shear force.

Chapter 3

- Describe one way in which gravity influences motor development.
- Demonstrate how the center of gravity is approximated.
- Perform the brief calculations and measurements necessary in the identification of an object's center of gravity.

- Determine the center of gravity of the entire body based on the segmental centers of gravity.
- Convert an object's mass (in kilograms) to its weight (in newtons), illustrating how mass is converted to force through the multiplication of mass by the constant for the acceleration of gravity.

Chapter 4

- Provide examples of each of Newton's three laws.
- Describe the conditions of force equilibrium when an individual is seated (at rest) in a chair.
- Demonstrate the three types of muscle contraction and describe the movements of the two muscle attachments in each.
- Describe the effect of excursion on muscle strength in a concentric contraction.
- Describe what is meant by the excursion requirements of movement at a joint.
- Describe what happens to a muscle when its antagonistic motion occurs.
- Describe the change in distance between the origin and insertion of a muscle in a concentric contraction and how this differs from that in an eccentric contraction.
- Describe what happens to the origin and insertion of a flexor muscle when the joint is pulled into extension by an outside force.
- Identify and briefly describe an example of each type of external force described in the chapter.
- Define and differentiate *force magnitude, force orientation,* and *internal (muscular) force direction.*
- Differentiate the determinants of muscle force and excursion.
- Explain how forces are combined through addition and subtraction to determine the resultant force in a tug-of-war game.
- Explain both the parallelogram and polygon methods for the combination of multiple forces when two individuals push a cart.

Chapter 5

- Differentiate rotary and linear motion based on (1) the velocity of points in a bar moving in a line versus in a circle and (2) the orientation of the bar.
- Describe the difference in the effect of the amount of force used in linear versus rotary motion.
- Provide a synonym for the term *torque.*
- Identify factors used in the determination of linear and rotary equilibrium.
- Identify the angle of pull at which all the muscle's force is used for the rotary movement of the joint.
- Identify the angle of pull at which the moment arm is the longest.
- Identify at which moment arm the movement is strongest.
- Provide everyday examples of each lever system.
- Explain why most musculoskeletal levers are class III levers.
- Explain how changing the force's angle of pull and the muscle length affect the tendency of the force to rotate the lever at the joint.
- Identify the lever and axis of various musculoskeletal segments.

Chapter 6

- Differentiate between open- and closed-chain hip movements.
- Describe the relationship between lumbar curve and hamstring length.
- Describe the three basic pairs of movements and the nature of vertebral column movement.
- Describe the normal and pathological curves of the vertebral column.
- Explain the effects of unilateral and bilateral contractions of vertebral muscles.
- Explain how movements differ in direction and plane according to the relationship of the force to the axis.
- Describe movements and muscle functions in the trunk that relate to and accompany upper-extremity movements.
- Describe how the trunk remains balanced against the downward pull of gravity.
- Describe the relationship between head and neck position and the force the position exerts on the cervical intervertebral disks.
- Explain the relationship between rotary force (extension) and compression force during activation of the back extensors.
- Explain the role of pelvic stabilization in seating.
- Describe the basic biomechanics of one common restraint system.

Chapter 7

- Describe the joints of the shoulder complex and the elbow in terms of their classifications and degrees of freedom, including the plane and axis associated with each degree of joint freedom.

- Differentiate scapular from glenohumeral movement.
- State the major movements and movers of the shoulder complex.
- Describe how arrows are used to demonstrate the analysis of muscle forces affecting the shoulder and elbow.
- Describe the scapular movement and stabilization that accompany glenohumeral movement.
- Describe the separate contributions of scapular rotation and glenohumeral abduction to shoulder abduction when an individual raises the hand above the head.
- Explain the main effect of the deltoid compared with that of the supraspinatus in early glenohumeral abduction.
- Explain the biomechanical basis for shoulder subluxation.
- List the various roles of the rotator cuff muscles.
- Describe how manual muscle testing is an example of an isometric torque curve.
- Describe how manual muscle testing is an example of equilibrium of torques.
- Describe how the biceps long head can "become" an abductor of the glenohumeral joint.
- List the combination of joints necessary for flexion and extension and pronation and supination of the forearm.
- Describe how the use of the biceps in elbow flexion can depend on the forearm's position.
- Explain the role of the biceps in supination.
- Describe the contribution of the wrist joint to forearm pronation and supination range of motion.

Chapter 8

- Describe the differential effects of the major wrist flexors in terms of their functions of wrist flexion with deviation and wrist extension with deviation.
- Identify the strongest function, based on moment arm, of each wrist flexor and extensor.
- Describe how synergistic actions of wrist flexors and extensors yield balanced wrist ulnar and radial deviation.
- Describe the various imbalances at the wrist resulting from radial, ulnar, and median nerve damage at the level of the elbow.
- Explain the basic functions of the extrinsic and intrinsic musculature of the hand.
- Describe the balancing effect of the intrinsics on the long digital extensors.
- List in sequence the intrinsic and extrinsic muscles involved in opening and closing of the hand.
- Describe the effects of ulnar and median nerve damage in opening and closing of the hand.
- Describe the various prehension patterns of the thumb.
- Describe the effects of median and ulnar nerve damage on prehension.
- Identify which grasps require the thumb (and in what capacity) and which do not.
- Describe the differential functions of the thumb carpometacarpal, metacarpophalangeal, and interphalangeal joints.
- Describe the differential uses of the thenar and intrinsic thumb adductor muscles in wide versus narrow grip-span grasps that use the thumb.
- Describe the pathokinesiology of ulnar drift, boutonniere, bowstringing, wrist drop with grip failure, and intrinsic minus hand.
- Differentiate between joint contracture and tendon adhesion, using differential movements of adjacent joints to create slack.
- Explain the basis of tenodesis grip (tendon action) and explain tenodesis using the concept of passive insufficiency.

Chapter 9

- List and describe the four factors in stability and identify the missing stability factor in an unstable situation.
- Describe the stability problem of an individual with recent bilateral lower-extremity amputations as the individual attempts to move a wheelchair.
- Identify the stability risks associated with recliner wheelchairs.
- Demonstrate a safe wheelchair-to-bed standing pivot transfer, identifying both the original and the new bases of support.
- Describe lower-extremity movements in the sagittal and frontal planes during normal gait.
- Describe the muscle activity responsible for the movements in the sagittal and frontal planes during normal gait.
- Describe two compensations that an individual with weak hip abductors can use during unilateral stance.

Laboratory Activities

The laboratory activities described in this appendix can be valuable learning experiences. These activities should serve as guides to laboratory learning sessions if the course for which this book is used includes a laboratory component. However, we also encourage students who do not have laboratory sessions with their classes to work through these activities in small groups to further their applied understanding of the concepts presented in each chapter.

Chapter 1

- Interview faculty members to determine the philosophy of the department and the models on which the departmental curriculum is based.

Chapter 2

- Identify various forces at work around the room. Identify three different forces by considering the following common activities:

1. The resistance encountered when you move objects by sliding them along the floor
2. The force involved when you pull up the window shades
3. The force that makes you tired at the end of the day

Chapter 3

- Identify various movements of the human musculoskeletal system and the positions this system holds that are caused by the force of gravity:
    - In the upright (standing) position, begin with a flexed shoulder, elbow, and wrist and hold the position. Next, relax one joint at a time, starting proximally and ending with the wrist. List each motion and position caused by gravity in the standing position. What movement does gravity cause at each joint in this standing position? Which joint positions are held by gravity?
    - In the supine position on a mat, leave the shoulder extended and flex the elbow slightly past 90 degrees. Next, allow the elbow to move by relaxing all muscle contractions. What is gravity's effect?

Chapter 4

- As in the activities in Chapter 2, identify various forces at work around the room. Consider a typical window shade with a drawstring in terms of equilibrium of forces. When the shade is pulled up and stays up, is this equilibrium? If so, how is it established? What are the forces involved?
- Compare the excursion of a long spring with a short one. Also compare the force of recoil of one bungee cord with the force of four identical bungee cords pulled simultaneously. Draw parallels to relationships between normal muscle excursion and force capability.

- Identify examples of force equilibrium around the room (for example, sitting in a chair or on a mat).
- Working with a partner, hook a bungee cord to the doorknob of a closed door and stretch the cord by backing from the door one or two steps. Instruct someone to turn the knob to allow the door to swing open. The same person should hold onto the door to allow it to swing only as far as the bungee shortens. Measure the distance the door travels when the bungee recoils and the distance through which the bungee contracts. Repeat this action but stand farther from the door the next time. What is the name of the distance through which the bungee contracts? What does the movement of the door represent?

Chapter 5

- In small groups discuss why each of the following statements actually says the same thing about the strongest movement of the musculoskeletal segment:
  - Elbow flexion is strongest when the joint is flexed to 90 degrees because the flexors pull from their best angles and the muscle length is good.
  - The torque produced by the elbow flexors is greatest at 90 degrees of flexion because the moment arm is at its longest length and the actin and myosin overlap is ideal for force production by the muscle fibers.
  - The torque produced by the elbow flexors is greatest at 90 degrees of flexion because the force of flexion is farthest from the axis (has the greatest perpendicular distance) and the actin and myosin overlap is optimal for force production.
- Working in pairs, use a dynamometer to generate your own isometric torque curve. Set it on the second grip-span setting and attempt three grip efforts, measuring grip strength at 40 degrees of wrist extension, neutral position, and full wrist flexion. For each effort, plot the force of grasp on one axis and the wrist position on the other, using an illustration similar to the graph below.

  Discuss the following points related to the graph:

  - What happens to the strength of the grasp as the wrist position changes?
  - Identify the specific effect on the finger flexors when the grip begins from different wrist positions.

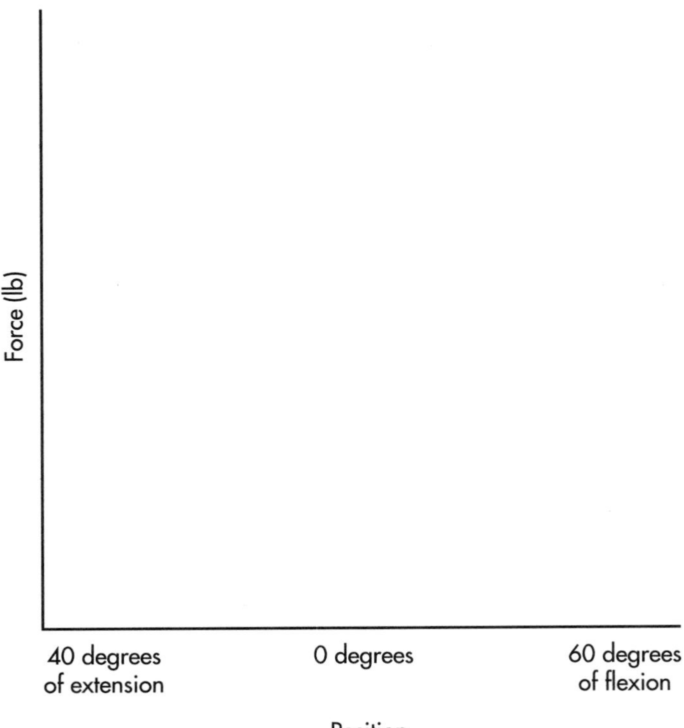

Chapter 6

- Draw the muscle masses (not individual portions) of the three erector spinae groups and the transversospinalis group onto a template of the trunk skeleton (see Figure 6-7), indicating the general direction of the fibers.
- Study your own upper extremity while performing (1) elbow and shoulder flexion to bring food to your mouth (self-feeding pattern) and (2) movement in which your hands rest on the front edge of the water fountain and you lower your head and upper trunk to take a drink:
  - Identify the joints and segments that make up the chain.
  - Describe the upper-extremity movement you observe, specifically the movement of the end of the chain. Is this movement linear or rotary?
  - Is the movement an example of open- or closed-chain movement?
- Using a skeleton of the trunk with the rod removed so that the curves are flexible, answer the following questions:
  - Identify the three normal curves. Describe each curve's location (superior to inferior) and type of convexity (anterior versus posterior).
  - Manipulate the pelvis to demonstrate the flattening of the lumbar curve. Which way must the pelvis be tilted to flatten this curve?
  - With one person loosely stabilizing the trunk in an upright position, carefully pull on four cords attached to the trunk. Attach three cords posteriorly to the vertebral column to simulate the extensor and the left and right lateral flexor muscle groups of the trunk. Also attach a cord anteriorly to the lower sternum to simulate the trunk flexors. Remember that these muscles originate largely from the pelvis. As you pull on the cords to balance or move the column, pull from the origin. Notice the large moment arm for the flexors and the short moment arm for the extensors and lateral flexors.
- Use your own bodies and observe movements in a partner. For each reach, identify (1) elbow and shoulder movements and positions held during the reach, (2) scapular movement and position held during the reach, and (3) trunk movement and position held during the reach:
  - Reach forward as far as possible with both arms, putting all your effort into the movement. In other words, reach with more than arm's length.
  - Reach directly to the left or right (again, in an extreme reach).
  - Reach as far as possible with the right arm for an object located in front of and to the left of the left shoulder.

Chapter 7

- To track scapular movement, observe various motions in a partner. Have your partner reach forward as far as possible with one arm, pushing the hand in front of the chest:
  - Identify the scapular motion, using proper terminology.
  - Return your partner to a resting position (seated upright). Palpate your partner's scapular spine, acromion, vertebral scapular border, and inferior scapular angle.
  - Instruct your partner to move again as before and palpate the movement of the scapula, paying close attention to the movement of the vertebral border from the vertebral column. How many centimeters would you estimate the scapula moved?
  - Instruct your partner to return to a resting position and to move through complete abduction, bringing the hand high into the air above the head. Palpate scapular movement, paying close attention to the inferior angle. How many centimeters did it move? What would you call this scapular motion? (What other terms have you heard used to describe this motion?)
- Using the goniometer, measure shoulder abduction to the midposition (halfway between full adduction and full abduction with the hand above the head). How many degrees of range of motion is this? What combination of movements are you actually measuring? Write instructions (as they would appear in a goniometry manual) for an OT practitioner who wants to measure humeral movement at the glenohumeral joint.
- Palpating muscular activity: To palpate muscle activity is to touch and examine with the hands (to "see" with the hands). Without experience, individuals lack the sensitivity to feel and discriminate between different "feels." Keep the following in mind as you develop skills in this area:
  - Always have the individual who is to be palpated relax.
  - Gently place your hands on the skin that lies over the structure you are trying to palpate.
  - Move your hands in a circular motion, in a sense "looking" for the structure of interest.

Now use the following tips as you work with a partner:

- For palpation of a muscle or tendon, have your partner move very slightly in a direction you know requires the use of the muscle. Actual movement is not necessary because the thought and intention to move causes a palpable muscle contraction.
- Immediately after the command to move, have your partner relax again. This change—from relaxation to contraction to relaxation—facilitates palpation. In other words, feeling one structure among many others is difficult until movement (contraction of the muscle fibers) defines the structure. Remember that our nervous systems function by differentiating—noticing change. Being aware of a constant stimulus is much more difficult.
- Now palpate the (1) middle deltoid during attempts to abduct the humerus at the glenohumeral joint, (2) the lower pectoralis major during attempts to adduct the humerus at the glenohumeral joint, (3) the upper pectoralis major during attempts to flex the humerus at the glenohumeral joint near 90 degrees of shoulder flexion, and (4) the anterior deltoid during attempts to flex the humerus at the glenohumeral joint.
- Draw the fibers of the middle deltoid, upper and lower trapezius, and serratus anterior as they abduct the humerus at the shoulder and hold it at 90 degrees of abduction. Draw arrows (vectors), beginning at the insertion and directing the arrow parallel to the fibers toward the origin. Remember, the arrowhead indicates direction. In this case, each force pulls its insertion toward its origin, but the deltoid fibers curve around the acromion. For the deltoid the arrow should start with the fibers from the insertion and continue straight past the point at which the fibers turn. The length of each arrow indicates the strength of contraction.

Chapter 8

- Measure metacarpophalangeal (MCP) hyperextension with traditional goniometry. Normal MCP hyperextension has the feel of a "stiff joint" even though it is normal. Work in a group of at least four and measure one person using a goniometer:
  - Measure the extent of hyperextension of the index finger's MCP joint. Each of the three measurers must keep their measurements a secret from the other members of the group.
  - Compare the three measurements, which most likely are different. What accounts for these differences? Ask the individual measured whether that individual noticed any difference in the manner in which each measurer performed.

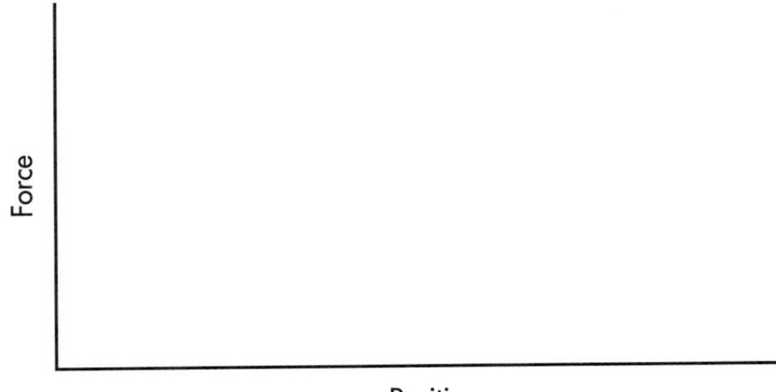

- For torque range of motion, work with a group of three students to measure MCP hyperextension. While one student uses a goniometer and a force gauge to perform the measurement on a second student, the third student charts the amount of force necessary to hyperextend the MCP to 5 and 10 degrees of hyperextension and to the end of its range if that range is beyond 10 degrees. The student should chart measurements on a graph similar to the one pictured above.
- Look around the classroom and find objects that require various grasp patterns—cylindrical, spherical, palmar, lateral, hook, power, scissor (thumb adduction), and tip prehension. Use a *T* to indicate which grasps require thumb use and indicate with a *T - O* which require thumb opposition.
- Discuss explanations for the following examples of function after nerve damage. Base your reasoning on a system of thought in which muscles are classified as either "working" or "not working":
  - Radial nerve damage at elbow, attempted radial deviation:
    Working: Flexor carpi radialis
    Not working: Extensor carpi radialis longus and brevis
    Result: Limited radial deviation with flexion because radial deviation is difficult to perform when the wrist flexes, which occurs when the flexor carpi radialis contracts
  - Radial nerve damage at elbow, attempted wrist flexion:
    Working: Flexor carpi radialis, flexor carpi ulnaris
    Not working: All extensors
    Result: Pure wrist flexion
  - Radial nerve damage above supinator, attempted slow supination without elbow flexion (that is,

attempted slow supination without intentional elbow flexion):
Working: Biceps as a supinator
Not working: Supinator, brachioradialis
Result: Forearm supination followed by elbow flexion because biceps is being used to supinate

- Ulnar nerve damage above elbow, attempted ulnar deviation:
Working: Extensor carpi ulnaris
Not working: Flexor carpi ulnaris
Result: Ulnar deviation with extension because the action of the extensor carpi ulnaris (which extends and ulnarly deviates) is unbalanced
- Median and ulnar nerves damaged at the wrist, attempted full digital extension:
Working: Extensor digitorum, which extends MCP and interphalangeal (IP) joints of digits
Not working: All lumbricals, all interossei
Result: "Clawing" of the digits (MCP hyperextension, slight IP flexion) because action of extensor digitorum is unbalanced without lumbricals or interossei to prevent MCP hyperextension at the end of the full extension sweep; slight IP flexion because interossei and lumbricals extend the IPs (or prevent slight flexion at the end of the sweep)
- Radial nerve damage above the level of the elbow, attempted digital extension:
Working: Interossei and lumbricals, wrist flexors (synergists for opening of the hand)
Not working: All extensors of the digits and wrist
Result: Hand in typical "wrist drop" position; IP extension possible through interossei and lumbricals but accompanied by MCP flexion; simultaneous IP and MCP extension impossible, preventing full hand opening; positioning of the hand to prepare to grasp an object also impossible without wrist extensors (wrist position normally extended to about 30 or 40 degrees when hand prepares to grasp)
- Median nerve at the elbow, attempted power grip:
Working: Interossei and lumbricals to digits 4 and 5, wrist extensors (as synergists), flexor digitorum profundus to digits 4 and 5, and adductor pollicis
Not working: Flexor digitorum superficialis, flexor digitorum profundus, and lumbricals to digits 2 and 3; abductor pollicis brevis, flexor pollicis brevis, and opponens pollicis (thenars)
Result: Weak grip using the ulnar side of the hand; digits 2 and 3 attempt to flex around object at MCPs; however, this action is via the interossei, so the IP is extended simultaneously; inability to bring the thumb around (oppose) to firmly lock the object into the palm (if the thumb *placed* passively, the adductors help hold the object into the palm)
- Median nerve at the wrist, attempted spherical or cylindrical grasp:
Working: Flexor digitorum superficialis to all digits, flexor digitorum profundus to all digits, all interossei, lumbricals to digits 4 and 5, flexor pollicis longus and adductor pollicis
Not working: Lumbricals to digits 2 and 3, all three thenar muscles
Result: No ability to position thumb in opposition (around the cylinder or ball); thumb in flat position on the plane of the palm; thumb adductor (adductor pollicis) able to adduct thumb against ball or cylinder if thumb is passively placed; slight tendency toward clawing of index and long fingers (digits 2 and 3) but interossei to these two digits preventing full claw; normal appearance in grasp of ulnar side of the hand (digits 4 and 5) but overall grip strength decreased because of failure of radial side of the hand (poorly balanced flexion of digits 2 and 3 accompanied by a lack of function of the thenar muscles)

Chapter 9

Please perform the following activities only if close supervision is available. You may want to wear bicycle helmets for the activities involving wheelchair stability. The publisher and authors do not endorse these activities unless they are performed under close supervision and exactly as described:

- Students should pair up and take turns with this activity. After securing a watchful partner, sit in a wheelchair; remove the legrests, footrests, and arm rests (if removable); and instruct your partner to stand behind you with hands on the handles (canes). Try the following exercises:
  - With your feet hanging toward the ground, push the wheels forward strongly enough that the front casters rise slightly off the ground. Make sure that your partner's hands remain on the handles and your partner is ready to catch you.
  - If you are unable to lift the front of the chair, instruct your partner to tilt you back slowly so that the front casters are in the air and try to balance the chair yourself. If you sense you are leaning too far backward, pull backward on the wheels (handrails) as if to back up. If you sense you are

falling forward (front casters moving toward the ground again), push the rear wheels (handrails) forward to put your chair "back in flight."

- After 5 minutes, switch roles.
- Identify the projection of the center of gravity of the seated individual when all four wheels are on the ground and when only the rear (large) wheels are on the ground.
- In terms of factors of stability, why is a wheelie so hard to achieve and maintain?

- Transfers: Students should pair up and use a wheelchair and a transfer belt to attempt both a sliding-board transfer and stand-pivot transfer. Describe each transfer in terms of base of support and center of gravity projection.
- Again, get in a wheelchair with your partner spotting you by holding onto the push handles:
  - Attempt a fast start by pushing hard on the rear-wheel rails.
  - Repeat the previous action but remove the footrests and fold your legs crossed in the seat so that they no longer hang down. Attempt a fast start (after ensuring that your partner is in place). What happens this second time with your legs folded?
- Wheel around in the chair and pull up to a spot. Stop without backing up first and lock the chair:
  - With your feet in the footrests and your partner in front of you, lean forward, bringing your chest to your knees as if to reach for something on the floor in front of you. What happens as you lean forward?
  - Wheel around again. This time stop and back up about 4 feet and put on the brakes. Lean forward as you did before, with your partner in place. What happens as you lean forward this time?
  - What accounts for the difference in the chair's stability as you lean forward? (HINT: Think about the front-to-back dimension of the base of support in each case.)
  - Based on this experience, what is the general rule for coming to a stop if you intend to lean forward?

Glossary

Abduction. Movement in a joint that brings the distal segment farther from the midline of the body

Acromioclavicular joint. A small synovial joint at which the clavicle articulates with the acromion process of the scapula

Active insufficiency. A condition in which shortened agonist muscles cannot move all possible joints through their full available ranges of motion

Adduction. Movement in a joint that brings the distal segment toward the midline of the body

Adductor brevis. One of the muscles in the hip adductor group that originates from the pubis and inserts along the linea aspera of the femur

Adductor group. Six muscles—the adductor magnus, adductor brevis, adductor longus, gracilis, obturator externus, and pectineus—that act primarily to adduct the thigh

Adductor longus. The most anterior muscle of the adductor group; originates from the pubis and inserts along the linea aspera of the femur

Adductor magnus. The largest of the adductor group of muscles; originates from the ischium and pubis and inserts linearly along the entire medial femur, with some fibers reaching to the tibial collateral ligament

Afferent nerves. Nerves that carry impulses from the body to the central nervous system

Agonist. A muscle that acts as the primary mover for a specific joint motion

Amphiarthrodial joint. A cartilaginous articulation between two or more adjacent bones that permits limited motion only

Antagonist. A muscle that opposes the agonist for a specific joint motion

Aponeurosis. Any fascial thickening where muscle fibers attach

Atlas. The first cervical vertebra

ATP. Adenosine triphosphate ($C_{10}H_{16}N_5O_{13}P_3$); stores large amounts of energy for various biochemical processes, including muscle contraction through its hydrolysis to ADP ($C_{10}H_{15}N_5O_{10}P_2$)

Autonomic nervous system. A system of efferent nerves and nerve fibers that allow the central nervous system to control organs and glands

Axis. *Physics:* The pivot point for an arc of motion or rotation *Anatomy:* The second cervical vertebra

Balance point. That part of a body upon which a force may act while the body remains in equilibrium

Ballistic movement. Strong, rapid contraction with movement completed primarily through momentum

Base of support. The amount of contact area that a body resting on a surface assumes

Belief. Mental acceptance and conviction in the truth, actuality, or validity of a particular tenet or body of tenets accepted by a group of people

Biceps femoris. One of the hamstring muscles that originates on the pelvis and proximal femur and inserts onto the head of the fibula and lateral tibia

Biomechanics. The science of internal and external forces acting on a living body

Bipennate muscle. A muscle whose fibers converge from opposite sides to attach onto a central tendon, like a feather

Body. A generic term in physics referring to a complete and entire mass or collection of material that is distinct from other masses

Camber. Tilting of wheels from a vertical position to make them more maneuverable

Carpal tunnel syndrome. Compression of the nerves, arteries, and veins that pass through a narrow anatomical compartment formed by the carpal bones and the flexor retinaculum (see page 98, A Closer Look Box 8-1)

Center of gravity. The balance point in or near a body located where the resultant force of the gravitational forces on the body's component particles acts

Center of gravity height. How high a body's center of gravity lies in relation to the surface upon which it stands

Center of gravity projection. A downward extension of the body's center of gravity outside the confines of the body itself

Center of rotation. The central point about which rotary motion occurs

Circumduction. Rotary movement that uses a combination of movements in various planes and involves more than one axis

Closed-chain movement. Movement that occurs at the proximal end of an extremity because the distal end is stabilized (see page 67, Figure 6-11, *B*)

Cocontraction. When agonist and antagonist muscles contract simultaneously to stabilize a joint

Compressive force. A normal force that pushes tissue surfaces closer together

Concentric contraction. Energy-expending process that results in shortening of the muscle fibers

Contracture. A condition in which skin, connective tissue, or muscle becomes shorter in its resting state and consequently limits movement

Coxa valga. A bowlegged appearance caused by an angle of more than 125 degrees between the head and neck and the shaft of the femur

Coxa vara. A knock-kneed appearance caused by an angle of less than 125 degrees between the head and neck and the shaft of the femur

CVA. Cerebral vascular accident, or stroke, caused when bleeding or clotting in the brain results in damage to surrounding neural tissue

Dens. A toothlike protuberance (odontoid process) of the axis on which the atlas rests

Diarthrodial joint. A joint in which a fluid-filled space occurs between two or more articulating bones, allowing freedom of motion

Displacement. Movement in a direction such that an object travels a quantifiable distance, for example, 60 miles north

Distensibility. Expansion or dilation inherent or caused by force experienced within tissue

Dorsal aponeurosis. A triangular-shaped widening of the extensor digitorum tendon over the metacarpophalangeal joint; serves as an attachment for intrinsic muscles; also known as the *extensor expansion, extensor hood,* or *dorsal hood*

Dorsal hood. See *dorsal aponeurosis*

Eccentric contraction. Energy-expending process that results in lengthening of the muscle fibers

Efferent nerves. Nerves that carry impulses from the central nervous system to the body

Elasticity. The inherent property of material to return to its original form or state after deformation

Epiphyseal plates. Centers of cartilaginous growth within bones

Equilibrium. The condition of an object at rest or in unaccelerated motion when acted on by two or more forces so that the resultant of all forces acting on it is zero ($\Sigma F = 0$) and the sum of all torques ($\Sigma T = 0$) about any axis is zero

Equilibrium of torques. The condition of an object in which all tendencies for rotation equal zero ($\Sigma T = 0$)

Erector spinae. Deep back muscles that run parallel to the vertebral column and consist of three major divisions—the spinalis (spine to spine), longissimus (transverse process to transverse process), and iliocostalis (rib to rib)

Eversion. A movement that rotates the sole of the foot from the midline of the body; associated with forefoot pronation

Excursion. The full extent that a muscle's fibers can elongate and shorten

Extension. Rotary movement at a joint that brings the skeletal segments farther from one another

Extensor digitorum longus. A pennate muscle originating on the lateral condyle of the tibia and the upper two-thirds of the fibula, its tendon splitting into four tendons that insert onto the lateral four toes

Extensor expansion. See *dorsal aponeurosis*

Extensor hallucis longus. Originates on the midfibula and inserts at the base of the distal phalanx of the great toe

Extensor hood. See *dorsal aponeurosis*

External abdominal oblique. One of four paired abdominal muscles; lies just lateral to the rectus abdominus and attaches medially onto the pelvis and the aponeurosis of the abdomen and laterally onto the ribs

External torque. A tendency toward rotation produced by forces outside the body

Factors in stability. The factors that determine whether individuals maintain balance—center of gravity height, base of support, center of gravity projection, and weight

False ribs. Five pairs of bones that lie inferior to the true ribs and articulate posteriorly with the vertebrae; have no bony anterior articulation

Fascia. Fibrous connective tissue that envelops, separates, or binds together muscles

Fast-twitch muscle fiber. Contains lower concentrations of myoglobin and predominates in muscles that contract rapidly for limited amounts of time

First-class lever. The axis of motion lies in between opposing forces of effort and resistance (see pages 51 through 52 and Table 5-1)

Flexion. Movement at a joint that brings the skeletal segments closer to one another

Flexion moment. A tendency to rotate that results in flexion

Flexor hallucis brevis. Originates on the plantar surface of the cuboid bone and inserts onto the base of the phalanx of the great toe

Flexor retinaculum. Fascia (also known as the *transverse carpal ligament*) that stretches from the hook of the hamate and pisiform bones to the scaphoid and trapezium and forms the fibrous "roof" of the carpal tunnel

Force. A vector quantity with the capacity to do work or cause physical change, such as acceleration of a body in the direction of its application

Frame of reference. Sources of existing philosophy, theory, practice, knowledge or research findings that are used by an individual or a group to determine how they judge, control, or direct action or expression

Friction. A force that resists movement when two bodies are in contact

Fusiform muscle. A cylindrical muscle in which all the fibers run parallel to one another from origin to insertion

Gait cycle. The normal walking pattern from the time one extremity makes contact with the floor until it swings and contacts the floor again

Ganglia. Collections of nerve-cell bodies that lie outside the central nervous system

Gastrocnemius. One of three muscles that comprises the triceps surae; originates on the medial and lateral condyles of the femur and inserts at the tendo calcaneus onto the calcaneus bone

Gemellus inferior. Originates on the ischial tuberosity and inserts onto the tendon of the obturator internus

Gemellus superior. Originates on the ischial spine and inserts onto the tendon of the obturator internus

Genu valga. A knock-kneed appearance caused by a pathological process of the knee, resulting in outward projection of the distal tibia

Genu vara. A bowlegged appearance caused by a pathological process of the knee, resulting in inward projection of the distal tibia

Glenohumeral joint. Synovial joint at which the head of the humerus articulates with the glenoid fossa of the scapula

Gluteus maximus. Heavy, coarse muscle that pads the ischial tuberosity; originates on the sacrum, coccyx, and ilium and inserts on the femur and iliotibial tract

Gluteus medius. A muscle lying beneath the gluteus maximus that originates on the ilium and inserts onto the greater trochanter of the femur

Gluteus minimus. A muscle lying beneath the gluteus medius that originates on the ilium and inserts onto the greater trochanter of the femur

Goniometer. An instrument used to measure joint angles of motion

Gracilis. One of the hip adductor group of muscles; originates on the pubis and inserts as a tendon onto the medial tibia

Gravitational attraction. The natural phenomenon of attraction between massive bodies so that all smaller masses around a larger mass are pulled toward the center of the large mass

Gravity environment. The natural force of attraction exerted by a celestial body, such as Earth, upon objects at or near its surface, tending to draw them toward the center of the body

Hamstrings. A group of muscles—the semitendinosus, semimembranosus, and biceps femoris—that comprise the back of the thigh; originating from the ischial tuberosity and inserting onto the proximal tibia

Hypertonia. Increased muscle tone or activity

Hypotonia. Less-than-normal muscle tone or activity

Iliacus. Originates on the pelvis and joins with the psoas major to form the iliopsoas tendon, which attaches to the lesser trochanter of the femur

Iliopsoas. Two muscles—the iliacus and psoas major—that originate on the pelvis and lumbar spine and insert as one tendon onto the lesser trochanter of the femur

Iliotibial tract. Fibrous fascia into which a number of muscles insert; runs down the lateral side of the thigh and blends into the joint capsule at the knee

Initial contact. The part of gait cycle at which the heel makes contact with the ground

Initial swing. The part of gait cycle at which the toes rise off the ground

Internal abdominal oblique. One of four paired abdominal muscles; lies just inferior and deep to the external abdominal oblique and attaches medially onto the lower ribs and laterally onto the pelvis

Internal torque. A tendency toward rotation produced by forces inside the body

Interossei. Seven small muscles of the foot or hand that originate on adjacent sides of the metatarsals or metacarpals and insert onto the extensor hood mechanism of the hand and the lateral side of the proximal phalanx and joint capsule

Intervertebral disk. A cartilaginous structure that lies between adjacent vertebral bodies in the spine

Intrinsic minus. Metacarpophalangeal hyperextension with incomplete interphalangeal extension caused by weakness of the intrinsic muscles in the hand (see page 16, Figure 2-6, page 108, Figure 8-10, and page 109, Figure 8-11)

Inversion. A movement that rotates the sole of the foot toward the midline of the body; associated with supination of the forefoot

Isometric contraction. Energy-expending process in which the length of the muscle fibers does not change

Joint force. The internal reaction force acting on contact surfaces when a joint is subjected to external loads

Kinesiology. Scientific study of the active and passive structures involved in movement

Kinetic model. Analysis of activity in terms of anatomy, physiology, pathology, and kinesiology to restore function via adaptive equipment or compensatory exercise techniques

Kyphosis. An exaggerated convexity in the thoracic curve of the spine

Labyrinthine reflexes. Motor responses caused or affected by the position of the head and consequently the effect of gravity acting on the inner ear (labyrinth)

Law of acceleration. Newton's second law of motion; states that forces are the product of a body's mass and its acceleration, or F = ma (see pages 32 through 33)

Law of action-reaction. Newton's third law of motion; states that if a force acts on an object and that object remains stationary, an equal force must be acting on the object in the opposite direction (see pages 33 through 35)

Law of inertia. Newton's first law of motion; states that a body at rest or in motion remains so unless acted on by an outside force (see page 32)

Lever arm. The rigid structure that spans the distance from an applied force to its center of motion, also known as the *moment arm of the force*

Leverage. Mechanical advantage produced by the length of the lever arm

Loading. The part of gait cycle in which the body's weight is shifted onto the lower extremity in contact with the ground

Longitudinal arch. A palmar arch that curves from the wrist to the fingertips, with its apex at the row of metacarpal heads

Lordosis. An exaggerated concavity in the lumbar curve of the spine

Lumbricals. Four small muscles of the foot or the hand that originate on the flexor tendons and insert onto the extensor hood mechanism of the digits

Manual muscle testing. A highly structured procedure of positioning and hand placement used to determine the degree of muscular weakness resulting from disease, injury, or disuse

Matter. A substance made up of atoms and molecules that exists as a solid, liquid, or gas

Mechanical advantage. The ratio of the output force produced to the applied input force, which is usually related to the length of the lever arm (see pages 48 through 49)

Mechanistic. Understanding of the world as a mechanism, especially a tendency to explain phenomena by reference to physical or biological causes only

Midstance. The part of gait cycle in which body weight is supported by the lower extremity in contact with the ground

Midswing. The part of gait cycle in which the leg is lifted off the ground and moves forward into terminal swing

MMT. Manual muscle testing

Model of practice. A unique means by which assumptions are organized and arranged to guide study and action within a profession

Moment arm. The perpendicular distance from an applied force to its axis of motion; also known as *lever arm*

Multijoint muscle. A muscle that crosses two or more joint axes, producing motion in more than one joint

Myoglobin. The primary source of oxygen in muscle tissue; has a higher affinity for oxygen than hemoglobin in the blood

Newton. The metric unit of force required to accelerate a mass of one kilogram one meter per second^2

Normal force. A force directed perpendicularly toward or from a surface area

Nucleus pulposus. Jellylike tissue that can be found at the center of intervertebral disks that absorbs forces on spinal segments

Obturator externus. One of the adductor group of muscles; originates on the pubis and ischium and inserts onto the greater trochanter

Obturator internus. Originates on the ischium and perineal fascia and inserts onto the greater trochanter of the femur

Open-chain movement. Movement that occurs at the distal end of an extremity because the proximal end is stabilized (see page 67, Figure 6-11, *A*)

Orthopedic model. Use of anatomy, physiology, pathology, and kinesiology in the design of restorative activities for specific muscle and joint problems

Pascal. The metric unit used to measure stress in materials, where $1 \text{ Pa} = 1 \text{ N/m}^2$

Passive insufficiency. A condition in which a multijoint muscle prevents full movement of joints in the opposite direction

Pectineus. One of the adductor group of muscles; originates on the pubis and inserts onto the lesser trochanter of the femur

Pelvic obliquity. Asymmetry of the pelvis in the frontal plane in which one side lies higher than the other in a resting position, usually due to pathological conditions of muscle shortening or bony deformities (see page 77, Figure 6-27)

Pelvic rotation. Asymmetry of the pelvis in the horizontal plane in which one side is anterior to the other in a resting position, usually due to pathological conditions of muscle shortening or bony deformities (see page 77, Figure 6-28)

Pelvic tilt. The angle of the pelvis in the sagittal plane in relationship to the spine

Pennate muscle. A muscle whose fibers originate on a bone and insert along the length of a tendon, like a feather

Percentile weight. The percentage assigned to body segments (such as the forearm or thigh) that represents the proportion of that segment to total body weight (see Appendix B)

Peroneus brevis. Originates on the lower two-thirds of the fibula and inserts onto the dorsum of the fifth metatarsal

Peroneus longus. Originates on the lateral condyle of the tibia and the upper two-thirds of the fibula and inserts onto the plantar surfaces of the cuneiform and base of the first metatarsal

Peroneus tertius. A partially separated portion of the extensor digitorum longus that originates on the lower fibula and inserts onto the base of the fifth metatarsal

Philosophy. A system of motivating concepts or principles used to critique and analyze fundamental beliefs as they are conceptualized or formulated

Piriformis. Originates on the sacrum and inserts onto the greater trochanter

Point of application. The exact place on a lever on which a force acts

Pound. A term, originating in England, for the unit of force equal to the weight of a standard one-pound mass, where the local acceleration of gravity is 32.174 feet per second^2

Preswing. The part of gait cycle in which the heel lifts off the ground

Psoas major. Originates on the lumbar spine and joins with the iliacus to form the iliopsoas tendon that attaches to the lesser trochanter of the femur

Quadriceps femoris. A muscle whose four distinct parts usually are considered as four separate muscles—the rectus femoris, vastus lateralis, vastus medialis, and vastus intermedius

Radial deviation. Movement of the hand or fingers toward the thumb and away from the midline of the body (in anatomical position); also known as *wrist abduction*

Rate of acceleration. The average rate at which final velocity (v) changes from initial velocity (u) with respect to time (t), or a = (v-u)/t; free-falling bodies under the influence of terrestrial gravity falling with an average rate of acceleration equal to approximately 9.81 meters (32 feet) per second^2

Reconstruction model. Use of voluntary activities that are graded and adapted to specific muscles and joints to restore physical function after illness or injury

Rectus abdominus. The most superficial layer of four paired abdominal muscles; attaches to the sternum superiorly and the pelvis inferiorly

Rectus femoris. One part of the quadriceps femoris that originates on the anterior inferior iliac spine and inserts onto the patella

Resultant force. A single force that is the sum of two or more forces with different orientations and a common point of application

Rotary motion. Movement in a circular arc around an immovable line or axis

Rotation. Joint movement around a longitudinal axis in a horizontal plane

Rotator cuff. Four muscles—the supraspinatus, infraspinatus, teres minor, and subscapularis—that secure the head of the humerus in the glenoid fossa of the scapula and help stabilize the glenohumeral joint

Sacrum. Five fused vertebrae at the caudal end of the spinal column

Sartorius. A long strap muscle originating on the lateral pelvis and inserting onto the medial surface of the tibia just below the knee joint

Scalar. A quantity, such as mass, length, or speed, defined by its magnitude and lacking direction

Scapulohumeral rhythm. Simultaneous glenohumeral and scapular movements that together produce full shoulder abduction and flexion

Scapulothoracic joint. The articulation between the scapula and the thorax (chest wall) that contributes about one third of shoulder motion as it repositions the glenohumeral joint; technically not a "joint"

Scoliosis. A pathological S-shaped curve of the spine that occurs in the frontal plane

Second-class lever. Lends mechanical advantage to the force of effort, which lies farther from the axis of motion than the force of resistance (see pages 51 through 52 and Table 5-1)

Segmental centers of gravity. The balance point in a segmental portion of the body, such as the forearm or thigh

Semimembranosus. One of the hamstring muscles that originates on the ischial tuberosity and inserts onto the posterior medial surface of the tibia

Semitendinosus. One of the hamstring muscles that originates on the ischial tuberosity and inserts via an aponeurosis onto the upper, medial surface of the tibia

Shear. Forces that operate in tangential or parallel directions to an object's surface

Slow-twitch muscle fiber. Contains higher concentrations of myoglobin and predominates in postural muscles that must work for prolonged periods without becoming fatigued

Slug. A British unit of measurement for a mass that is accelerated at the rate of one foot per second^2 when acted on by a 1-pound force (A slug equalling 32 pounds in Earth's gravity, where a 1-pound force accelerates at 32 feet per second^2)

Soleus. One of three muscles that forms the triceps surae; originates on the proximal tibia and fibula and inserts as the tendo calcaneus onto the calcaneus bone

Spasticity. Extreme hypertonicity of muscles exhibited as resistance to movement and increased reflexes

Stance phase. The part of gait cycle from the point at which the heel makes contact with the ground to the point at which the heel rises above the ground in preswing

Sternoclavicular joint. A small, freely moveable synovial joint at which the clavicle articulates with the sternum

Sternocleidomastoid. Most prominent anterior neck muscle originating on the sternum and proximal clavicle and inserting onto the mastoid process of the skull

Stress. A vector quantity found within the material on which forces act and measured by division of the amount of force by the amount of tissue, for example, N/m^2

Stroke. See CVA

Subluxation. Displacement or partial dislocation of joint components

Swing phase. The part of gait cycle in which the toe leaves the ground, accelerates into midswing, and decelerates into terminal swing

Synarthrodial joint. An immobile fibrous interface between two or more bones

Synergy. Muscles acting together to produce specific movements

Tangential. A force that operates superficially on an object's surface; also known as a *shear force*

Temporomandibular joint. The synovial joint at which the jaw articulates with the skull

Tendency to rotate. The ability of a force to cause rotation; also known as *torque* (see pages 48 through 49)

Tendinitis. Inflammation of the tendon and its muscular attachments

Tenodesis grasp. Passive tension present in the finger flexors caused by wrist extension because of passive insufficiency of the finger flexor tendons

Tenodesis release. A condition in which wrist flexion causes passive stretching of the extensor digitorum communis to allow sufficient finger extension to release objects held in the hand

Tenosynovitis. Inflammation of the tendon sheath

Tensile. Forces that pull tissues apart

Tensile force. A normal force that pulls two surfaces apart

Tensor fascia lata. A muscle that originates on the iliac crest of the pelvis and inserts onto the iliotibial tract just below the greater trochanter

Terminal stance. The part of gait cycle in which body weight shifts onto the inside of the foot in preparation for preswing

Terminal swing. The part of gait cycle in which the swing's momentum is slowed in preparation for initial contact

Third-class lever. Allows resistance to be moved at great speed and through great distance because the force of resistance lies farther from the axis than the force of effort (see pages 51 and 52 and Table 5-1)

Tibialis anterior. Originates on the lateral condyle and upper two-thirds of the tibia and inserts onto the medial sides of the cuneiform and the base of the first metatarsal

Tibialis posterior. The deepest muscle of the leg; originates on the lateral and posterior surface of the upper tibia and the posterior tibia and inserts onto the plantar navicular and cuneiform

Torque. The tendency of a force to cause rotation, as determined by the product of its force and distance from the axis of motion (moment arm), T = F x MA

Torque-angle curve. A curve documenting the amount of torque needed to bring a joint into different positions or joint angles (see pages 115 and 116 and Figures 8-20, 8-21, and 8-22)

Tracts. A bundle of nerve fibers with a common origin, termination, and function; convey impulses within the central nervous system

Transformative. Understanding of the world as a dynamic system in which change is a constant opportunity for evolution and diversification

Transverse arch. A palmar arch that curves from the radial to the ulnar side of the hand, with its apex near the head of the third metacarpal

Transversospinalis. Deep back muscles that run upward and medial to the spinal column and consist of three major divisions—the semispinalis (transverse process below to spinous process above), multifidus (in the furrow between spines and transverse processes), and rotatores (transverse process below to lamina above)

Transversus abdominis. The deepest of four paired abdominal muscles; fibers run horizontally from the ribs and vertebral fascia to an aponeurosis at the midline of the abdomen

Triceps surae. Three muscles—the gastrocnemius, soleus, and plantaris—that form the calf of the lower leg

True ribs. The seven pairs of bones that articulate posteriorly with the vertebrae and anteriorly with the sternum to form the rib cage

Ulnar deviation. Movement of the hand or fingers toward the little finger and closer to the midline of the body (in anatomical position); also known as *wrist adduction*

Ulnar drift. A pathological condition occurring when the extensor digitorum communis tendon slips to the ulnar side of the metacarpophalangeal joint

Vastus intermedius. A part of the quadriceps femoris that originates on the upper two thirds of the femur and inserts onto the other tendons of the quadriceps and the joint capsule of the knee

Vastus lateralis. A part of the quadriceps femoris that originates from the joint capsule of the hip and inserts onto the patella and the lateral joint capsule of the knee

Vastus medialis. A part of the quadriceps femoris that originates on the proximal femur and inserts onto the patella and the medial joint capsule of the knee

Vector. A force or an influence that can be described completely by magnitude and direction

Velocity. Displacement that occurs over a specific amount of time, for example, 60 miles per hour

Weight. A force (equal to the product of the object's mass and the acceleration of gravity) representing the attraction of a body to Earth or another celestial body

Work. The transfer of energy to a body by the application of a force that moves the body in the direction of the force; calculated through multiplication of the force by the distance through which the body moves and expressed in joules, ergs, and foot-pounds

Index

C

I